ESAP™ 2019

Endocrine Society's
Endocrine Self-Assessment Program
Questions, Answers, and Discussions

Lisa R. Tannock, MD, Program Chair
Professor of Medicine
Chief, Division of Endocrinology
and Molecular Medicine
University of Kentucky and
Department of Veterans Affairs

Kristien Boelaert, MD
Reader in Endocrinology
Center for Endocrinology, Diabetes,
and Metabolism
University of Birmingham

Barbara Gisella Carranza Leon, MD
Assistant Professor of Medicine
Division of Diabetes, Endocrinology,
and Metabolism
Vanderbilt University Medical Center

Alice Y. Chang, MD, MSc
Assistant Professor
Division of Endocrinology, Diabetes,
and Nutrition
Mayo Clinic

Stephen Clement, MD
Medical Director, Endocrine Services
Inova Fairfax Hospital

Dima Lutfi Diab, MD
Associate Professor of Clinical Medicine
University of Cincinnati

Marie Freel, MB, ChB, PhD
Consultant Endocrinologist
Queen Elizabeth University Hospital
Glasgow, United Kingdom

Michael S. Irwig, MD
Associate Professor of Medicine
Division of Endocrinology
George Washington University

Jacqueline Jonklaas, MD, PhD
Professor
Division of Endocrinology and Metabolism
Georgetown University

Steven B. Magill, MD, PhD
Associate Clinical Professor of Medicine
Endocrinology, Diabetes, and Metabolism
Medical College of Wisconsin

Deepika Reddy, MD
Assistant Professor
Division of Diabetes, Endocrinology,
and Metabolism
University of Utah Healthcare

Roberto Salvatori, MD
Professor of Medicine
Medical Director, Johns Hopkins
Pituitary Center
Johns Hopkins University

Aniket Sidhaye, MD
Assistant Professor of Medicine
Johns Hopkins University

Savitha Subramanian, MD
Associate Professor of Medicine
University of Washington

Anand Vaidya, MD, MMSC
Assistant Professor of Medicine
Brigham and Women's Hospital
Harvard Medical School

Thomas J. Weber, MD
Associate Professor of Medicine
Division of Endocrinology, Metabolism,
and Nutrition
Duke University Medical Center

Abbie L. Young, MS, CGC, ELS(D)
Medical Editor

Endocrine Society
2055 L Street NW, Suite 600, Washington, DC 20036
1-888-ENDOCRINE • www.endocrine.org

ENDOCRINE
SOCIETY
Hormone Science to Health

ENDOCRINE
SOCIETY
Hormone Science to Health

The Endocrine Society is the world's largest, oldest, and most active organization working to advance the clinical practice of endocrinology and hormone research. Founded in 1916, the Society now has more than 18,000 global members across a range of disciplines. The Society has earned an international reputation for excellence in the quality of its peer-reviewed journals, educational resources, meetings, and programs that improve public health through the practice and science of endocrinology.

Visit us at:
education.endocrine.org
endocrine.org

Other Publications:
https://www.endocrine.org/publications

On the Cover:
Left: Noncontrast brain MRI showing a diffusely enlarged pituitary gland in a patient with ipilimumab-induced hypophysitis.
Upper right: Abdominal CT showing a 5.8-cm right-sided adrenal mass with a precontrast density of −44 Hounsfield units determined to be a myelolipoma.
Lower right: Pelvis x-ray demonstrating diffuse sclerosis involving the pelvis and proximal femurs, which was determined to be due to metastatic prostate cancer to bone.

OVERVIEW

The Endocrine Self-Assessment Program (ESAP™) is a self-study curriculum aimed at physicians wanting a self-assessment and a broad review of endocrinology. The ESAP Reference Edition consists of 120 brand-new multiple-choice questions in all areas of endocrinology, diabetes, and metabolism. There is extensive discussion of each correct answer, a comprehensive syllabus, and references. ESAP is updated annually with new questions.

The ESAP reference book is intended primarily for consultation and self-assessment of knowledge relating to endocrinology. As a reference book, educational credits are not available upon completion of the multiple-choice questions included. For information on educational products that include educational credit, please visit endocrine.org/store.

LEARNING OBJECTIVES

ESAP 2019 will allow learners to assess their knowledge of all aspects of endocrinology, diabetes, and metabolism.

Upon completion of this educational activity, learners will be able to:

- Recognize clinical manifestations of endocrine and metabolic disorders and select among current options for diagnosis, management, and therapy.
- Identify risk factors for endocrine and metabolic disorders and develop strategies for prevention.
- Evaluate endocrine and metabolic manifestations of systemic disorders.
- Use existing resources pertaining to clinical guidelines and treatment recommendations for endocrine and related metabolic disorders to guide diagnosis and treatment.

TARGET AUDIENCE

ESAP is a self-study curriculum aimed at physicians seeking initial certification or recertification in endocrinology, program directors interested in a testing and training instrument, and clinicians simply wanting a self-assessment and a broad review of endocrinology.

STATEMENT OF INDEPENDENCE

The Endocrine Society has a policy of ensuring that the content and quality of this educational activity are balanced, independent, objective, and scientifically rigorous. The scientific content of this activity was developed under the supervision of the Endocrine Society's ESAP Faculty Working Group.

DISCLOSURE POLICY

The faculty, committee members, and staff who are in position to control the content of this activity are required to disclose to the Endocrine Society and to learners any relevant financial relationship(s) of the individual or spouse/partner that have occurred within the last 12 months with any commercial interest(s) whose products or services are related to the content. Financial relationships are defined by remuneration in any amount from the commercial interest(s) in the form of grants; research support; consulting fees; salary; ownership interest (eg, stocks, stock options, or ownership interest excluding diversified mutual funds); honoraria or other payments for participation in speakers' bureaus, advisory boards, or boards of directors; or other financial benefits. The intent of this disclosure is not to prevent planners with relevant financial relationships from planning or delivering content, but rather to provide learners with information that allows them to make their own judgments of whether these financial relationships may have influenced the educational activity with regard to exposition or conclusion. The Endocrine Society has reviewed all disclosures and resolved or managed all identified conflicts of interest, as applicable.

The following faculty reported relevant financial relationship(s): **Barbara Gisella Carranza Leon, MD,** has received research support from Amgen. **Michael S. Irwig, MD,** served as male hypogonadism faculty for MedScape. **Roberto Salvatori, MD**, received grant support from National Institutes of Health and Department of Defense; serves on the advisory board for Pfizer; and is a clinical trial investigator for Novartis, Chiasma, and Strongbridge. **Savitha Subramanian, MD**, serves on the advisory board for Akcea Therapeutics and Intarcia. **Anand Vaidya, MD**, received grant support from National Institutes of Health and Doris Duke Charitable Foundation.

The following committee members reported no relevant financial relationships: **Lisa R. Tannock, MD; Kristien Boelaert, MD; Alice Y. Chang, MD, MSc; Stephen Clement, MD; Dima L. Diab, MD; Marie Freel, MD; Jacqueline Jonklaas, MD, PhD; Steven B. Magill, MD; Deepika Reddy, MD; Aniket Sidhaye, MD;** and **Thomas J. Weber, MD**.

The medical editor for this program, **Abbie L. Young, MS, CGC, ELS(D),** reported no relevant financial relationships.

The Endocrine Society staff associated with the development of content for this activity reported no relevant financial relationships.

DISCLAIMERS

The information presented in this activity represents the opinion of the faculty and is not necessarily the official position of the Endocrine Society.

USE OF PROFESSIONAL JUDGMENT:

The educational content in this self-assessment test relates to basic principles of diagnosis and therapy and does not substitute for individual patient assessment based on the health care provider's examination of the patient and consideration of laboratory data and other factors unique to the patient. Standards in medicine change as new data become available.

DRUGS AND DOSAGES:

When prescribing medications, the physician is advised to check the product information sheet accompanying each drug to verify conditions of use and to identify any changes in drug dosage schedule or contraindications.

POLICY ON UNLABELED/OFF-LABEL USE

The Endocrine Society has determined that disclosure of unlabeled/off-label or investigational use of commercial product(s) is informative for audiences and therefore requires this information to be disclosed to the learners at the beginning of the presentation. Uses of specific therapeutic agents, devices, and other products discussed in this educational activity may not be the same as those indicated in product labeling approved by the Food and Drug Administration (FDA). The Endocrine Society requires that any discussions of such "off-label" use be based on scientific research that conforms to generally accepted standards of experimental design, data collection, and data analysis. Before recommending or prescribing any therapeutic agent or device, learners should review the complete prescribing information, including indications, contraindications, warnings, precautions, and adverse events.

ACKNOWLEDGMENT OF COMMERCIAL SUPPORT

This activity is not supported by educational grant(s) or other funds from any commercial supporter.

PUBLICATION DATE: November 2018

Laboratory Reference Ranges

Reference ranges vary among laboratories. The listed reference ranges should be used when interpreting laboratory values presented in ESAP™. Conventional units are listed first with SI units in parentheses.

Lipid Values

High-density lipoprotein (HDL) cholesterol

Optimal --------------------------- >60 mg/dL (>1.55 mmol/L)

Normal ---------------------- 40-60 mg/dL (1.04-1.55 mmol/L)

Low ------------------------------ <40 mg/dL (<1.04 mmol/L)

Low-density lipoprotein (LDL) cholesterol

Optimal ------------------------- <100 mg/dL (<2.59 mmol/L)

Low ---------------------- 100-129 mg/dL (2.59-3.34 mmol/L)

Borderline-high ------------ 130-159 mg/dL (3.37-4.12 mmol/L)

High --------------------- 160-189 mg/dL (4.14-4.90 mmol/L)

Very high ----------------------- ≥190 mg/dL (≥4.92 mmol/L)

Non-HDL cholesterol

Optimal ------------------------- <130 mg/dL (<3.37 mmol/L)

Borderline-high ------------ 130-159 mg/dL (3.37-4.12 mmol/L)

High --------------------------- ≥240 mg/dL (≥6.22 mmol/L)

Total cholesterol

Optimal ------------------------- <200 mg/dL (<5.18 mmol/L)

Borderline-high ------------ 200-239 mg/dL (5.18-6.19 mmol/L)

High --------------------------- ≥240 mg/dL (≥6.22 mmol/L)

Triglycerides

Optimal ------------------------- <150 mg/dL (<1.70 mmol/L)

Borderline-high ------------ 150-199 mg/dL (1.70-2.25 mmol/L)

High --------------------- 200-499 mg/dL (2.26-5.64 mmol/L)

Very high ----------------------- ≥500 mg/dL (≥5.65 mmol/L)

Lipoprotein (a) ------------------------- ≤30 mg/dL (≤1.07 µmol/L)

Apolipoprotein B ----------------------- 50-110 mg/dL (0.5-1.1 g/L)

Hematologic Values

Erythrocyte sedimentation rate -------------------------- 0-20 mm/h

Haptoglobin ------------------------ 30-200 mg/dL (300-2000 mg/L)

Hematocrit --------------------------- 41%-50% (0.41-0.51) (male); 35%-45% (0.35-0.45) (female)

Hemoglobin A$_{1c}$ ---------------------- 4.0%-5.6% (20-38 mmol/mol)

Hemoglobin -------------------- 13.8-17.2 g/dL (138-172 g/L) (male); 12.1-15.1 g/dL (121-151 g/L) (female)

International normalized ratio -------------------------------- 0.8-1.2

Mean corpuscular volume (MCV) ----------- 80-100 µm^3 (80-100 fL)

Platelet count ------------------- 150-450 × 10^3/µL (150-450 × 10^9/L)

Protein (total) ------------------------------ 6.3-7.9 g/dL (63-79 g/L)

Reticulocyte count ------ 0.5%-1.5% of red blood cells (0.005-0.015)

White blood cell count ----------- 4500-11,000/µL (4.5-11.0 × 10^9/L)

Thyroid Values

Thyroglobulin ------------- 3-42 ng/mL (3-42 µg/L) (after surgery and radioactive iodine treatment: <1.0 ng/mL [<1.0 µg/L])

Thyroglobulin antibodies -------------------- ≤4.0 IU/mL (≤4.0 kIU/L)

Thyrotropin (TSH) ------------------------------------- 0.5-5.0 mIU/L

Thyrotropin-receptor antibodies ------------------------- ≤1.75 IU/L

Thyroid-stimulating immunoglobulin --------- ≤120% of basal activity

Thyroperoxidase (TPO) antibodies ----------- <2.0 IU/mL (<2.0 kIU/L)

Thyroxine (T$_4$) (free) -------------- 0.8-1.8 ng/dL (10.30-23.17 pmol/L)

Thyroxine (T$_4$) (total) ----------- 5.5-12.5 µg/dL (94.02-213.68 nmol/L)

Free thyroxine (T$_4$) index --------------------------------------- 4-12

Triiodothyronine (T$_3$) (free) --------- 2.3-4.2 pg/mL (3.53-6.45 pmol/L)

Triiodothyronine (T$_3$) (total) -------- 70-200 ng/dL (1.08-3.08 nmol/L)

Triiodothyronine (T$_3$), reverse -------- 10-24 ng/dL (0.15-0.37 nmol/L)

Triiodothyronine uptake, resin --------------------------- 25%-38%

Radioactive iodine uptake ----- 3%-16% (6 hours); 15%-30% (24 hours)

Endocrine Values

Serum

Aldosterone ----------------------- 4-21 ng/dL (111.0-582.5 pmol/L)

Alkaline phosphatase ----------------- 50-120 U/L (0.84-2.00 µkat/L)

Alkaline phosphatase (bone-specific) --------- ≤20 µg/L (adult male); ≤14 µg/L (premenopausal female); ≤22 µg/L (postmenopausal female)

Androstenedione ------ 65-210 ng/dL (2.27-7.33 nmol/L) (adult male); 80-240 ng/dL (2.79-8.38 nmol/L) (adult female)

Antimullerian hormone ----------- 0.7-19.0 ng/mL (5.0-135.7 pmol/L) (male, >12 years); 0.9-9.5 ng/mL (6.4-67.9 pmol/L) (female, 13-45 years); <1.0 ng/mL (<7.1 pmol/L) (female, >45 years)

Calcitonin ------------------ <16 pg/mL (<4.67 pmol/L) (basal, male); <8 pg/mL (<2.34 pmol/L) (basal, female); ≤130 pg/mL (≤37.96 pmol/L) (peak calcium infusion, male); ≤90 pg/mL (≤26.28 pmol/L) (peak calcium infusion, female)

Carcinoembryonic antigen ------------------- <2.5 ng/mL (<2.5 µg/L)

Chromogranin A ----------------------------- <93 ng/mL (<93 µg/L)

Corticosterone ------- 53-1560 ng/dL (1.53-45.08 nmol/L) (>18 years)

Corticotropin (ACTH) ---------------- 10-60 pg/mL (2.2-13.2 pmol/L)

Cortisol (8 AM) --------------------- 5-25 µg/dL (137.9-689.7 nmol/L)

Cortisol (4 PM) --------------------- 2-14 µg/dL (55.2-386.2 nmol/L)

C-peptide ------------------------ 0.9-4.3 ng/mL (0.30-1.42 nmol/L)

C-reactive protein ------------------- 0.8-3.1 mg/L (7.62-29.52 nmol/L)

Cross-linked N-telopeptide of type 1 collagen --------------------- 5.4-24.2 nmol BCE/mmol creat (male); 6.2-19.0 nmol BCE/mmol creat (female)

Dehydroepiandrosterone sulfate (DHEA-S)

	Female	Male
Age 18-29 years	44-332 µg/dL (1.19-9.00 µmol/L)	89-457 µg/dL (2.41-12.38 µmol/L)
Age 30-39 years	31-228 µg/dL (0.84-6.78 µmol/L)	65-334 µg/dL (1.76-9.05 µmol/L)

	Female	Male
Age 40-49 years	18-244 µg/dL	48-244 µg/dL
	(0.49-6.61 µmol/L)	(1.30-6.61 µmol/L)
Age 50-59 years	15-200 µg/dL	35-179 µg/dL
	(0.41-5.42 µmol/L)	(0.95-4.85 µmol/L)
Age ≥60 years	15-157 µg/dL	25-131 µg/dL
	(0.41-4.25 µmol/L)	(0.68-3.55 µmol/L)

Deoxycorticosterone ---------- <10 ng/dL (<0.30 nmol/L) (>18 years)

1,25-Dihydroxyvitamin D_3 --------- 16-65 pg/mL (41.6-169.0 pmol/L)

Estradiol ------------------- 10-40 pg/mL (36.7-146.8 pmol/L) (male);
10-180 pg/mL (36.7-660.8 pmol/L) (follicular, female);
100-300 pg/mL (367.1-1101.3 pmol/L) (midcycle, female);
40-200 pg/mL (146.8-734.2 pmol/L) (luteal, female);
<20 pg/mL (<73.4 pmol/L) (postmenopausal, female)

Estrone ------------------- 10-60 pg/mL (37.0-221.9 pmol/L) (male);
17-200 pg/mL (62.9-739.6 pmol/L) (premenopausal female);
7-40 pg/mL (25.9-147.9 pmol/L) (postmenopausal female)

α-Fetoprotein ------------------------------- <6 ng/mL (<6 µg/L)

Follicle-stimulating hormone (FSH) --------------------------------
1.0-13.0 mIU/mL (1.0-13.0 IU/L) (male);
<3.0 mIU/mL (<3.0 IU/L) (prepuberty, female);
2.0-12.0 mIU/mL (2.0-12.0 IU/L) (follicular, female);
4.0-36.0 mIU/mL (4.0-36.0 IU/L) (midcycle, female);
1.0-9.0 mIU/mL (1.0-9.0 IU/L) (luteal, female);
>30 mIU/mL (>30 IU/L) (postmenopausal, female)

Free fatty acids ------------------- 10.6-18.0 mg/dL (0.4-0.7 nmol/L)

Gastrin ----------------------------------- <100 pg/mL (<100 ng/L)

Growth hormone (GH) ------ 0.01-0.97 ng/mL (0.01-0.97 µg/L) (male);
0.01-3.61 ng/mL (0.01-3.61 µg/L) (female)

Homocysteine --------------------------- ≤1.76 mg/L (≤13 µmol/L)

β-Human chorionic gonadotropin (β-hCG) -------------------------
<3.0 mIU/mL (<3.0 IU/L) (nonpregnant female);
>25 mIU/mL (>25 IU/L) indicates a positive pregnancy test

β-Hydroxybutyrate ----------------------- <3.0 mg/dL (<300 µmol/L)

17-Hydroxypregnenolone ---------- 29-189 ng/dL (0.87-5.69 nmol/L)

17α-Hydroxyprogesterone ---- <220 ng/dL (<6.67 nmol/L) (adult male);
<80 ng/dL (<2.42 nmol/L) (follicular, female);
<285 ng/dL (<8.64 nmol/L) (luteal, female);
<51 ng/dL (<1.55 nmol/L) (postmenopausal, female)

25-Hydroxyvitamin D --------- <20 ng/mL (<49.9 nmol/L) (deficiency);
21-29 ng/mL (52.4-72.4 nmol/L) (insufficiency); 30-80 ng/mL
(74.9-199.7 nmol/L) (optimal levels); >80 ng/mL (>199.7 nmol/L)
(toxicity possible)

Inhibin B --------------------------- 15-300 pg/mL (15-300 ng/L)

Insulinlike growth factor 1 (IGF-1)

	Female	Male
Age 18 years	162-541 ng/mL	170-640 ng/mL
	(21.2-70.9 nmol/L)	(22.3-83.8 nmol/L)
Age 19 years	138-442 ng/mL	147-527 ng/mL
	(18.1-57.9 nmol/L)	(19.3-69.0 nmol/L)
Age 20 years	122-384 ng/mL	132-457 ng/mL
	(16.0-50.3 nmol/L)	(17.3-59.9 nmol/L)

	Female	Male
Age 21-25 years	116-341 ng/mL	116-341 ng/mL
	(15.2-44.7 nmol/L)	(15.2-44.7 nmol/L)
Age 26-30 years	117-321 ng/mL	117-321 ng/mL
	(15.3-42.1 nmol/L)	(15.3-42.1 nmol/L)
Age 31-35 years	113-297 ng/mL	113-297 ng/mL
	(14.8-38.9 nmol/L)	(14.8-38.9 nmol/L)
Age 36-40 years	106-277 ng/mL	106-277 ng/mL
	(13.9-36.3 nmol/L)	(13.9-36.3 nmol/L)
Age 41-45 years	98-261 ng/mL	98-261 ng/mL
	(12.8-34.2 nmol/L)	(12.8-34.2 nmol/L)
Age 46-50 years	91-246 ng/mL	91-246 ng/mL
	(11.9-32.2 nmol/L)	(11.9-32.2 nmol/L)
Age 51-55 years	84-233 ng/mL	84-233 ng/mL
	(11.0-30.5 nmol/L)	(11.0-30.5 nmol/L)
Age 56-60 years	78-220 ng/mL	78-220 ng/mL
	(10.2-28.8 nmol/L)	(10.2-28.8 nmol/L)
Age 61-65 years	72-207 ng/mL	72-207 ng/mL
	(9.4-27.1 nmol/L)	(9.4-27.1 nmol/L)
Age 66-70 years	67-195 ng/mL	67-195 ng/mL
	(8.8-25.5 nmol/L)	(8.8-25.5 nmol/L)
Age 71-75 years	62-184 ng/mL	62-184 ng/mL
	(8.1-24.1 nmol/L)	(8.1-24.1 nmol/L)
Age 76-80 years	57-172 ng/mL	57-172 ng/mL
	(7.5-22.5 nmol/L)	(7.5-22.5 nmol/L)
>Age 80 years	53-162 ng/mL	53-162 ng/mL
	(6.9-21.2 nmol/L)	(6.9-21.2 nmol/L)

Insulinlike growth factor binding protein 3 -------------- 2.5-4.8 mg/L

Insulin ------------------------- 1.4-14.0 µIU/mL (9.7-97.2 pmol/L)

Islet-cell antibody assay ------- 0 Juvenile Diabetes Foundation units

Luteinizing hormone (LH) ------- 1.0-9.0 mIU/mL (1.0-9.0 IU/L) (male);
<1.0 mIU/mL (<1.0 IU/L) (prepuberty, female);
1.0-18.0 mIU/mL (1.0-18.0 IU/L) (follicular, female);
20.0-80.0 mIU/mL (20.0-80.0 IU/L) (midcycle, female);
0.5-18.0 mIU/mL (0.5-18.0 IU/L) (luteal, female);
>30 mIU/mL (>30 IU/L) (postmenopausal, female)

Metanephrines (plasma fractionated)
Metanephrine ------------------------ <99 pg/mL (<0.50 pmol/L)
Normetanephrine -------------------- <165 pg/mL (<0.90 pmol/L)

75-g oral glucose tolerance test ----- 60-100 mg/dL (3.3-5.6 mmol/L) (fasting)
Blood glucose values ------- <200 mg/dL (<11.1 mmol/L) (1 hour);
<140 mg/dL (<7.8 mmol/L) (2 hour)
Between 140-200 mg/dL (7.8-11.1 mmol/L) is considered
impaired glucose tolerance or prediabetes. Greater than
200 mg/dL (11.1 mmol/L) is a sign of diabetes mellitus.

50-g oral glucose tolerance test for gestational diabetes ------------
<140 mg/dL (<7.8 mmol/L) (1 hour)

100-g oral glucose tolerance test for gestational diabetes -----------
<95 mg/dL (<5.3 mmol/L) (fasting);
<180 mg/dL (<10.0 mmol/L) (1 hour);
<155 mg/dL (<8.6 mmol/L) (2 hour);
<140 mg/dL (<7.8 mmol/L) (3 hour)

Osteocalcin --------------------- 9.0-42.0 ng/mL (9.0-42.0 µg/L)

Parathyroid hormone, intact (PTH) -------- 10-65 pg/mL (10-65 ng/L)

Parathyroid hormone–related protein (PTHrP) ----------- <2.0 pmol/L

Progesterone ---------------------- ≤1.2 ng/mL (≤3.8 nmol/L) (male);

   ≤1.0 ng/mL (≤3.2 nmol/L) (follicular, female);

   2.0-20.0 ng/mL (6.4-63.6 nmol/L) (luteal, female);

   ≤1.1 ng/mL (≤3.5 nmol/L) (postmenopausal, female);

   >10.0 ng/mL (>31.8 nmol/L) (evidence of ovulatory adequacy)

Proinsulin ---------------------- 26.5-176.4 pg/mL (3.0-20.0 pmol/L)

Prolactin --------------------- 4-23 ng/mL (0.17-1.00 nmol/L) (male);

   4-30 ng/mL (0.17-1.30 nmol/L) (nonlactating female);

   10-200 ng/mL (0.43-8.70 nmol/L) (lactating female)

Prostate-specific antigen (PSA) ---- <2.0 ng/mL (<2.0 µg/L) (≤40 years);

   <2.8 ng/mL (<2.8 µg/L) (≤50 years);

   <3.8 ng/mL (<3.8 µg/L) (≤60 years);

   <5.3 ng/mL (<5.3 µg/L) (≤70 years);

   <7.0 ng/mL (<7.0 µg/L) (≤79 years);

   <7.2 ng/mL (<7.2 µg/L) (≥80 years)

Renin activity, plasma, sodium replete, ambulatory - - - 0.6-4.3 ng/mL
   per h

Renin, direct concentration ------------ 30-40 pg/mL (0.7-1.0 pmol/L)

Sex hormone–binding globulin (SHBG) - - 1.1-6.7 µg/mL (10-60 nmol/L)
(male);

   2.2-14.6 µg/mL (20-130 nmol/L) (female)

α-Subunit of pituitary glycoprotein hormones - - <1.2 ng/mL (<1.2 µg/L)

Testosterone (bioavailable) --------- 0.8-4.0 ng/dL (0.03-0.14 nmol/L)

   (20-50 years, female on oral estrogen);

   0.8-10.0 ng/dL (0.03-0.35 nmol/L)

   (20-50 years, female not on oral estrogen);

   83.0-257.0 ng/dL (2.88-8.92 nmol/L) (male 20-29 years);

   72.0-235.0 ng/dL (2.50-8.15 nmol/L) (male 30-39 years);

   61.0-213.0 ng/dL (2.12-7.39 nmol/L) (male 40-49 years);

   50.0-190.0 ng/dL (1.74-6.59 nmol/L) (male 50-59 years);

   40.0-168.0 ng/dL (1.39-5.83 nmol/L) (male 60-69 years)

Testosterone (free) --------- 9.0-30.0 ng/dL (0.31-1.04 nmol/L) (male);

   0.3-1.9 ng/dL (0.01-0.07 nmol/L) (female)

Testosterone (total) -------- 300-900 ng/dL (10.4-31.2 nmol/L) (male);

   8-60 ng/dL (0.3-2.1 nmol/L) (female)

Vitamin B$_{12}$ ---------------------- 180-914 pg/mL (133-674 pmol/L)

Chemistry Values

Alanine aminotransferase -------------- 10-40 U/L (0.17-0.67 µkat/L)

Albumin ------------------------------------ 3.5-5.0 g/dL (35-50 g/L)

Amylase --------------------------- 26-102 U/L (0.43-1.70 µkat/L)

Aspartate aminotransferase ------------ 20-48 U/L (0.33-0.80 µkat/L)

Bicarbonate ------------------------- 21-28 mEq/L (21-28 mmol/L)

Bilirubin (total) ---------------------- 0.3-1.2 mg/dL (5.1-20.5 µmol/L)

Blood gases

   Po$_2$, arterial blood ---------------- 80-100 mm Hg (10.6-13.3 kPa)

   Pco$_2$, arterial blood ----------------- 35-45 mm Hg (4.7-6.0 kPa)

Blood pH --- 7.35-7.45

Calcium ------------------------- 8.2-10.2 mg/dL (2.1-2.6 mmol/L)

Calcium (ionized) ------------------ 4.60-5.08 mg/dL (1.2-1.3 mmol/L)

Carbon dioxide ---------------------- 22-28 mEq/L (22-28 mmol/L)

CD$_4$ cell count ----------------------- 500-1400/µL (0.5-1.4 × 10^9/L)

Chloride ------------------------ 96-106 mEq/L (96-106 mmol/L)

Creatine kinase ---------------------- 50-200 U/L (0.84-3.34 µkat/L)

Creatinine ---------------- 0.7-1.3 mg/dL (61.9-114.9 µmol/L) (male);

   0.6-1.1 mg/dL (53.0-97.2 µmol/L) (female)

Ferritin --------------------------- 15-200 ng/mL (33.7-449.4 pmol/L)

Folate ------------------------------------ ≥4.0 ng/mL (≥4.0 µg/L)

Glucose ----------------------------- 70-99 mg/dL (3.9-5.5 mmol/L)

γ-Glutamyltransferase -------------------- 2-30 U/L (0.03-0.50 µkat/L)

Iron ------------------------- 50-150 µg/dL (9.0-26.8 µmol/L) (male);

   35-145 µg/dL (6.3-26.0 µmol/L) (female)

Lactate dehydrogenase ---------------- 100-200 U/L (1.7-3.3 µkat/L)

Lactic acid ----------------------- 5.4-20.7 mg/dL (0.6-2.3 mmol/L)

Lipase ----------------------------- 10-73 U/L (0.17-1.22 µkat/L)

Magnesium ------------------------- 1.5-2.3 mg/dL (0.6-0.9 mmol/L)

Osmolality ------------------- 275-295 mOsm/kg (275-295 mmol/kg)

Phosphorus ------------------------- 2.3-4.7 mg/dL (0.7-1.5 mmol/L)

Potassium ------------------------ 3.5-5.0 mEq/L (3.5-5.0 mmol/L)

Prothrombin time -- 8.3-10.8 s

Serum urea nitrogen ------------------- 8-23 mg/dL (2.9-8.2 mmol/L)

Sodium ------------------------- 136-142 mEq/L (136-142 mmol/L)

Transferrin saturation ------------------------------------ 14%-50%

Troponin I ---------------------------------- <0.6 ng/mL (<0.6 µg/L)

Tryptase -------------------------------- <11.5 ng/mL (<11.5 µg/L)

Uric acid ----------------------- 3.5-7.0 mg/dL (208.2-416.4 µmol/L)

Urine

Albumin ----------------- 30-300 µg/mg creat (3.4-33.9 µg/mol creat)

Albumin-to-creatinine ratio ------------------------- <30 mg/g creat

Aldosterone ------------------------- 3-20 µg/24 h (8.3-55.4 nmol/d)

   (should be <12 µg/24 h [<33.2 nmol/d] with oral sodium loading—

   confirmed with 24-hour urinary sodium >200 mEq)

Calcium ----------------------- 100-300 mg/24 h (2.5-7.5 mmol/d)

Catecholamine fractionation

   Normotensive normal ranges:

     Dopamine ---------------------- <700 µg/24 h (<4567 nmol/d)

     Epinephrine ---------------------- <35 µg/24 h (<191 nmol/d)

     Norepinephrine ----------------- <170 µg/24 h (<1005 nmol/d)

Citrate ---------------------- 320-1240 mg/24 h (16.7-64.5 mmol/d)

Cortisol ----------------------------- 4-50 µg/24 h (11-138 nmol/d)

Cortisol following dexamethasone suppression test (low-dose: 2 day,

   2 mg daily) ------------------------- <10 µg/24 h (<27.6 nmol/d)

Creatinine ------------------------ 1.0-2.0 g/24 h (8.8-17.7 mmol/d)

Glomerular filtration rate (estimated) -------- >60 mL/min per 1.73 m^2

5-Hydroxyindole acetic acid --------- 2-9 mg/24 h (10.5-47.1 µmol/d)

Iodine (random) --- >100 µg/L

17-Ketosteroids --------- 6.0-21.0 mg/24 h (20.8-72.9 µmol/d) (male);

   4.0-17.0 mg/24 h (13.9-59.0 µmol/d) (female)

Metanephrine fractionation

   Metanephrine ---------------------- <400 µg/24 h (<2028 nmol/d)

   Normetanephrine ------------------- <900 µg/24 h (<4914 nmol/d)

   Total metanephrine ---------------- <1000 µg/24 h (<5260 nmol/d)

Osmolality ---------------- 150-1150 mOsm/kg (150-1150 mmol/kg)

Oxalate ----------------------------- <40 mg/24 h (<456 mmol/d)

Phosphate ---------------------- 0.9-1.3 g/24 h (29.1-42.0 mmol/d)
Potassium ----------------------- 17-77 mEq/24 h (17-77 mmol/d)
Sodium ------------------------- 40-217 mEq/24 h (40-217 mmol/d)
Uric acid ----------------------------- <800 mg/24 h (<4.7 mmol/d)

Saliva

Cortisol (salivary), midnight -------------- <0.13 µg/dL (<3.6 nmol/L)

Semen

Semen analysis --------------- >20 million sperm/mL; >50% motility

T$_3$ --- triiodothyronine
T$_4$ --- thyroxine
TPO antibodies ------------------------- thyroperoxidase antibodies
TRH ------------------------------------ thyrotropin-releasing hormone
TRAb ------------------------------ thyrotropin-receptor antibodies
TSH --- thyrotropin
VLDL ------------------------------------ very low-density lipoprotein

Abbreviations

ACTH --- corticotropin
ACE inhibitor --------------- angiotensin-converting enzyme inhibitor
ALT -- alanine aminotransferase
AST -- aspartate aminotransferase
BMI -- body mass index
CNS -- central nervous system
CT -- computed tomography
DHEA ------------------------------------ dehydroepiandrosterone
DHEA-S --------------------------- dehydroepiandrosterone sulfate
DNA ------------------------------------ deoxyribonucleic acid
DPP-4 inhibitor ----------------------- dipeptidyl-peptidase 4 inhibitor
DXA ----------------------------- dual-energy x-ray absorptiometry
FDA ---------------------------------- Food and Drug Administration
FGF-23 ----------------------------- fibroblast growth factor 23
FNA ------------------------------------ fine-needle aspiration
FSH ---------------------------------- follicle-stimulating hormone
GH --- growth hormone
GHRH ------------------------- growth hormone–releasing hormone
GLP-1 receptor agonist ----- glucagonlike peptide 1 receptor agonist
GnRH ------------------------------ gonadotropin-releasing hormone
hCG ---------------------------------- human chorionic gonadotropin
HDL -- high-density lipoprotein
HIV ------------------------------- human immunodeficiency virus
HMG-CoA reductase inhibitor ------------ 3-hydroxy-3-methylglutaryl
    coenzyme A reductase inhibitor
IGF-1 ------------------------------------ insulinlike growth factor 1
LDL -- low-density lipoprotein
LH -- luteinizing hormone
MCV -------------------------------------- mean corpuscular volume
MRI ---------------------------------- magnetic resonance imaging
NPH insulin --------------------- neutral protamine Hagedorn insulin
PCSK9 inhibitor - - - - proprotein convertase subtilisin/kexin 9 inhibitor
PET ------------------------------- positron emission tomography
PSA -- prostate-specific antigen
PTH -- parathyroid hormone
PTHrP ----------------------- parathyroid hormone–related protein
SGLT-2 inhibitor ----------- sodium-glucose cotransporter 2 inhibitor
SHBG --------------------------------- sex hormone–binding globulin

ENDOCRINE SELF-ASSESSMENT PROGRAM 2019

Part I

1 A 59-year-old woman attends your clinic for advice regarding her blood pressure. She has had hypertension for 10 years and is currently treated with enalapril and amlodipine. She has a history of a transient ischemic attack and rate-controlled atrial fibrillation for which she is on atorvastatin and apixaban. She smokes 10 cigarettes per day. Given her medical history, she would like to avoid surgical operations unless deemed necessary.

On physical examination, her blood pressure is 138/85 mm Hg (mean of 3 seated readings) and pulse rate is 72 beats/min. The rest of her physical examination findings are normal.

Laboratory test results:
  Sodium = 138 mEq/L (136-142 mEq/L) (SI: 138 mmol/L [136-142 mmol/L])
  Potassium = 3.2 mEq/L (3.5-5.0 mEq/L) (SI: 4.0 mmol/L [3.5-5.0 mmol/L])
  Chloride = 99 mEq/L (96-106 mEq/L) (SI: 99 mEq/L [96-106 mmol/L])
  Serum urea nitrogen = 11 mg/dL (8-23 mg/dL) (SI: 3.9 mmol/L [2.9-8.2 mmol/L])
  Creatinine = 0.75 mg/dL (0.6-1.1 mg/dL) (SI: 66.3 μmol/L [53.0-97.2 μmol/L])
  Aldosterone = 30 ng/dL (4-21 ng/dL) (SI: 832.2 pmol/L [111.0-582.5 pmol/L])
  Plasma renin activity (sodium replete) = 0.1 ng/mL per h (0.6-4.3 ng/mL per h)
  Urinary aldosterone = 38 μg/24 h (3-20 μg/24 h) (SI: 105.3 nmol/d [8.3-55.4 nmol/d])
  Urinary sodium = 300 mEq/24 h (40-217 mEq/24 h) (SI: 300 mmol/d [40-217 mmol/d])

Adrenal CT shows an 11-mm left-sided adrenal nodule with a density of −10 Hounsfield units and greater than 50% washout 10 minutes after contrast administration.

In addition to advising smoking cessation, which of the following is the best next step?
  A. Continue current therapy; no further investigations
  B. Refer for adrenal venous sampling
  C. Arrange for a saline suppression test
  D. Add spironolactone to the current regimen
  E. Repeat laboratory testing after discontinuing enalapril

2 A 61-year-old woman with hypertension and history of esophageal carcinoma sustains a fracture of her right hip after falling. DXA scan reveals T-scores of −3.0 in the spine and −3.4 in the left femoral neck. She went through natural menopause at age 48 years and has not taken estrogen. She underwent esophagogastrectomy and chemoradiation in 2007. She has no history of kidney stones or parathyroid disease.

She has limited dietary calcium intake and does not take any calcium supplements, but she does take over-the-counter cholecalciferol, 1000 IU daily. She relies on a proton-pump inhibitor and calcium carbonate as needed for reflux.

Her physical examination findings are unremarkable.

Laboratory test results (12 weeks after her hip fracture):
  Serum calcium = 8.7 mg/dL (8.2-10.2 mg/dL) (SI: 2.2 mmol/L [2.1-2.6 mmol/L])
  Serum phosphate = 3.0 mg/dL (2.3-4.7 mg/dL) (SI: 1.0 mmol/L [0.7-1.5 mmol/L])
  Serum creatinine = 1.8 mg/dL (0.6-1.1 mg/dL) (SI: 159.1 μmol/L [53.0-97.2 μmol/L])
  Glomerular filtration rate (estimated) = 34 mL/min per 1.73 m^2 (>60 mL/min per 1.73 m^2)
  Serum intact PTH = 80 pg/mL (10-65 pg/mL) (SI: 80 ng/L [10-65 ng/L])
  Serum 25-hydroxyvitamin D = 25 ng/mL (30-80 ng/mL [optimal]) (SI: 62.4 nmol/L [74.9-199.7 nmol/L])
  Serum albumin = 3.8 g/dL (3.5-5.0 g/dL) (SI: 38 g/L [35-50 g/L])
  Serum alkaline phosphatase = 150 U/L (50-120 U/L) (SI: 2.51 μkat/L [0.84-2.00 μkat/L])
  Urinary calcium = 60 mg/24 h (100-300 mg/24 h) (SI: 1.5 mmol/d [2.5-7.5 mmol/d])

Which of the following should be recommended in addition to adequate calcium and vitamin D supplementation?
A. Alendronate
B. Zoledronic acid
C. Denosumab
D. Teriparatide
E. Abaloparatide

3 A 37-year-old man with type 1 diabetes mellitus returns for follow-up. Diabetes complications include microalbuminuria and mild symptoms of peripheral neuropathy. He reports ongoing difficulty with glucose control despite improvements to his lifestyle and self-management routine over the past year. He has no worrisome symptoms. Review of his glucometer download shows that he checks blood glucose by fingerstick 4 to 5 times per day with a mean glucose value of 212 mg/dL (11.8 mmol/L). The data confirm that 67% of values are above the target range and 12% of values are below the target range. His point-of-care hemoglobin A_{1c} level today is 9.1% (76 mmol/mol).

He is currently on a multiple daily injection regimen. Basal insulin is detemir, 21 units daily at bedtime. Insulin aspart is dosed for meals at 1 unit per 10 g of carbohydrate and to correct for high blood glucose with a sensitivity factor of 1 unit per 25 mg/dL (1.4 mmol/L), with a glucose target of 110 mg/dL (6.1 mmol/L). He eats at restaurants 5 to 6 times per week, and while he is disciplined about portion sizes, he finds it difficult to judge the carbohydrate content of these meals in particular. He exercises 3 times per week, with a mixture of cardio and weight lifting, and he frequently experiences either high or low glucose values afterwards. He retains hypoglycemia awareness. He works both night and day shifts on a schedule that frequently changes. His only additional medication is lisinopril, 20 mg daily.

On physical examination, his blood pressure is 125/78 mm Hg, and pulse rate is 88 beats/min. There are no signs of hypertrophy at insulin injection sites. He has loss of Achilles tendon reflexes but intact sensation to vibratory and monofilament testing.

In addition to nutritional counseling, which of the following is the best next step to improve his glycemic management?
A. Insulin pump with 2 different basal patterns to account for his variable work schedule
B. Real-time continuous glucose monitor
C. Integrated insulin pump and continuous glucose monitor with "threshold suspend" feature
D. Hybrid closed-loop insulin pump and continuous glucose monitoring system
E. Flash continuous glucose monitoring system

4 A 31-year-old woman with polycystic ovary syndrome seeks advice on improving her fertility while trying to conceive. She stopped birth control 6 months ago. Initially, her periods were monthly, but over the past 3 months, she has had only 1 period. Polycystic ovary syndrome was diagnosed in her early 20s when she developed significant hirsutism. Menarche was at age 13 years, and thereafter she had irregular menses (about 6 periods per year). Her family history is notable for type 2 diabetes in her father and a paternal aunt. Her paternal uncle had a myocardial infarction in his 50s.

On physical examination, her height is 62 in (157.5 cm) and weight is 123 lb (55.9 kg) (BMI = 22.5 kg/m^2). Her blood pressure is 124/72 mm Hg. She has terminal hair growth on her upper lip, chin, abdomen, and inner thighs with a Ferriman-Gallwey score of 15. She has no acanthosis nigricans.

Laboratory test results:
Total testosterone = 48 ng/dL (8-60 ng/dL) (SI: 1.7 nmol/L [0.3-2.1 nmol/L])
TSH = 2.1 mIU/L (0.5-5.0 mIU/L)
Prolactin = 12.1 ng/mL (4-30 ng/mL) (SI: 0.5 nmol/L [0.17-1.30 nmol/L])
17-Hydroxyprogesterone = 73 ng/dL (<80 ng/dL) (SI: 2.2 nmol/L [<2.42 nmol/L])
FSH = 5.2 mIU/mL (2.0-12.0 mIU/mL) (SI: 5.2 IU/L [2.0-12.0 IU/L])
Fasting glucose = 94 mg/dL (70-99 mg/dL) (SI: 5.2 mmol/L [3.9-5.5 mmol/L])

Which of the following is the best option to improve her fertility?
A. Clomiphene
B. Gonadotropins
C. Metformin
D. Laparoscopic ovarian drilling
E. Diet and lifestyle modification

5 A 65-year-old man with type 2 diabetes mellitus is hospitalized for severe hypoglycemia. Diabetes was diagnosed at age 50 years. He was treated with metformin and glyburide for 10 years, after which insulin glargine was initiated. At age 60, he experienced the first of 3 myocardial infarctions, resulting in stage III heart failure with reduced ejection fraction. Over the next 4 years, his diabetes control deteriorated.

The heart transplant team had recommended that he receive a left ventricular assist device (LVAD). Before placement of the device, the patient's insulin regimen consisted of glargine, 65 units in the morning, and lispro, 10 units with each meal. Nine days ago, the patient was hospitalized for LVAD placement, and he was discharged 7 days later. He was instructed to resume his usual insulin regimen at discharge.

Two days after hospital discharge, the patient was found unresponsive in his kitchen with an open carton of fruit juice. A fingerstick glucose measurement performed by the emergency medical team was 44 mg/dL (2.4 mmol/L). The patient regained consciousness after treatment with intravenous glucose, and he was transported to your hospital. When you interview the patient, he does not recall walking to the kitchen or having any symptoms of hypoglycemia. According to his hospital records from the previous admission, his regimen was transitioned from an insulin drip to correction dose insulin after LVAD placement. His postoperative course was unremarkable.

On physical examination, his blood pressure is 140/80 mm Hg, pulse rate is 80 beats/min, and temperature is 96.8°F (36°C). His height is 70 in (177.8 cm), and weight is 200 lb (90.9 kg) (BMI = 28.7 kg/m^2) (unchanged from values recorded during his previous hospitalization). His examination findings are normal, except for the presence of a driveline cable exiting his chest and attached to a suitcase device.

Laboratory test results:
Serum urea nitrogen, normal
Creatinine, normal
Liver function, normal
Hemoglobin A$_{1c}$ = 8.5% (4.0%-5.6%) (69 mmol/mol [20-38 mmol/mol])
Serum cortisol (AM) = 14 µg/dL (5-25 µg/dL) (SI: 386.2 nmol/L [137.9-689.7 nmol/L])
Fasting glucose = 152 mg/dL (70-99 mg/dL) (SI: 8.4 mmol/L [3.9-5.5 mmol/L])

Which of the following is the most important next step in this patient's management?
A. Perform an ACTH stimulation test and initiate glucocorticoids
B. Change insulin glargine to insulin degludec
C. Start continuous glucose monitoring for hypoglycemia unawareness
D. Screen for sepsis by measuring lactate and drawing blood cultures
E. Reduce his insulin glargine and prandial insulin dosages by 50%

6 A 31-year-old man presents with abdominal pain near his umbilicus. He describes symptoms of bloating, central abdominal pain, and daily diarrhea for several months. He takes no medications, and he does not smoke cigarettes. He has a history of testicular cancer and has been in remission for more than 5 years.

On physical examination, he is afebrile, blood pressure is 122/80 mm Hg, and pulse rate is 70 beats/min. His height is 69 in (175 cm), and weight is 148 lb (67.3 kg) (BMI = 21.9 kg/m^2). He has no signs of Cushing syndrome and there is no palpable abdominal pain or mass.

Abdominal CT with intravenous contrast documents a heterogeneously enhancing right adrenal mass measuring 3.4 x 3.2 cm (*see images, arrows*). The mass is relatively round and confined to the right adrenal gland. The left adrenal gland appears normal.

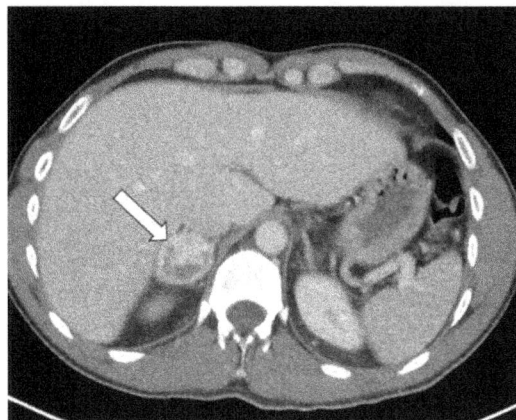 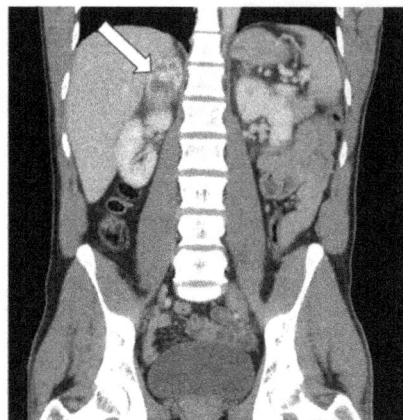

Axial view.   Coronal view.

A specific adrenal-related review of systems reveals that he has no history of episodic spells of adrenergic symptoms, including no sensations of palpitations, sweating, anxiety, tremors, pallor, flushing, headaches, or vision changes. He has had no known episodes of hypertension or orthostasis and no history of weight gain, weight loss, excessive virilization, or feminization.

Laboratory test results:
    Serum cortisol following 1-mg dexamethasone suppression test = 0.7 µg/dL (SI: 19.3 nmol/L)
    Plasma ACTH following 1-mg dexamethasone suppression test = <5.0 pg/mL (SI: 1.1 pmol/L)
    Plasma renin activity = 1.5 ng/mL per h (0.6-4.3 ng/mL per h)
    Serum aldosterone = 5.0 ng/dL (4-21 ng/dL) (SI: 138.7 pmol/L [111.0-582.5 pmol/L])
    Plasma metanephrine = <39 pg/mL (<99 pg/mL) (SI: <0.20 nmol/L [<0.50 nmol/L])
    Plasma normetanephrine = 720 pg/mL (<165 pg/mL) (SI: 3.93 nmol/L [<0.90 nmol/L])
    Urinary free cortisol = 37 µg/24 h (4-50 µg/24 h) (SI: 102 nmol/d [11-138 nmol/d])

Which of the following is the most likely diagnosis?
    A. Adrenocortical carcinoma
    B. Hyperfunctioning adrenocortical adenoma
    C. Nonfunctional lipid-poor adrenocortical adenoma
    D. Testicular cancer metastasis to the adrenal gland
    E. Pheochromocytoma

7 A 69-year-old man with a history of craniopharyngioma is seen in follow-up for panhypopituitarism and diabetes insipidus. He underwent surgical resection 9 months ago with subsequent adjuvant radiation therapy. He has since been on a regimen of hydrocortisone, 15 mg in the morning and 5 mg in afternoon; levothyroxine, 125 mcg daily; testosterone gel, 1.62% 2 applicators per day; and desmopressin, 1 spray (10 mcg) at bedtime (10 PM) and 1 spray in the morning. He feels well, with no excessive urination during the night. He reports that the morning desmopressin effect lasts about 10 hours, and he experiences polyuria in the late evening before taking the bedtime dose. He had a seizure recently, and his neurologist recommended starting oxcarbazepine therapy. Although the patient filled the prescription, he has not yet started the drug. Recent measurements of sodium, free T_4, and testosterone are normal.

Which of the following is the most important next step in this patient's management?
- A. Increase the hydrocortisone dosage
- B. Decrease the testosterone dosage
- C. Decrease the levothyroxine dosage
- D. Measure sodium again in 2 weeks
- E. Measure free T_4 and testosterone again in 2 weeks

8   A 57-year-old postmenopausal woman is referred for management of cardiovascular risk. Eleven months ago, she had advanced lipid testing through her naturopathic primary care provider's office and was found to have elevated lipoprotein (a) levels. At the time, she was told that her cardiovascular risk was very high and was prescribed a medication, which she did not start. Recently, she developed chest tightness; cardiac workup was unrevealing with no evidence of clinical cardiovascular disease. She takes alprazolam for generalized anxiety disorder and several dietary supplements, but no other medications. She does not smoke cigarettes, and she drinks 2 to 4 alcoholic beverages a week. She exercises regularly. Her father had a stroke at age 57 years, and a paternal uncle had a stroke at age 60 years. Her paternal grandmother underwent 2-vessel coronary bypass surgery and aortic valve replacement at age 72 years.

On physical examination, she is a healthy, anxious-appearing woman. Her blood pressure is 106/68 mm Hg. Her height is 68 in (172.7 cm), and weight is 163 lb (74 kg) (BMI = 24.8 kg/m^2). The rest of her examination findings are normal.

Laboratory test results (sample drawn while fasting, no treatment):
    Total cholesterol = 197 mg/dL (<200 mg/dL [optimal]) (SI: 5.10 mmol/L [<5.18 mmol/L])
    Triglycerides = 65 mg/dL (<150 mg/dL [optimal]) (SI: 0.73 mmol/L [<1.70 mmol/L])
    HDL cholesterol = 86 mg/dL (>60 mg/dL [optimal]) (SI: 2.23 mmol/L [>1.55 mmol/L])
    LDL cholesterol = 98 mg/dL (<100 mg/dL [optimal]) (SI: 2.54 mmol/L [<2.59 mmol/L])
    Non-HDL cholesterol = 111 mg/dL (<130 mg/dL [optimal]) (SI: 2.87 mmol/L [<3.37 mmol/L])
    Apolipoprotein B = 83 mg/dL (50-110 mg/dL) (SI: 0.83 g/dL [0.5-1.1 g/dL])
    Lipoprotein (a) = 150 mg/dL (≤30 mg/dL) (>95th percentile for Caucasians) (SI: 5.36 µmol/L [≤1.07 µmol/L])
    Hemoglobin A_{1c} = 5.5% (4.0%-5.6%) (37 mmol/mol [20-38 mmol/mol])
    TSH = 2.38 mIU/L (0.5-5.0 mIU/L)
    Fasting plasma glucose = 90 mg/dL (70-99 mg/dL) (SI: 5.0 mmol/L [3.9-5.5 mmol/L])

Her 10-year atherosclerotic cardiovascular disease risk is 1.1% based on the American College of Cardiology/ American Heart Association cardiovascular risk calculator.

Which of the following is the best next step in this patient's management?
- A. Start low-dosage aspirin
- B. Start a statin
- C. Start niacin
- D. Start a PCSK9 inhibitor
- E. No therapy is necessary now

9   A 42-year-old black man returns to the endocrinology clinic for follow-up of diabetes mellitus. Diabetes was diagnosed 8 years ago. His hemoglobin A_{1c} level measured 2 weeks ago was 6.8% (4.0%-5.6%) (51 mmol/mol [20-38 mmol/mol]). He is being treated with metformin, 1000 mg twice daily, and pioglitazone, 45 mg daily. He checks his blood glucose 1 to 2 times per day, and his 2-week glucose average is 187 mg/dL (10.4 mmol/L). Fasting glucose measurements range from 127 to 173 mg/dL (7.0-9.6 mmol/L), and postdinner glucose measurements range from 167 to 223 mg/dL (9.3-12.4 mmol/L). He has no microvascular complications.

He has a history of hypertension and is treated with losartan and metoprolol. Three months ago, atorvastatin, 80 mg daily, was prescribed to treat dyslipidemia. He has sickle cell trait. His hemoglobin value measured 9 months ago was 15.5 g/dL (13.8-17.2 g/dL) (155 g/L [138-172 g/L]). He has never had a blood transfusion. He does not smoke cigarettes and has 2 servings of alcohol per week. On review of his family history, his paternal grandmother has diabetes mellitus. His mother and sister have sickle cell anemia.

On physical examination, he appears well. His height is 70.5 in (179 cm) and weight is 206 lb (93.6 kg), (BMI = 29.1 kg/m^2). His blood pressure is 142/84 mm Hg, and pulse rate is 82 beats/min. Findings on cardiac, lung, and abdominal examinations are normal. There is no evidence of neuropathy.

Laboratory test results:
    Creatinine = 1.4 mg/dL (0.7-1.3 mg/dL) (SI: 123.8 µmol/L [61.9-114.9 µmol/L])
    Estimated glomerular filtration rate = 72 mL/min per 1.73 m^2 (>60 mL/min per 1.73 m^2)
    Fasting glucose = 139 mg/dL (70-99 mg/dL) (SI: 7.7 mmol/L [3.9-5.5 mmol/L])
    Electrolytes, normal

Which of the following is the best next step in this patient's management?
    A. Stop the atorvastatin and measure hemoglobin A$_{1c}$ again in 3 months
    B. Order a complete blood cell count and differential
    C. Order hemoglobin electrophoresis
    D. Start a third antihyperglycemic medication
    E. Refer to a dietician to review a diabetic meal plan

10 A 73-year-old woman presents to the emergency department with a 2-day history of generalized weakness, drowsiness, and fever. Her family members have noted her to have loss of appetite, weight loss of 6.6 lb (3 kg), and lethargy. The patient has a history of hyperlipidemia, hypertension, and a right-sided subcortical lacunar infarct 2 months earlier. She has made a full functional recovery from her cerebrovascular accident and is on treatment with simvastatin, aspirin, and amlodipine.

On physical examination, her height is 65 in (165.1 cm) and weight is 114 lb (51.7 kg) (BMI = 19.0 kg/m^2). She is lethargic, and her Glasgow Coma Scale score is 15. Her temperature is 102.9°F (39.4°C), blood pressure is 163/77 mm Hg, and pulse rate is 120 beats/min and regular. Her mucous membranes are dry. Her cardiovascular examination reveals a soft, pansystolic murmur, but findings on the rest of her respiratory and abdominal examination are normal. She is not jaundiced. She has a fine tremor of the hands, and a small diffuse goiter is noted along with a thyroid bruit. Neurologic examination reveals generalized weakness, with a power grade of 5/5 on the right, and 3/5 on the left. A Babinski response is present on the left foot; the other reflexes are normal. Findings on cranial nerve examination are normal, and her neck is supple. She has no rash and is not hyperpigmented.

Laboratory test results:
    Hemoglobin = 12.3 g/dL (12.1-15.1 g/dL) (SI: 123 g/L [121-151 g/L])
    White blood cell count = 13,500/µL (4500-11,000/µL) (SI: 13.5 x 10^9/L [4.5-11.0 x 10^9/L])
    Platelet count = 154 x 10^3/µL (150-450 x 10^3/µL) (SI: 154 x 10^9/L [150-450 x 10^9/L])
    Renal function and calcium, normal
    Liver function, normal except for elevated ALT = 63 U/L (10-40 U/L) (SI: 1.05 µkat/L [0.17-0.67 µkat/L])
    C-reactive protein = 6.2 mg/L (0.8-3.1 mg/L) (SI: 59.05 nmol/L [7.62-29.52 nmol/L])
    TSH = <0.01 mIU/L (0.5-5.0 mIU/L)
    Urine dip stick and microscopy = normal

Electrocardiography shows sinus tachycardia. Findings on chest radiography are normal. Brain CT shows a right-sided subcortical lacunar infarct but no other abnormalities.

Which of the following is the most appropriate next investigation?
    A. Measure serum cortisol
    B. Measure free T$_4$
    C. Perform brain MRI
    D. Perform lumbar puncture
    E. Perform thyroid ultrasonography

11 A 25-year-old man is referred to the endocrine clinic for management of hypogonadism. The patient reports abnormal pubertal development with a lack of secondary sexual characteristics, including genital growth, voice changes, and appearance of facial and body hair. He grew up in a developing country where access to medical care was limited. He has had no trauma or illnesses involving his testes such as torsion, trauma, or mumps. Upon moving to the United States, he established medical care with a primary care physician and was told that he had a low testosterone level and a normal pituitary MRI.

On physical examination, his height is 75 in (191 cm) and weight is 217 lb (99 kg) (BMI = 26.7 kg/m^2). His blood pressure is 113/75 mm Hg, and pulse rate is 68 beats/min. His physical examination findings are notable for testicular volumes of 3 mL bilaterally, sparse body and pubertal hair, and bilateral gynecomastia.

Which of the following tests would be best to assess his androgen status?
  A. Total testosterone by equilibrium dialysis
  B. Total testosterone by liquid chromatography–tandem mass spectrometry
  C. Total testosterone by automated immunoassay
  D. Free testosterone by direct radioimmunoassay using a labeled testosterone analogue
  E. Free testosterone by ammonium sulfate precipitation

12 A 67-year-old woman with end-stage renal disease secondary to polycystic kidney disease presents for evaluation of low bone density. She sustained a Colles fracture of her left wrist after a fall. DXA scan revealed T-scores of –3.1 (Z-score, –1.2) in the spine and –3.7 (Z-score, –2.4) in the left total hip. She undergoes hemodialysis every Monday, Wednesday, and Friday and is on calcium acetate and vitamin D supplementation per her nephrologist. She has no history of kidney stones. She has no history of long-term glucocorticoid exposure. Her mother has osteoporosis. The patient underwent surgical menopause at age 44 years. She has breast cancer with a history of radiation therapy and currently takes letrozole.

Her physical examination findings are unremarkable.

Laboratory test results:
  Serum calcium = 9.1 mg/dL (8.2-10.2 mg/dL) (SI: 2.3 mmol/L [2.1-2.6 mmol/L])
  Serum phosphate = 5.2 mg/dL (2.3-4.7 mg/dL) (SI: 1.7 mmol/L [0.7-1.5 mmol/L])
  Serum creatinine = 7.9 mg/dL (0.6-1.1 mg/dL) (SI: 698.4 μmol/L [53.0-97.2 μmol/L])
  Glomerular filtration rate (estimated) = 5 mL/min per 1.73 m^2 (>60 mL/min per 1.73 m^2)
  Serum intact PTH = 85 pg/mL (10-65 pg/mL) (SI: 85 ng/L [10-65 ng/L])
  Serum 25-hydroxyvitamin D = 32 ng/mL (30-80 ng/mL [optimal]) (SI: 79.9 nmol/L [74.9-199.7 nmol/L])
  Serum 1,25-dihydroxyvitamin D = 28 pg/mL (16-65 pg/mL) (SI: 83.2 pmol/L [41.6-169.0 pmol/L])
  Serum albumin = 4.3 g/dL (3.5-5.0 g/dL) (SI: 43 g/L [35-50 g/L])
  Serum bone-specific alkaline phosphatase = 18 μg/L (≤20 μg/L)

In addition to counseling on fall prevention, which of the following should be recommended as the best next step with regard to this patient's bone health?
  A. Start bisphosphonate therapy
  B. Start denosumab
  C. Start teriparatide
  D. Measure serum C-telopeptide
  E. Perform a transiliac bone biopsy

13 An 86-year-old man with a 30-year history of diabetes mellitus is admitted to the psychiatry unit for suicidal ideation after the unexpected death of his spouse 4 weeks ago. You are consulted on the second hospital day after he is found confused, with a fingerstick glucose value of 42 mg/dL (2.3 mmol/L). His blood glucose and his mental status improved after ingesting oral glucose. For the past 10 years, he has been treated with a combination tablet consisting of metformin, 500 mg, and glyburide, 5 mg (2 tablets twice daily). He describes feeling extremely despondent, and he has no urge to eat. He reports a 20-lb (9.1-kg) weight loss over the past 4 months, stating that he simply has no appetite. He has no diabetes-related complications.

On physical examination, he is a thin man with poor muscle mass and a cachectic appearance. His clothes and appearance are unkempt. His height is 70 in (177.8 cm), and weight is 125 lb (56.8 kg) (BMI = 17.9 kg/m^2). His blood pressure is 130/80 mm Hg, and pulse rate is 80 beats/min. Sensation in his feet is intact to monofilament testing. He uses a walker for ambulation. Examination findings are otherwise unremarkable.

Laboratory test results:
    Hemoglobin A$_{1c}$ = 7.5% (4.0%-5.6%) (58 mmol/mol [20-38 mmol/mol])
    Serum urea nitrogen = 12 mg/dL (8-23 mg/dL) (SI: 4.3 mmol/L [2.9-8.2 mmol/L])
    Creatinine = 0.9 mg/dL (0.7-1.3 mg/dL) (SI: 79.6 μmol/L [61.9-114.9 μmol/L])
    Chemistry panel, normal
    Liver function, normal
    Serum lactate, undetectable
    Albumin = 2.5 g/dL (3.5-5.0 g/dL) (SI: 25 g/L [35-50 g/L])
    Urinalysis, normal except for trace ketones

Which of the following is the most important next step in this patient's management?
    A. Reduce the dosage of the metformin and glyburide combination by half
    B. Discontinue all diabetes medications and order a nutrition consult
    C. Discontinue glyburide and maintain the metformin dosage at 500 mg twice daily
    D. Discontinue metformin and glyburide and start an SGLT-2 inhibitor
    E. Discontinue metformin and glyburide and start a DPP-4 inhibitor

14 A 55-year-old man with hypothyroidism, chronic back pain, and obstructive sleep apnea is interested in weight-loss medications. His weight has been a problem since he was in his early 30s. His highest weight was 250 lb (113.4 kg), and his current weight is 244 lb (110.8 kg). The patient has never participated in a commercial weight-loss program, but he has followed self-administered diets. He regularly skips breakfast, as he is not hungry when he wakes up, and lunch is usually a sandwich. His evening meal is the largest of the day, and it typically includes a protein, a vegetable, and a carbohydrate. Before bedtime, he usually has a large portion of cake, a peanut butter and jelly sandwich, or a big bowl of ice cream with cookies. He reports that 5 to 6 nights a week he wakes around 1 to 3 AM because of hunger, which he satisfies by eating a meal (typically a sandwich and chips). He is active during the day, walking close to 10,000 steps daily.

He uses continuous positive airway pressure for sleep apnea. His medications include levothyroxine, a multivitamin, and acetaminophen as needed.

On physical examination, his height is 72 in (182.9 cm) and weight is 244 lb (110.9 kg) (BMI = 33.1 kg/m^2). His blood pressure is 134/80 mm Hg, and pulse rate is 67 beats/min. He has mild thyromegaly, his lungs are clear to auscultation, and his heart sounds are regular. His abdomen is soft and nontender, and he has no lower-extremity edema.

If you were to prescribe a medication for this patient, which of the following would you recommend?
    A. Phentermine
    B. Sertraline
    C. Lorcaserin
    D. Amitriptyline
    E. Bupropion/naltrexone

15 You are asked to consult on a 31-year-old man in the neurosurgical ward. He underwent transsphenoidal surgery for management of a nonfunctional pituitary macroadenoma 36 hours ago. The neurosurgical resident is concerned that he has developed diabetes insipidus. The patient reports feeling thirsty but otherwise has no complaints. His fluid balance chart suggests an average urine output of 220 mL/h and fluid intake of 5 L over the past 24 hours.

On physical examination, he is alert and appears euvolemic with moist mucous membranes. His blood pressure is 112/72 mm Hg, and resting pulse rate is 84 beats/min.

Laboratory test results:

Sodium = 141 mEq/L (136-142 mEq/L) (SI: 141 mmol/L [136-142 mmol/L])

Potassium = 4.2 mEq/L (3.5-5.0 mEq/L) (SI: 4.2 mmol/L [3.5-5.0 mmol/L])

Chloride = 103 mEq/L (96-106 mEq/L) (SI: 103 mmol/L [96-106 mmol/L])

Serum urea nitrogen = 15 mg/dL (8-23 mg/dL) (SI: 5.4 mmol/L [2.9-8.2 mmol/L])

Creatinine = 0.92 mg/dL (0.7-1.3 mg/dL) (SI: 81.3 µmol/L [61.9-114.9 µmol/L])

Serum osmolality = 295 mOsm/kg (275-295 mOsm/kg) (SI: 295 mmol/kg [275-295 mmol/kg])

Glucose = 96 mg/dL (70-99 mg/dL) (SI: 5.3 mmol/L [3.9-5.5 mmol/L])

Calcium = 9.1 mg/dL (8.2-10.2 mg/dL) (SI: 2.3 mmol/L [2.1-2.6 mmol/L])

Urine osmolality = 190 mOsm/kg (150-1150 mOsm/kg) (SI: 190 mmol/kg [150-1150 mmol/kg])

In addition to regular monitoring of fluid balance and plasma sodium and osmolality, how would you manage this patient?

A. A single dose of subcutaneous desmopressin

B. A single dose of intranasal desmopressin

C. Scheduled subcutaneous desmopressin for 48 hours

D. Reduced fluid intake

E. No treatment required

16 You are consulted regarding the discovery of a goiter in an inpatient on the neurosurgical service. The patient is a 27-year-old woman who is scheduled for transsphenoidal surgery for a pituitary adenoma in the morning. Her admission was scheduled the evening before her surgery and the admitting resident noted her goiter and requested an endocrinology opinion.

The patient describes amenorrhea and galactorrhea of approximately 9 months' duration. She also notes weight gain, fatigue, and constipation.

On physical examination, her vital signs are normal and her BMI is 30 kg/m^2. She has some mild bilateral upper- and lower-extremity swelling and dry skin. Her thyroid gland is approximately twice normal size. The enlargement is symmetric and the gland is firm and nontender to palpation. Her physical examination findings are otherwise unremarkable.

Laboratory test results:

Complete metabolic panel, normal

Complete blood cell count, normal

Serum pregnancy test, negative

Serum prolactin:

4 months ago = 80 ng/mL (4-30 ng/mL) (SI: 3.5 nmol/L [0.17-1.30 nmol/L])

1 week ago = 150 ng/mL (4-30 ng/mL) (SI: 6.5 nmol/L [0.17-1.30 nmol/])

The patient has normal formal testing of her visual fields. Her pituitary MRI is shown (*see images*).

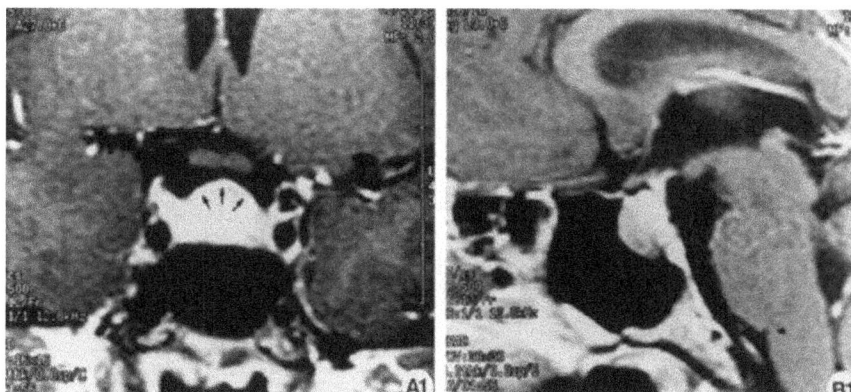

Reprinted from Sarlis NJ, Brucker-Davis F, Doppman JL, Skarulis MC. *J Clin Endocrinol Metab*. 1997; 82(3):808-811.

Which of the following would you recommend to the neurosurgical team as the best next step in this patient's management?

A. Further endocrinology evaluation after the patient has undergone transsphenoidal pituitary surgery
B. Thyrotropin-releasing hormone stimulation test
C. Cancellation of pituitary surgery until the results of serum TSH measurement are available
D. Empiric treatment with levothyroxine before pituitary surgery
E. Cancellation of pituitary surgery and initiation of a dopamine agonist

17 A 57-year-old man comes for metabolic bone evaluation after recently documented bone loss. Osteoporosis was diagnosed 13 months ago based on a DXA study that showed a right femoral neck T-score of –2.6. A previous metabolic bone workup revealed no clear contributing etiology according to medical history or biochemical studies. Given no history of previous low-trauma fractures and a low absolute risk of fracture by FRAX calculation (2.2% and 8.3% for 10-year risk of hip and major osteoporotic fracture, respectively), he opted for conservative management with supplemental calcium and vitamin D and weight-bearing exercise.

Thirteen months after his first DXA, he underwent another assessment on the same instrument. The lumbar spine bone mineral density was stable, but the right total proximal femur bone mineral density was reported to be significantly lower (absolute bone mineral density decline of 0.069 g/cm^2 or –7.6%).

Given these findings, which of the following is the best next step in this patient's management?

A. Start teriparatide daily injections
B. Start an oral bisphosphonate
C. Order another DXA scan to confirm the decline in proximal femur bone mineral density
D. Review the DXA images to ensure valid assessment of the hip regions of interest
E. Repeat the workup for secondary causes of osteoporosis

18 A 67-year-old woman was diagnosed with type 2 diabetes mellitus 13 years ago. She has no known diabetes-related complications. Her current hemoglobin A_{1c} level is 8.6% (70 mmol/mol) despite taking metformin, 1000 mg twice daily. She also has hypertension. Menopause was at age 53 years. A bone density scan performed 1 year ago documented a spine T-score of –2.2 and left total hip T-score of –2.6. Weekly alendronate was prescribed. She does not smoke cigarettes, but does report drinking 1 to 2 glasses of red wine each day. Her mother has diabetes and osteoporosis, and her father has diabetes and coronary artery disease.

On physical examination, her weight is 192 lb (82.5 kg) and height is 66 in (167.5 cm) (BMI = 31.0 kg/m^2). Her pulse rate is 72 beats/min, and blood pressure is 136/64 mm Hg. She has acanthosis nigricans on her neck and under her arms. Findings on dental, cardiac, pulmonary, and abdominal examination are normal. There is no focal tenderness on palpation of the spine, and spinal curvature appears normal.

In addition to metformin, current medications include lisinopril, 30 mg daily; atorvastatin, 40 mg daily; alendronate, 70 mg weekly; calcium carbonate, 1200 mg daily; and ergocalciferol, 2000 IU daily.

Laboratory test results:
  Serum urea nitrogen = 21 mg/dL (8-23 mg/dL) (SI: 7.5 mmol/L [2.9-8.2 mmol/L])
  Creatinine = 1.1 mg/dL (0.6-1.1 mg/dL) (SI: 97.2 μmol/L [53.0-97.2 μmol/L])
  25-Hydroxyvitamin D = 31 ng/mL (30-80 ng/mL [optimal]) (SI: 77.4 nmol/L [74.9-199.7 nmol/L])
  Calcium = 9.1 mg/dL (8.2-10.2 mg/dL) (SI: 2.3 mmol/L [2.1-2.6 mmol/L])

You counsel her to limit consumption of alcohol and to increase weight-bearing exercise.

Which of the following is the best next step in this patient's diabetes management?

A. Add liraglutide
B. Add canagliflozin
C. Add sitagliptin
D. Add pioglitazone
E. Maintain current regimen

19 A 25-year-old transgender patient assigned female at birth who identifies as male initiated masculinizing testosterone injections 9 months ago for gender dysphoria. He had regular monthly bleeding before initiation of testosterone. He had no bleeding for 4 months after the third month of hormone therapy. However, for the past 2 months, bleeding has recurred intermittently and this has markedly increased dysphoria.

Laboratory test result (assessment just before the current visit, midway between injections):
    Total testosterone = 343 ng/dL (300-900 ng/dL [male]; (0.3-1.9 ng/dL [female]) (SI: 11.9 nmol/L [10.4-31.2 nmol/L (male)]; [0.01-0.07 nmol/L (female)])

His testosterone dosage is 50 mg subcutaneously weekly. He has already had a gynecologic examination and ultrasonography, and there is no evidence of infection or uterine abnormality. In considering his options to stop the bleeding, he is most concerned about worsening dysphoria.

Which of the following is the best option to stop the bleeding and avoid worsening this patient's gender dysphoria?
    A. Prescribe a short course of estrogen
    B. Prescribe oral progesterone
    C. Switch from subcutaneous to intramuscular testosterone therapy
    D. Recommend a copper intrauterine device
    E. Increase the testosterone dosage

20 A 75-year-old woman presents to the emergency department with abdominal pain. She has no personal history of malignancy, and she is a lifelong nonsmoker. Recent colonoscopy and mammography screenings were negative. The patient takes no medications and has no history of foreign travel or sick exposures. Abdominal CT with intravenous contrast is performed. CT findings reveal diverticulitis, but also an incidentally discovered right adrenal mass. The mass is 3.5 cm x 2.5 cm in diameter and described as lobular, largely enhancing with contrast, and containing components of microscopic fat. One week later, the patient undergoes a dedicated adrenal washout protocol CT scan, which documents that the adrenal mass has an unenhanced density of 23 Hounsfield units and less than 50% absolute washout of contrast after 15 minutes.

Laboratory test results:
    Serum cortisol following 1-mg dexamethasone suppression test = 1.1 µg/dL (30.3 nmol/L)
    Plasma metanephrine = 91 pg/mL (<99 pg/mL) (SI: 0.46 nmol/L [<0.50 nmol/L])
    Plasma normetanephrine = 141 pg/mL (<165 pg/mL) (SI: 0.77 nmol/L [<0.90 nmol/L])
    DHEA-S = 118 µg/dL (15-157 µg/dL) (SI: 3.2 µmol/L [0.41-4.25 µmol/L])

A CT-guided biopsy of the mass reveals cells with no marked mitotic index and no malignant-appearing cells.

Which of the following is the most reasonable next step in this patient's management?
    A. Referral for adrenalectomy
    B. Measurement of late-night salivary cortisol
    C. Repeated imaging in 1 year
    D. Repeated biopsy in 1 year
    E. No need for further imaging surveillance

21 A 25-year-old medical student presents to discuss whether he could have a pituitary tumor. The patient saw his primary care physician for an evaluation of possible gynecomastia that has been present for approximately 1 to 2 years. He is self-conscious about the physical appearance of his chest. He has no relevant medical history but does admit to smoking marijuana a few times each month. He has no symptoms such as headaches, galactorrhea, or low libido. He has a family history of a pituitary tumor in a maternal aunt and is worried about this possibility. He takes no medications.

On physical examination, he is anxious. His height is 69 in (175 cm) and weight is 193 lb (88 kg) (BMI = 28 kg/m^2). His blood pressure is 143/77 mm Hg, and pulse rate is 83 beats/min. Visual fields are normal by confrontation examination. He may have mild bilateral gynecomastia or pseudogynecomastia. Testicular volume is 20 mL bilaterally.

Laboratory test results (1 PM):
 Total testosterone = 275 ng/dL (300-900 ng/dL) (SI: 9.54 nmol/L [10.4-31.2 nmol/L])
 LH = 3.8 mIU/mL (1.0-9.0 mIU/mL) (SI: 3.8 IU/L [1.0-9.0 IU/L])
 FSH = 5.1 mIU/mL (1.0-13.0 mIU/mL) (SI: 5.1 IU/L [1.0-13.0 IU/L])
 Free T$_4$ = 1.1 ng/dL (0.8-1.8 ng/dL) (SI: 14.2 pmol/L [10.30-23.17 pmol/L])
 Prolactin = 12 ng/mL (4-23 ng/mL) (SI: 0.52 nmol/L [0.17-1.00 nmol/L])
 Complete blood cell count, normal
 Chemistry panel, normal

Which of the following is the best next step in this patient's management?
 A. Morning measurement of serum cortisol, IGF-1, and TSH
 B. Mammography
 C. Pituitary MRI with gadolinium
 D. Testicular ultrasonography
 E. α-Subunit measurement

22 A 61-year-old black woman presents to her primary care clinic with polyuria, polydipsia, and lightheadedness and is admitted to the hospital for symptomatic hyperglycemia. She was recently diagnosed with type 2 diabetes mellitus and metformin was initiated. However, after 5 months, her regimen was transitioned to NPH insulin and regular insulin due to poor glycemic control. The outpatient total daily insulin dose was 170 units. Her history is notable for a 55.5-lb (27-kg) weight loss since the diagnosis of diabetes.

On physical examination, she has temporal wasting and extensive acanthosis nigricans, including on the palms and tongue. Her height is 64 in (162.5 cm), and weight is 116 lb (52.7 kg) (BMI = 19.9 kg/m^2).

Laboratory test results are notable for a normal anion gap and a triglyceride value of 39 mg/dL (<150 mg/dL [optimal]) (SI: 0.44 mmol/L [<1.70 mmol/L]).

Her hospital course is characterized by the persistence of hyperglycemia without ketosis or fasting hypoglycemia. Intravenous insulin is initiated, peaking at 11,650 units daily.

Which of the following is the underlying cause of this patient's presentation?
 A. Antiinsulin antibodies
 B. Antiinsulin receptor antibodies
 C. An underlying infection
 D. Partial lipodystrophy
 E. Occult malignancy

23 A 44-year-old man is referred by his primary care physician for management of a lipid disorder. Your clinic's policy is to obtain fasting lipid testing before visits. However, 1 week before his scheduled visit with you, the patient calls and states that he is unable to fast prior to testing because he works graveyard shifts from 11 PM to 7 AM 6 days a week. A quick review of his chart suggests that he has hypertension treated with a β-adrenergic blocker. He also has treated hypothyroidism and does not smoke cigarettes or drink alcohol. Family history documentation is limited. At his last clinic visit, his blood pressure was 138/90 mm Hg and BMI was 34 kg/m^2.

Laboratory test results from 4 months ago (nonfasting):

Total cholesterol = 227 mg/dL (<200 mg/dL [optimal]) (SI: 5.88 mmol/L [<5.18 mmol/L])

Triglycerides = 525 mg/dL (<150 mg/dL [optimal]) (SI: 5.93 mmol/L [<1.70 mmol/L])

HDL cholesterol = 37 mg/dL (>60 mg/dL [optimal]) (SI: 0.96 mmol/L [>1.55 mmol/L])

Non-HDL cholesterol = 190 mg/dL (<130 mg/dL [optimal]) (SI: 4.92 mmol/L [<3.37 mmol/L])

Hemoglobin A_{1c} = 5.7% (4.0%-5.6%) (39 mmol/mol [20-38 mmol/mol])

TSH = 2.1 mIU/L (0.5-5.0 mIU/L)

Which of the following do you suggest as the best next step in this patient?
- A. Perform nonfasting lipid testing on the day of the visit
- B. Perform fasting lipid testing after a 10- to 12-hour fast at the end of shift
- C. Start statin without repeat lipid testing
- D. Start fibrate
- E. Start fish oil

24 A 61-year-old man with a 12-year history of diabetes mellitus is seen in the endocrinology clinic for follow-up. He is being treated with metformin, 2000 mg daily, and glipizide, 10 mg daily. He has a history of microalbuminuria and hypertension and is being treated with lisinopril, chlorthalidone, and amlodipine. He takes furosemide, 60 mg, in a divided dose daily. He also takes simvastatin.

He has peripheral neuropathy and developed a Charcot joint involving the left foot 2 years ago. He was initially treated with off-loading of the foot. He was fitted for a custom left shoe and has been followed closely by his podiatrist. He has a history of coronary artery disease, peripheral arterial disease, and a silent myocardial infarction. Previous echocardiography demonstrated diastolic dysfunction. He underwent stenting of a popliteal artery lesion in the left leg 18 months ago. He takes clopidogrel and aspirin. He has a 38 pack-year cigarette smoking history, but he quit smoking 4 years ago. He rarely drinks alcohol.

On physical examination, he appears well. His height is 69 in (175 cm) and weight is 227 lb (103.2 kg) (BMI = 33.5 kg/m^2). His blood pressure is 126/81 mm Hg, and pulse rate is 87 beats/min. He has central adiposity. Findings on cardiac, lung, and abdominal examinations are normal. The distal pulses are mildly reduced. He has significant pedal edema. There is a Charcot joint involving the left foot. He has absent sensation to 10-g monofilament distal to each ankle. The Achilles reflexes are absent, and vibrational sense is reduced in both feet.

Laboratory test results:

Hemoglobin A_{1c} = 8.7% (4.0%-5.6%) (72 mmol/mol [20-38 mmol/mol])

Creatinine = 1.5 mg/dL (0.7-1.3 mg/dL) (SI: 132.6 μmol/L [61.9-114.9 μmol/L]

Estimated glomerular filtration rate = 56 mL/min per 1.73 m^2 (>60 mL/min per 1.73 m^2)

TSH = 2.73 mIU/mL (0.5-5.0 mIU/L)

Electrolytes, normal

After referral to a dietician, which of the following medications would you recommend to improve this patient's glycemic control?
- A. Pioglitazone
- B. Liraglutide
- C. Saxagliptin
- D. Canagliflozin
- E. Acarbose

25 Acromegaly is diagnosed in a 47-year-old man, and laboratory test results are as follows:

Random GH = 18.9 ng/mL (0.01-0.97 ng/mL) (SI: 18.9 μg/L [0.01-0.97 μg/L])

IGF-1 = 893 ng/mL (91-246 ng/mL) (SI: 117 nmol/L [11.9-32.2 nmol/L])

Pituitary MRI shows a 1.2-cm intrasellar macroadenoma, with no obvious cavernous sinus invasion. He undergoes operation, and the neurosurgeon tells you that he "got it all."

Postoperatively, the patient does well and reports reduced swelling of his hands and feet. You see him before hospital discharge, and he is discharged on no medications. He returns for follow-up 12 weeks later and lab work shows the following:

Random GH = 1.4 ng/mL (0.01-0.97 ng/mL) (SI: 1.4 µg/L [0.01-0.97 µg/L])

IGF-1 = 389 ng/mL (91-246 ng/mL) (SI: 51 nmol/L [11.9-32.2 nmol/L])

Which of the following is the best next step?
A. Perform pituitary MRI and refer him back to neurosurgery
B. Start somatostatin analogue therapy
C. Measure GH after an oral glucose load
D. Start cabergoline therapy
E. Measure IGFBP-3

26 A 48-year-old man attends his first postoperative visit after adrenalectomy for a pheochromocytoma 6 weeks ago. He had presented with episodes of headache, tachycardia, and hypertension and was found to have elevated urinary metanephrine excretion. Abdominal CT revealed an 8-cm right-sided pheochromocytoma with no evidence of metastatic spread. He has been feeling well since his operation and his "spells" have resolved. He currently takes no medication. No genetic cause for his pheochromocytoma has been identified.

On physical examination, his blood pressure is 128/72 mm Hg and resting pulse rate is 68 beats/min. Other than healing laparoscopic incision scars, examination findings are normal.

Laboratory test results (postoperative):

Urinary metanephrine = 284 µg/24 h (<400 µg/24 h) (SI: 1440 nmol/d [<2028 nmol/d])

Urinary normetanephrine = 469 µg/24 h (<900 µg/24 h) (SI: 2561 nmol/d [<4914 nmol/d])

Urinary total metanephrine = 720 µg/24 h (<1000 µg/24 h) (SI: 3787 nmol/d [<5260 nmol/d])

The pathology report summary states, "Pheochromocytoma with extensive central necrosis, focal capsular invasion, and early invasion into the adrenal vein. There is no extension into surrounding fat. The Ki67 proliferation index is 2.5%."

On the basis of these results, which of the following is the best next step in this patient's management?
A. Refer for ^{131}I-MIBG radionuclide therapy
B. Measure chromogranin A
C. Measure urinary metanephrine in 6 months
D. Refer for platinum-based adjuvant chemotherapy
E. Perform ^{123}I-MIBG scan in 6 months

27 A 39-year-old woman presents with progressive substernal chest pain of approximately 1-month duration, as well as a 2-month history of dyspnea on exertion, palpitations, tremor, night sweats, and weight loss of 30 lb (13.6 kg). She does not smoke cigarettes. Her mother has autoimmune hypothyroidism.

On physical examination, her height is 68 in (172.7 cm) and weight is 137 lb (62.3 kg) (BMI = 20.8 kg/m^2). Her blood pressure is 134/76 mm Hg, pulse rate is 104 beats/min and regular, and pulse oximetry is 98% on room air. Findings on cardiovascular, respiratory, and abdominal examinations are unremarkable. She has a symmetric, diffusely enlarged thyroid gland to approximately twice its normal size. There is no cervical lymphadenopathy. She has no signs of Graves-related ophthalmopathy or dermopathy.

Laboratory test results:

    TSH = <0.01 mIU/L (0.5-5.0 mIU/L)

    Free T$_4$ = 6.5 ng/dL (0.8-1.8 ng/dL) (SI: 83.7 pmol/L [10.30-23.17 pmol/L])

    TRAb = 34.2 IU/L (≤1.75 IU/L)

    Calcium = 9.3 mg/dL (8.2-10.2 mg/dL) (SI: 2.3 mmol/L [2.1-2.6 mmol/L])

    Lactate dehydrogenase = 172 U/L (100-200 U/L) (SI: 2.9 μkat/L [1.7-3.3 μkat/L])

    β-hCG = 2.8 mIU/mL (<3.0 mIU/mL) (SI: 2.8 IU/L [<3.0 IU/L])

A ^{99m}Tc technetium scan and chest CT are shown (*see images*).

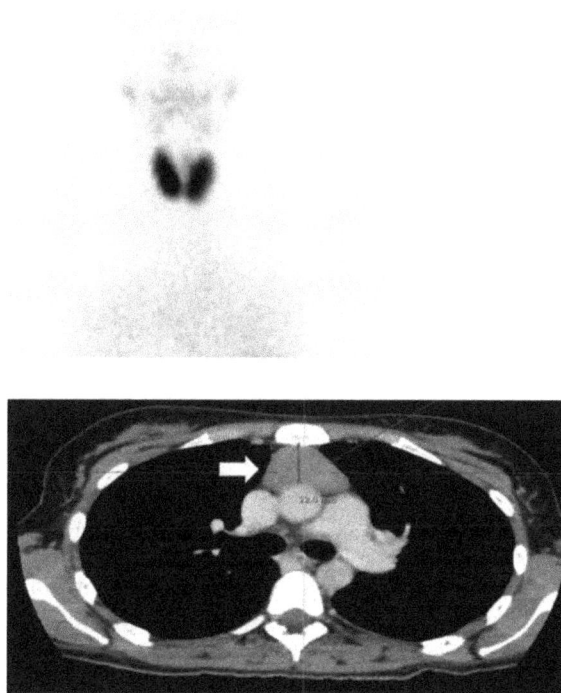

Which of the following most likely explains the mediastinal mass?

    A. Lymphoma

    B. Germinoma

    C. Parathyroid mass

    D. Thymoma

    E. Ectopic thyroid tissue

28 A 21-year-old woman presents for evaluation of secondary amenorrhea. Menarche occurred at age 13 years. Menses were regular and monthly until age 15 when they stopped for a year. Her pediatrician thought it was due to low body fat percentage from running cross-country. At age 17 years, oral contraceptives were prescribed. Recently she decided to stop oral contraceptives. In the past 6 months she has had no menses, so she sought evaluation by her gynecologist. Micronized progesterone (for 10 days) was prescribed on 2 separate occasions at a lower and higher dose, and she had no withdrawal bleeding. Pelvic ultrasonography revealed ovarian volume of 5 mL bilaterally with a uterine lining thickness of 3 mm. The patient has no hot flashes, vaginal dryness, or galactorrhea. She runs 2 to 4 miles 3 to 5 times a week. There is no history of eating disorders, and

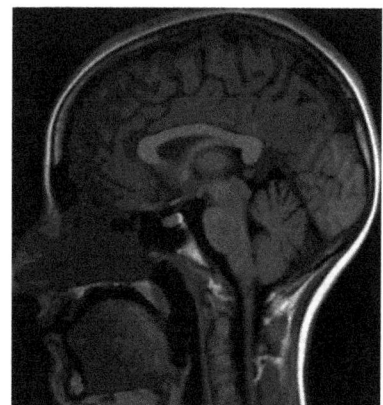

she is doing well in nursing school. She has never been pregnant and has never had a pelvic infection or gynecologic procedure.

On physical examination, her blood pressure is 110/74 mm Hg. Her height is 65 in (165 cm), and weight is 115 lb (52.3 kg) (BMI = 19.1 kg/m^2). She has no terminal hair growth or acne. The thyroid gland is normal in size without nodules. The rest of her examination findings are unremarkable.

Recent laboratory test results:
    TSH = 2.3 mIU/L (0.5-5.0 mIU/L)
    Prolactin = 12 ng/mL (4-30 ng/mL [nonlactating female]) (SI: 0.17-1.30 nmol/L)
    LH = 13.0 mIU/mL (1.0-18.1 mIU/mL) (SI: 13.0 IU/L [1.0-18.1 IU/L])
    FSH = 6.6 mIU/mL (2.0-12.0 mIU/mL) (SI: 6.6 IU/L [2.0-12.0 IU/L])
    Estradiol = 62 pg/mL (10-180 pg/mL) (SI: 227.6 pmol/L [36.7-660.8 pmol/L])
    Androstenedione = 322 ng/dL (80-240 ng/dL) (SI: 11.2 nmol/L [2.79-8.38 nmol/L])
    Cortisol (8 AM) = 12 μg/dL (5-25 μg/dL) (SI: 331.1 nmol/L [137.9-689.7 nmol/L])
    Antimullerian hormone = 10.0 ng/mL (0.9-9.5 ng/mL) (SI: 71.4 pmol/L [6.4-67.9 pmol/L])

Head MRI is performed (*see image*), and she is now referred to endocrinology for a question of secondary hypogonadism.

Which of the following is the most likely diagnosis?
    A. Premature ovarian insufficiency
    B. Polycystic ovary syndrome
    C. Functional hypothalamic amenorrhea
    D. Partial empty sella syndrome
    E. Asherman syndrome

29 A 40-year-old woman seeks evaluation of hypocalcemia due to hypoparathyroidism that occurred as a result of thyroidectomy for thyroid lymphoma 1 year ago. Despite treatment with 4 g of elemental calcium daily in divided doses and calcitriol, 1 mcg daily, she continues to have intermittent mild to moderate symptoms of hypocalcemia. She reports no diarrhea, nausea, or vomiting. She is adherent to her regimen of supplements and medications. She tried hydrochlorothiazide in the past, but this resulted in significant hypokalemia despite potassium supplementation, with minimal benefit in terms of her calcium level. She has no history of kidney stones.

On physical examination, she has a positive Chvostek sign. Neck exam reveals a surgically absent thyroid gland with an intact scar. Her examination findings are otherwise unremarkable.

Laboratory test results:
    Serum calcium = 7.3 mg/dL (8.2-10.2 mg/dL) (SI: 1.8 mmol/L [2.1-2.6 mmol/L])
    Serum phosphate = 5.5 mg/dL (2.3-4.7 mg/dL) (SI: 1.8 mmol/L [0.7-1.5 mmol/L])
    Serum creatinine = 0.7 mg/dL (0.6-1.1 mg/dL) (SI: 61.9 μmol/L [53.0-97.2 μmol/L])
    Serum intact PTH = 3 pg/mL (10-65 pg/mL) (SI: 3 ng/L [10-65 ng/L])
    Serum 25-hydroxyvitamin D = 43 ng/mL (30-80 ng/mL [optimal]) (SI: 107.3 nmol/L [74.9-199.7 nmol/L])
    Serum albumin = 3.9 g/dL (3.5-5.0 g/dL) (SI: 39 g/L [35-50 g/L])
    Serum magnesium = 1.9 mg/dL (1.5-2.3 mg/dL) (SI: 0.8 mmol/L [0.6-0.9 mmol/L])
    Urinary calcium = 420 mg/24 h (100-300 mg/24 h) (SI: 10.5 mmol/d [2.5-7.5 mmol/d])

Which of the following is the most appropriate next step in the management of this patient's hypocalcemia?
    A. Increase the calcitriol dosage
    B. Increase elemental calcium intake
    C. Start a phosphate-binding agent
    D. Start rhPTH (1-84) injections once daily
    E. No changes to her current medications

30 A 58-year-old woman is diagnosed with a neuroendocrine tumor after an extensive workup for abdominal discomfort. The patient has no history of diabetes mellitus. Her symptoms of abdominal pain prompted abdominal ultrasonography, which revealed liver lesions. Biopsy confirmed neuroendocrine tumor.

Now, 2 weeks later, she presents to a local hospital with persistent symptomatic hypoglycemia and syncopal episodes. D10 infusion is initiated, and you are consulted for further management and recommendations.

On interviewing the patient, she describes no significant weight gain over the past 6 months, but since recently increasing her frequency of oral food intake, she thinks she may have gained a couple pounds. She currently has no appetite, and she was nauseated this morning. She has not vomited. She has no family history of pituitary disease, hypercalcemia, parathyroid disease, or pancreatic lesions. Findings on physical examination are normal.

Abdominal CT shows a possible lesion in the tail of the pancreas; a CT cut through the liver is shown (see image).

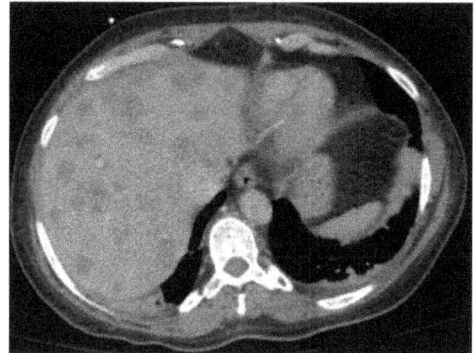

Laboratory test results:
    Proinsulin, markedly elevated
    Insulin, markedly elevated
    C-peptide, markedly elevated
    Glucose = 40 mg/dL (70-99 mg/dL) (SI: 2.2 mmol/L [3.9-5.5 mmol/L])

In addition to starting octreotide, which of the following additional medical therapies or interventions would have the most impact in treating her hypoglycemia?
    A. Hepatic embolization of liver metastases
    B. Pancreatectomy
    C. Initiation of diazoxide
    D. Initiation of continuous glucose monitoring
    E. Chemotherapy with everolimus

31 A 57-year-old woman with a history of psoriatic arthritis treated with multiple courses of high-dosage glucocorticoids in the past is admitted to the hospital with fevers and shortness of breath. Her medications include conjugated estrogen tablets, 0.625 mg daily, and prednisone, 5 mg daily. Following admission, her respiratory status deteriorates, necessitating intubation and initiation of antibiotic therapy for pneumonia. Stress-dosage hydrocortisone is also provided for presumed secondary adrenal insufficiency. Her estrogen therapy is also continued at her family's request and is administered via a feeding tube. One week after admission, her condition has improved and weaning from the ventilator is being considered.

On physical examination, her temperature is 95.9°F (35.5°C), blood pressure is 154/76 mm Hg, and pulse rate is 105 beats/min. Her thyroid gland is nonpalpable.

Additional laboratory evaluation (including thyroid function testing) is performed before weaning her from the ventilator:
    TSH = 0.15 mIU/L (0.5-5.0 mIU/L)
    Total T$_4$ = 12.0 µg/dL (5.5-12.5 µg/dL) (SI: 154.5 nmol/L [94.02-213.68 nmol/L])
    Comprehensive metabolic panel, normal
    Serum albumin, normal

Additional information is provided by the patient's primary care physician indicating that a screening serum TSH value 6 months ago was 3.0 mIU/L.

Which of the following is the most likely explanation for the pattern of this patient's thyroid function test results?
  A. Subclinical hyperthyroidism
  B. Central hypothyroidism
  C. Recovery from nonthyroidal illness
  D. Combined effect of nonthyroidal illness and steroid therapy
  E. Glucocorticoid therapy

32 A 20-year-old transgender woman presents for a follow-up visit for management of gender dysphoria. She describes herself as being a girly kid in childhood and identifying with girls. She has always been envious of women in terms of their appearance, dating men, and female roles in society. She has been under the care of a therapist regarding gender identity and has attended a transgender support group. At her last clinic visit 3 months ago, her oral estradiol dosage was increased from 2 to 4 mg daily and her spironolactone dosage was increased from 50 to 100 mg twice daily.

On physical examination, her height is 71 in (180 cm) and weight is 185 lb (84 kg) (BMI = 26 kg/m^2). Her blood pressure is 134/90 mm Hg, and pulse rate is 99 beats/min. Her physical examination findings are normal, and bilateral breast tissue is present.

Laboratory test results:
  Three months ago:
    Total testosterone = 116 ng/dL (8-60 ng/dL) (SI: 4.0 nmol/L [0.3-2.1 nmol/L])
    Estradiol = 56 pg/mL (10-180 pg/mL) (SI: 206 pmol/L [36.7-660.8 pmol/L])
  Today's visit:
    Total testosterone = 8 ng/dL (SI: 0.3 nmol/L)
    Estradiol = 538 pg/mL (SI: 1975 pmol/L)

Which of the following is the most likely explanation for her laboratory findings?
  A. A missed dose of estrogen at the time of the blood draw 3 months ago
  B. Self-titration of her estradiol dosage to 6 mg daily
  C. A switch in the mode of estradiol delivery from oral to sublingual
  D. Pharmacy error with the type of estrogen dispensed
  E. Laboratory error with today's estradiol measurement

33 A 70-year-old woman is referred to you for an opinion on management of her osteoporosis. Her pertinent history is notable for a vertebral fracture 5 years ago, which prompted DXA imaging that showed osteoporosis in the lumbar spine (T-score = –3.0) and osteopenia within both proximal femurs. She underwent natural menopause at age 50 years and did not take hormone therapy. She does take calcium citrate, 600 mg twice daily, and vitamin D, 2000 IU daily. She has a history of rate-controlled atrial fibrillation. After an appropriate workup for secondary causes of osteoporosis, which was normal, she was prescribed risedronate, 150 mg monthly, which she did not tolerate because of severe gastroesophageal reflux. Given that she had no overt dental disorders or concerns, her regimen was then switched to denosumab, 60 mg twice yearly, which she tolerated well initially. However, she has developed significant erythema with pruritis at the injection site following the last 2 injections. Nonetheless, follow-up DXA studies after 3 years of therapy show improvement in lumbar spine bone mineral density, such that her lumbar spine T-score is now in the osteopenic range (T-score, –1.9). She returns to discuss the best approach to her osteoporosis management.

Current laboratory test results:
  Creatinine = 0.8 mg/dL (0.6-1.1 mg/dL) (SI: 70.7 µmol/L [53.0-97.2 µmol/L])
  Calcium adjusted for albumin = 9.5 mg/dL (8.2-10.2 mg/dL) (SI: 2.4 mmol/L [2.1-2.6 mmol/L])
  25-Hydroxyvitamin D = 45 ng/mL (30-80 ng/mL [optimal]) (SI: 112.3 nmol/L [74.9-199.7 nmol/L])

The rest of her relevant chemistry and hematology profiles are unremarkable.

In light of her clinical history, which of the following is the most appropriate recommendation regarding management of her osteoporosis now?
- A. Continue denosumab twice yearly
- B. Continue denosumab, but decrease the dosing to once yearly
- C. Discontinue denosumab, but continue supplemental calcium and vitamin D
- D. Discontinue denosumab and start raloxifene
- E. Discontinue denosumab and start zoledronic acid once yearly

34 A 41-year-old man with type 2 diabetes mellitus, hypertension, obstructive sleep apnea, and kidney stones comes for a follow-up visit. You have been managing his type 2 diabetes and weight problem for the last 8 months. His most recent hemoglobin A_{1c} measurement was 6.4% (46 mmol/mol). The patient reports that he gained most of his excess weight in the past 5 years. At his initial appointment, his weight was 222 lb (100.9 kg), and you recommended a 2000-calorie per day meal plan. Since then, he has also been participating in an exercise program. These efforts have thus far resulted in a 6-lb (2.7-kg) weight loss. His current medications include metformin, empagliflozin, lisinopril, and hydrochlorothiazide.

Other relevant medical history includes an episode of acute pancreatitis 1 year ago. He has a family history of type 2 diabetes, but no other notable diagnoses.

On physical examination, his height is 69 in (175.3 cm) and weight is 230 lb (104.5 kg) (BMI = 34 kg/m^2). His blood pressure is 149/95 mm Hg, pulse rate is 84 beats/min, and respiratory rate is 18 breaths/min. Lungs are clear to auscultation bilaterally, heart sounds are regular, and his abdomen is soft and nontender.

During your visit, you review his food diary. After a long discussion, you decide to prescribe a weight-loss medication.

Which of the following weight-loss medications would you recommend?
- A. Phentermine
- B. Liraglutide
- C. Phentermine/topiramate
- D. Naltrexone/bupropion
- E. Lorcaserin

35 You are asked to consult on a 52-year-old man who has been on hemodialysis for 6 months. Before initiation of dialysis, his hemoglobin A_{1c} level was 6.6% (49 mmol/mol) with lifestyle intervention alone. Following the initiation of dialysis, his appetite improved. Blood glucose levels are now in the range of 200 to 250 mg/dL (11.1-13.9 mmol/L), and his hemoglobin A_{1c} level is 7.8% (62 mmol/mol).

In addition to type 2 diabetes and end-stage renal disease, his medical history includes hypertension, retinopathy, and lower-extremity neuropathy.

On physical examination, he is a thin man in no distress. His height is 68 in (172.7 cm), and weight is 160 lb (72.7 kg) (BMI = 24.3 kg/m^2). His blood pressure is 138/64 mm Hg, and pulse rate is 80 beats/min. Dialysis access is noted on the left forearm. He has decreased sensation to monofilament testing bilaterally on the lower extremities. The rest of his examination findings are unremarkable.

You suggest initiation of insulin for management of hyperglycemia, which he refuses. He is willing to start oral therapy.

Which of the following medications would be safest to improve glycemic control in this patient?
- A. Glyburide
- B. Pioglitazone
- C. Repaglinide
- D. Exenatide
- E. Dapagliflozin

36   A 62-year-old man was diagnosed with a 1.9-cm macroprolactinoma 10 years ago. At that time, his prolactin level was 389 ng/mL (4-23 ng/mL) (SI: 16.9 nmol/L [0.17-1.00 nmol/L]). He was treated with cabergoline. After an initial decline in serum prolactin, his levels started to increase despite a progressive increase in the cabergoline dosage. MRI showed the mass to be enlarging, and he therefore underwent surgery about 5 years ago. However, because of extensive cavernous sinus invasion, surgery was not curative. Two years ago, he received 5040 cGy of fractionated radiation therapy.

At his appointment today, his prolactin concentration is 1670 ng/mL (72.6 nmol/L), up from 982 ng/mL (42.9 nmol/L) 3 months ago. The maximal size of the mass is 2.3 cm, with invasion of the left cavernous sinus and abutment of the left side of the optic chiasm. Comparison with last year's MRI shows tumor enlargement. He takes cabergoline, 3.5 mg weekly.

On physical examination, he has no heart murmur. Findings on neuro-ophthalmology exam are normal.

Which of the following is the best next step in this patient's management?

A. Switch from cabergoline to bromocriptine
B. Switch from cabergoline to temozolomide
C. Add octreotide
D. Add pasireotide
E. Refer for stereotactic radiosurgery

37   A 60-year-old woman is referred to you for recommendations regarding possible surgical management of primary hyperparathyroidism. She has no history of fractures, renal stones, or craniocervical radiation. She underwent menopause at age 49 years and never took hormone therapy. She does not take calcium supplements, but she does consume 3 servings of dairy products daily, as well as cholecalciferol, 1000 IU daily. Her family history is negative for history of osteoporosis, nephrolithiasis, or endocrine tumors, including known parathyroid disease. Review of systems is noncontributory.

On physical examination, she measures 2 in (5 cm) shorter than her self-reported maximal height. She has mild lower thoracic kyphosis. The rest of her examination findings, including exam of the anterior neck, are unremarkable.

DXA results are shown (*see images and tables*):

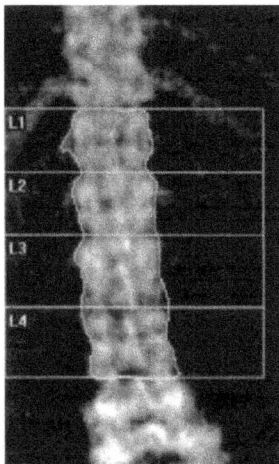

Radius	BMD, g/cm²	T-Score
One-third	0.618	−1.3
Mid	0.547	−1.1
UD	0.382	−1.0
Total	0.520	−1.1

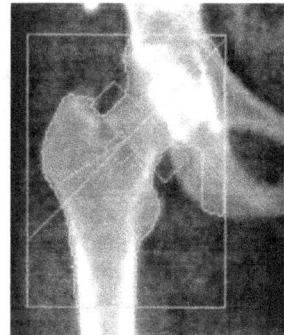

Region	BMD, g/cm²	T-Score
Neck	0.686	−1.5
Troch	0.613	−0.9
Inter	0.892	−1.3
Total	0.795	−1.2

Region	BMD, g/cm²	T-Score
L1	0.778	−1.9
L2	0.880	−1.3
L3	0.955	−1.2
L4	0.867	−1.8
Total	0.874	−1.6

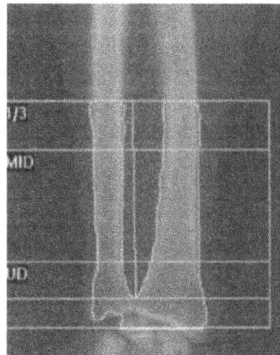

Laboratory test results:

    Serum calcium = 10.7 mg/dL (8.2-10.2 mg/dL) (SI: 2.7 mmol/L [2.1-2.6 mmol/L])

    Serum phosphate = 3.2 mg/dL (2.3-4.7 mg/dL) (SI: 1.0 mmol/L [0.7-1.5 mmol/L])

    Serum intact PTH = 80 pg/mL (10-65 pg/mL) (SI: 80 ng/L [10-65 ng/L])

    Serum creatinine = 0.9 mg/dL (0.6-1.1 mg/dL) (SI: 79.6 μmol/L [53.0-97.2 μmol/L])

    Serum albumin = 4.4 mg/dL (3.5-5.0 g/dL) (SI: 44 g/L [35-50 g/L])

    Urinary calcium = 290 mg/24 h (100-300 mg/24 h) (SI: 7.3 mmol/d [2.5-7.5 mmol/d])

    Urinary creatinine = 1.2 g/24 h (1.0-2.0 g/24 h) (SI: 10.6 mmol/d [8.8-17.7 mmol/d])

    Fractional excretion of calcium = 0.02

Which of the following is the best next step to determine this patient's candidacy for parathyroidectomy?

    A. Anteroposterior and lateral radiographs of the thoracic and lumbar spine

    B. Measurement of plasma ionized calcium

    C. Genetic testing for pathogenic variants in the calcium-sensing receptor gene (*CASR*)

    D. Technetium ^{99m}Tc parathyroid scan

    E. Thyroid ultrasonography

38 A 19-year-old woman is referred to the endocrinology clinic for evaluation and treatment of diabetes mellitus. The patient was born at 37 weeks' gestation with a birth weight of 4.0 lb (1800 g). At age 8 weeks, the patient presented in diabetic ketoacidosis. She was initially treated with intravenous insulin and subsequently with subcutaneous insulin. She has since remained on insulin therapy.

She has had poor glycemic control, and over the last 2 years her hemoglobin A_{1c} measurements have ranged from 8.5% to 10.1% (69-87 mmol/mol). She administers 16 units of insulin glargine at bedtime. She uses a carbohydrate ratio of 1 unit insulin aspart to 12 g carbohydrate with meals (the total bolus amount ranges from 14 to 16 units of insulin aspart per day). She has had no subsequent hospitalizations for uncontrolled diabetes or hypoglycemia. She has mild peripheral neuropathy, but does not have hypertension or dyslipidemia. She has a levonorgestrel implant for birth control. She does not smoke cigarettes and occasionally drinks alcohol. No family members have diabetes.

On physical examination she appears well. Her height is 65 in (165 cm), and weight is 127 lb (57.7 kg) (BMI = 21.1 kg/m^2). Her blood pressure is 106/72 mm Hg, and pulse rate is 74 beats/min. Examination findings are normal except for reduced sensation to 10-g monofilament in both feet.

Laboratory test results:

    Hemoglobin A_{1c} = 8.9% (4.0%-5.6%) (74 mmol/mol [20-38 mmol/mol])

    Creatinine = 0.8 mg/dL (0.6-1.1 mg/dL) (SI: 70.7 μmol/L [53.0-97.2 μmol/L])

    Estimated glomerular filtration rate = >90 mL/min per 1.73 m^2 (>60 mL/min per 1.73 m^2)

    Glucose = 134 mg/dL (70-99 mg/dL) (SI: 7.4 mg/dL [3.9-5.5 mmol/L])

    C-peptide = 1.8 ng/mL (0.9-4.3 ng/mL) (SI: 0.6 nmol/L [0.30-1.42 nmol/L])

    Electrolytes, normal

    Glutamic acid decarboxylase antibodies, undetectable

    Islet-cell antibodies, undetectable

Which of the following is the best next step in this patient's management?

    A. Switch to insulin pump therapy

    B. Start glyburide

    C. Start metformin

    D. Start empagliflozin

    E. Switch to insulin degludec and insulin lispro

39 A 20-year-old woman seeks a second opinion for the evaluation and treatment of delayed puberty. She was first evaluated at age 16 years when she did not have breast development or start menses. She has been managed for the past few years by pediatrics and is now transitioning to adult endocrinology. Her initial evaluation included a head MRI that showed no pituitary abnormality, as well as the laboratory results shown in the table. No hormone therapy was started in the year after her initial evaluation. At age 17 years, her examination findings were still consistent with Tanner stage 1 development and test results showed no change in gonadotropin or estradiol concentrations. She began taking estradiol, 0.5 mg every other day. Every 6 months, therapy was discontinued for 3 months to see if spontaneous pubertal progression might occur. The initial 2 years of therapy were associated with development of pubic hair only. At her follow-up visit 6 months ago, the estradiol dosage was increased to 0.5 mg daily. She has noticed initial breast development with this most recent dosage change. She has no difficulty with sense of smell.

On physical examination, her height is 62 in (157.5 cm) and weight is 105 lb (47.7 kg) (BMI = 19.2 kg/m^2). Maternal height is 66 in (167.6 cm) and paternal height is 72 in (182.9 cm). Her thyroid gland is palpable with swallowing, without nodules or enlargement. Breasts and pubic hair distribution are consistent with Tanner stage 2 development. Pelvic ultrasonography shows a smaller-than-normal uterus and ovaries with tiny follicles.

	Age		
Measurement	16 Years (before treatment)	17 Years (estradiol, 0.5 mg every other day)	20 Years (estradiol, 0.5 mg daily)
FSH	1.6 mIU/mL (SI: 1.6 IU/L)	1.5 mIU/mL (SI: 1.5 IU/L)	1.0 mIU/mL (SI: 1.0 IU/L)
LH	0.5 mIU/mL (SI: 0.5 IU/L)	0.4 mIU/mL (SI: 0.4 IU/L)	0.5 mIU/mL (SI: 0.5 IU/L)
Estradiol	17 pg/mL (SI: 62.4 pmol/L)	2 pg/mL (SI: 7.3 pmol/L)	29 pg/mL (SI: 106.5 pmol/L)
Prolactin	6.8 ng/mL (SI: 0.30 nmol/L)	8.0 ng/mL (SI: 0.35 nmol/L)	...
TSH	2.1 mIU/L	2.0 mIU/L	...
Total T$_4$	...	6.7 µg/dL (SI: 86.2 nmol/L)	...
ACTH	...	...	23 pg/mL (SI: 5.1 pmol/L)
Cortisol (8 AM)	...	...	12 µg/dL (SI: 331.1 nmol/L)
IGF-1	...	...	132 ng/mL (SI: 17.3 nmol/L)
Bone age	13 years	13 years	14 years

Reference ranges: FSH (prepuberty), <3.0 mIU/mL (<3.0 IU/L); LH (prepuberty) <1.0 mIU/mL (<1.0 IU/L); estradiol (follicular, premenopausal), 10-180 pg/mL (36.7-660.8 pmol/L); prolactin, 4-30 ng/mL (0.17-1.30 nmol/L); TSH, 0.5-5.0 mIU/L; total T$_4$, 5.5-12.5 µg/dL (94.02-213.68 nmol/L); ACTH, 10-60 pg/mL (2.2-13.2 pmol/L); cortisol (8 AM), 5-25 µg/dL (137.9-689.7 nmol/L); IGF-1, 122-384 ng/mL (16.0-50.3 nmol/L).

Which of the following is the best next step in this patient's management?
- A. Start an oral contraceptive
- B. Add micronized progesterone, 100 mg daily
- C. Start growth hormone
- D. Increase the estradiol dosage
- E. Discontinue estradiol and observe for 3 months before the next estradiol dosage increase

40 A 21-year-old woman with a history of optic nerve glioma diagnosed at age 11 years presents for follow-up. At diagnosis, the optic nerve glioma was treated surgically and she had postoperative radiotherapy (cumulative dose, 40 Gy). She also developed complex partial epilepsy, which is now well controlled. She was treated with recombinant human GH from age 12 to 19 years. She feels well and has no concerns. Her periods are regular. She takes lamotrigine for epilepsy, but is on no other medications.

On physical examination, her height is 61 in (155 cm) and weight is 110 lb (50 kg) (BMI = 20.8 kg/m^2). Breasts and pubic hair are Tanner stage 4. Her blood pressure is 102/68 mm Hg.

Laboratory test results:

    TSH = 0.8 mIU/L (0.5-5.0 mIU/L)

    Free T$_4$ = 1.0 ng/dL (0.8-1.8 ng/dL) (SI: 12.3 pmol/L [10.30-23.17 pmol/L])

    Serum cortisol (8 AM) = 15.0 µg/dL (5-25 µg/dL) (SI: 413.8 nmol/L [137.9-689.7 nmol/L])

    IGF-1 = 72 ng/mL (116-341 ng/mL) (SI: 9.4 nmol/L [15.2-44.7 nmol/L])

    FSH = 8.0 mIU/mL (2.0-12.0 mIU/mL [follicular]) (SI: 8.0 IU/L [2.0-12.0 IU/L])

    LH = 12.0 mIU/mL (1.0-18.0 mIU/mL [follicular]) (SI: 12.0 IU/L [1.0-18.0 IU/L])

    Estradiol = 110 pg/mL (10-180 pg/mL [follicular]) (SI: 403.8 pmol/L [36.7-660.8 pmol/L])

Which of the following management strategies would you advise for this patient?

    A. Annual evaluation of full pituitary function indefinitely
    B. Evaluation of pituitary function if symptomatic of hormonal deficiency
    C. Annual screening of gonadotropins only
    D. Thyrotropin-releasing hormone stimulation test
    E. Insulin tolerance test

41   A 67-year-old man is referred for evaluation of Paget disease of bone after he presented to his orthopedist with right-sided hip pain. He was found to have an elevated alkaline phosphatase level, and an x-ray of his right hip confirmed the diagnosis. His bony pain has somewhat improved with taking ibuprofen as needed. He also reports fatigue, decreased appetite, and a 15-lb (6.8-kg) weight loss over the past couple of months. He has not had any fractures. He has no history of thyroid disease. His father had Paget disease. The patient takes a daily supplement containing 800 mg of calcium and 1000 IU of cholecalciferol.

He was recently evaluated by a urologist for symptoms of benign prostatic hyperplasia, but he has not started taking medication for this yet.

On physical examination, his vital signs are unremarkable, but he appears ill. Examination of his pelvis and hips does not reveal any palpable bony abnormalities and there is no tenderness to palpation.

His imaging results are shown (*see images*).

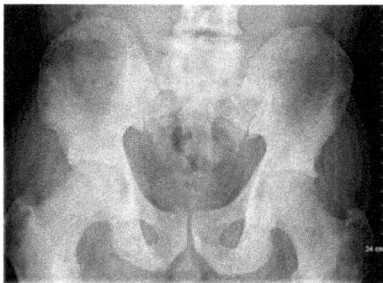

Plain x-ray of the pelvis (*anteroposterior view*).

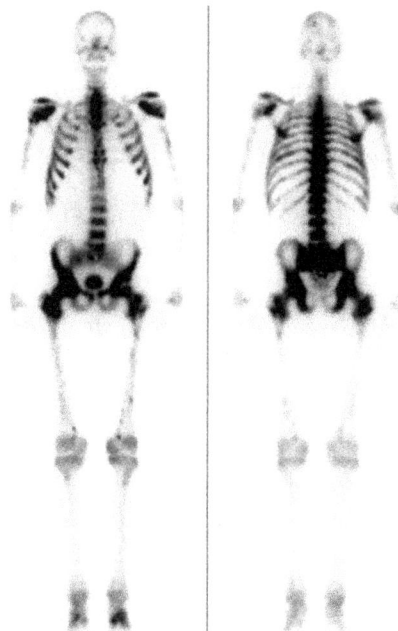

Bone scan.

Laboratory test results:

Serum calcium = 8.9 mg/dL (8.2-10.2 mg/dL) (SI: 2.2 mmol/L [2.1-2.6 mmol/L])

Serum phosphate = 2.7 mg/dL (2.3-4.7 mg/dL) (SI: 0.9 mmol/L [0.7-1.5 mmol/L])

Serum creatinine = 0.9 mg/dL (0.7-1.3 mg/dL) (SI: 79.6 μmol/L [61.9-114.9 μmol/L])

Serum 25-hydroxyvitamin D = 30 ng/mL (30-80 ng/mL [optimal]) (SI: 74.9 nmol/L [74.9-199.7 nmol/L])

Serum albumin = 3.7 g/dL (3.5-5.0 g/dL) (SI: 37 g/L [35-50 g/L])

Serum total alkaline phosphatase = 2328 U/L (50-120 U/L) (SI: 38.88 μkat/L [0.84-2.00 μkat/L])

Serum bone-specific alkaline phosphatase = 668.7 μg/L (≤20 μg/L)

Which of the following is the most appropriate next step?
- A. Serum protein electrophoresis
- B. Serum PSA measurement
- C. Serum intact PTH measurement
- D. Serum FGF-23 measurement
- E. Iliac crest bone biopsy

42 A 49-year-old man presents for management of cardiovascular risk. One year ago, he developed a syncopal episode while training for a triathlon and underwent an extensive cardiac workup. Electrocardiography and stress echocardiography were unrevealing for cardiac ischemia. Coronary artery calcium testing was performed, and the patient had a coronary artery calcium score of 220 corresponding to the 80th percentile. He does not smoke cigarettes and drinks 1 alcoholic beverage per week. He continues to train for marathons without problems. His family history is unremarkable for premature atherosclerotic cardiovascular disease, and both of his parents are alive and well in their 70s.

On physical examination, his blood pressure is 126/78 mm Hg. His height is 75 in (190.5 cm), and weight is 195 lb (88.5 kg) (BMI = 24.4 kg/m^2). No hepatosplenomegaly or xanthomas are noted on examination.

Laboratory test results (sample drawn while fasting):

Total cholesterol = 175 mg/dL (<200 mg/dL [optimal]) (SI: 4.53 mmol/L [<5.18 mmol/L])

Triglycerides = 49 mg/dL (<150 mg/dL [optimal]) (SI: 0.55 mmol/L [<1.70 mmol/L])

HDL cholesterol = 63 mg/dL (>60 mg/dL [optimal]) (SI: 1.63 mmol/L [>1.55 mmol/L])

LDL cholesterol = 102 mg/dL (<100 mg/dL [optimal]) (SI: 2.64 mmol/L [<2.59 mmol/L])

Non-HDL cholesterol = 112 mg/dL (<130 mg/dL [optimal]) (SI: 2.90 mmol/L [<3.37 mmol/L])

Hemoglobin A$_{1c}$ = 5.4% (4.0%-5.6%) (36 mmol/mol [20-38 mmol/mol])

TSH = 1.28 mIU/L (0.5-5.0 mIU/L)

Fasting plasma glucose = 91 mg/dL (70-99 mg/dL) (SI: 5.05 mmol/L [3.9-5.5 mmol/L])

His 10-year atherosclerotic cardiovascular disease risk is 1.7% based on the American College of Cardiology/American Heart Association cardiovascular risk calculator. He prefers to not start medication but will do so if it is recommended.

Which of the following is the best next step to guide your decision about the need for therapy?
- A. Reassess the coronary artery calcium score now; start statin therapy if the score has increased
- B. Assess high-sensitivity C-reactive protein; start statin therapy if elevated
- C. Measure LDL particle number; initiate statin therapy if elevated
- D. No further testing needed; initiate statin therapy now
- E. No further testing needed; no therapy is indicated

43 A 50-year-old woman with type 2 diabetes mellitus seeks advice regarding continued poor glycemic control. Her medical history is notable for Crohn disease diagnosed at age 35 years, a small-bowel resection, and hypothyroidism. Diabetes was diagnosed 15 months ago on the basis of blood work done around the time of small-bowel resection. She had no excessive thirst or urination. She was initially treated with metformin, and her current regimen includes metformin, 1500 mg once daily at night, and glimepiride, 4 mg once daily in the morning.

Her hemoglobin A_{1c} level was 7.6% (60 mmol/mol) at diagnosis, rising to 8.6% (70 mmol/mol) after 11 months and to greater than 10.0% (>86 mmol/mol) after 15 months. She checks her glucose once daily and reports both fasting hyperglycemia and postprandial hyperglycemia, with a mean glucose value of 250 mg/dL (13.9 mmol/L). She seldom consumes sweets or sugary beverages. While she has no specific exercise routine, she walks 2 miles 5 days per week.

On physical examination, her blood pressure is 112/79 mm Hg and pulse rate is 98 beats/min. Her height is 63 in (160 cm), and weight is 165.3 lb (75 kg) (BMI = 29.2 kg/m^2). There is no evidence of acanthosis nigricans, Cushing syndrome, or acromegaly.

Which of the following tests would best guide future management?
A. Fasting C-peptide measurement
B. Fasting insulin measurement
C. Glutamic acid decarboxylase antibody assessment
D. Ferritin measurement
E. Genetic testing for maturity-onset diabetes of the young

44 A 57-year-old man is diagnosed with Graves disease and mild orbitopathy after developing weight loss, palpitations, and dry, itchy eyes. He has no proptosis, and his thyroid gland is approximately twice normal size. He does not smoke cigarettes. He routinely wears dark glasses and likes to sleep with the head of his bed raised.

Laboratory test results:
  TSH = <0.01 mIU/L (0.5-5.0 mIU/L)
  Free T_4 = 5.1 ng/dL (0.8-1.8 ng/dL) (SI: 65.6 pmol/L [10.30-23.17 pmol/L])
  Total T_3 = 600 ng/dL (70-200 ng/dL) (SI: 9.2 nmol/L [1.08-3.08 nmol/L])
  TRAb = 5.0 IU/L (<1.75 IU/L)

He is initially treated with methimazole and rendered euthyroid. He elects to receive radioactive iodine therapy. He does not return for follow-up until about 5 months after his therapy. He now has fatigue, constipation, and worsening orbitopathy, and he has experienced marked weight gain. These symptoms have been ongoing for the last 2 months. His weight has increased from 189 to 229 lb (86-104 kg) (current BMI = 30 kg/m^2).

Chemosis and proptosis are noted on eye examination with a clinical activity score of 6/10. His thyroid is slightly enlarged and firm to palpation.

Laboratory test results:
  TSH = 80 mIU/L (0.5-5.0 mIU/L)
  Free T_4 = 0.3 ng/dL (0.8-1.8 ng/dL) (SI: 3.9 pmol/L [10.30-23.17 pmol/L])
  Total T_3 = 60 ng/dL (70-200 ng/dL) (SI: 0.9 nmol/L [1.08-3.08 nmol/L])

In addition to treatment with radioactive iodine, which of the following is most likely to have triggered this patient's worsening orbitopathy?
A. Use of sunglasses
B. Pretreatment with methimazole
C. Raising the head of his bed
D. Development of hypothyroidism
E. Age older than 45 years

45 A 69-year-old man with hypertension and erectile dysfunction is self-referred for a second opinion regarding testosterone replacement therapy. The patient has experienced a gradual decline in his erectile function over the past 4 years, and his libido is present but "not what it once was." His primary care physician recommended testosterone supplementation based on his symptoms and 2 low testosterone measurements. His fraternal twin brother had a cardiac stent placed for coronary artery disease at age 67 years. The patient is inclined to try testosterone therapy but would like to discuss the possible benefits vs risks. Current medications include metoprolol, hydrochlorothiazide, and verapamil.

On physical examination, his height is 69 in (175 cm) and weight is 177 lb (80 kg) (BMI = 26 kg/m^2). His blood pressure is 132/85 mm Hg, and pulse rate is 74 beats/min. Examination findings are normal. Testicular volume is 15 mL bilaterally, and no gynecomastia is present.

Laboratory test results:

Total testosterone (8 AM measurements on 2 occasions) = 228 and 241 ng/dL (300-900 ng/dL) (SI: 7.9 and 8.4 nmol/L [10.4-31.2 nmol/L])

Free testosterone (8 AM measurements on 2 occasions) = 4.2 and 4.5 ng/dL (9.0-30.0 ng/dL) (SI: 0.15 and 0.16 nmol/L [0.31-1.04 nmol/L])

LH = 6.7 mIU/mL (1.0-9.0 mIU/mL) (SI: 6.7 IU/L [1.0-9.0 IU/L])

FSH = 7.1 mIU/mL (1.0-13.0 mIU/mL) (SI: 7.1 IU/L [1.0-13.0 IU/L])

TSH = 4.1 mIU/mL (0.5-5.0 mIU/L)

PSA = 2.2 ng/mL (<5.3 ng/mL) (SI: 2.2 µg/L [<5.3 µg/L])

Complete blood cell count, normal

Chemistry panel, normal

Which of the following is the best next step in this patient's management?
   A. Start testosterone replacement therapy
   B. Start testosterone plus an aromatase inhibitor
   C. Start testosterone plus tadalafil
   D. Start yohimbine
   E. Avoid testosterone because of risk of cardiovascular disease

46 A 61-year-old woman undergoes CT imaging of the chest after accidentally swallowing a metal object while eating. The scan shows multiple bilateral pulmonary nodules and hilar lymphadenopathy. Subsequent abdominal imaging reveals retroperitoneal adenopathy and normal adrenal glands. A mediastinal lymph node biopsy confirms the diagnosis of mantle-cell lymphoma, and she is treated with rituximab and bendamustine.

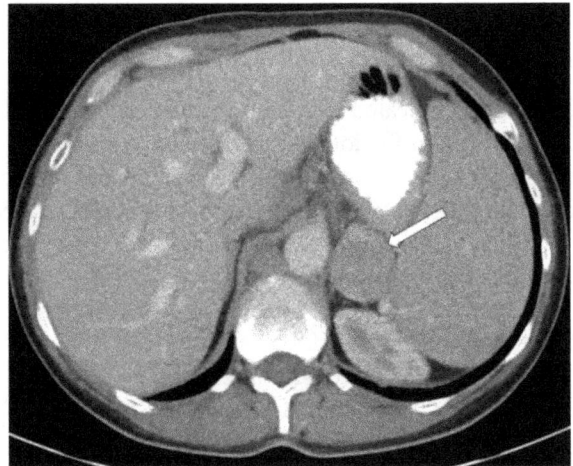

Now, 2 years later, all of her known adenopathy has regressed in size on surveillance CT imaging. However, there is an enlarging left adrenal mass that is described as heterogeneous and 4.8 x 3.9 x 5.0 cm in size with an unenhanced density of greater than 10 Hounsfield units (*see image, arrow*). The right adrenal gland appears normal. Plasma metanephrines are normal, and the patient has normal blood pressure and no signs or symptoms of Cushing syndrome.

Which of the following is the best next step to distinguish whether this enlarging adrenal mass represents lymphoma or a primary adrenal malignancy?
   A. MRI imaging
   B. PET-CT imaging
   C. Biopsy of the adrenal mass
   D. Laparoscopic adrenalectomy
   E. Radical adrenalectomy

47 A 51-year-old postmenopausal woman presents with a 6-month history of progressively worsening hirsutism. Before menopause, she had hair growth on her face, abdomen, and upper thighs and regularly used electrolysis to treat hair growth. She went through menopause at age 49 years. For the past 6 months, she has required more frequent electrolysis treatments, and there are new areas of hair growth on her body.

On physical examination, she has terminal hair growth on her face, chin, center of her chest, upper back, buttocks, and inner thighs with a Ferriman-Gallwey score of 22. There is no clitoromegaly.

Laboratory test results:
    Total testosterone = 71 ng/dL (8-60 ng/dL) (SI: 2.5 nmol/L [0.3-2.1 nmol/L])
    DHEA-S = 193 µg/dL (15-200 µg/dL) (SI: 5.2 µmol/L [0.41-5.42 µmol/L])
    LH = 19.6 mIU/mL (>30.0 mIU/mL [postmenopausal]) (SI: 19.6 IU/L [>30.0 IU/L])
    FSH = 26.1 mIU/mL (>30.0 mIU/mL [postmenopausal]) (SI: 26.1 IU/L [>30.0 IU/L])
    Androstenedione = 106 ng/dL (80-240 ng/dL) (SI: 3.70 nmol/L [2.79-8.38 nmol/L])

Ovarian ultrasonography does not show any evidence of tumor. Left ovarian volume is 6 cc with a 1-cm ovarian cyst, and right ovarian volume is 7 cc.

She is very tearful and discouraged by her appearance. Which of the following is the best next step in this patient's management?
    A. Oral contraceptive
    B. Spironolactone
    C. Reassurance that her symptoms are due to menopause
    D. Ovarian and adrenal venous sampling
    E. Referral to gynecology for bilateral oophorectomy

48 A 56-year-old woman is referred to you by the bariatric surgery team for assistance with weight loss. She has been overweight since age 38 years. Her highest recorded weight was 235 lb (106.8 kg) 6 years ago, and at that time she underwent Roux-en-Y gastric bypass. She initially lost 100 lb (45.5 kg), but over the past 2 years she regained 80 lb (36.4 kg). Her current weight is 208 lb (94.5 kg). The patient has been working with a dietitian on a monthly basis, and for the past 6 months her weight has remained stable. During this time, she has focused on eating 3 meals a day and decreasing her carbohydrate intake. She works with a fitness trainer 3 days a week. The patient feels hungry all the time on her current meal plan.

Other medical history includes obstructive sleep apnea, depression, hypertension, hyperlipidemia, and chronic back pain. Her medications consist of a multivitamin, iron, hydrochlorothiazide, fluoxetine, rosuvastatin, and omeprazole. She regularly takes opioids for her back pain. She has no family history of glaucoma or cancer.

On physical examination, her blood pressure is 150/89 mm Hg and pulse rate is 77 beats/min. Her height is 62.5 in (158.8 cm), and weight is 208 lb (94.5 kg) (BMI = 37.4 kg/m^2). She does not look cushingoid. She has multiple white stretch marks on her abdomen. She does not have thyromegaly, her lungs are clear to auscultation bilaterally, and her heart sounds are regular.

During the visit, you make changes to her meal plan and ask her to increase her activity level.

Which of the following medications would you recommend to help this patient lose weight?
    A. Lorcaserin
    B. Phentermine
    C. Metformin
    D. Naltrexone/bupropion
    E. Liraglutide

49 A 28-year-old man is seen in the endocrinology clinic for evaluation of hypoglycemia. He has had 3 episodes of severe hypoglycemia in the last 3 and one-half weeks, which necessitated paramedic calls for treatment. He was evaluated twice in the emergency department for treatment of hypoglycemia, after which he was stabilized and discharged home. He has a history of hypoxic brain injury in childhood and is disabled. He takes an anticonvulsant medication and resides in a group home. He has lost about 12 lb (5.5 kg) in the last 2 years but does not have a history of malabsorption. He has no history of diabetes mellitus. Other residents in the group home are being treated for diabetes.

On physical examination, he is lean but appears well. His height is 69 in (175 cm), and weight is 137 lb (62.3 kg) (BMI = 20.3 kg/m^2). His blood pressure is 106/71 mm Hg, and pulse rate is 82 beats/min. He responds to some questions. He is alert but is not aware of the time or date. Examination findings are unremarkable.

Laboratory test results:
Hemoglobin A$_{1c}$ = 5.0% (4.0%-5.6%) (31 mmol/mol [20-38 mmol/mol])
TSH = 1.97 mIU/L (0.5-5.0 mIU/L)
Electrolytes, normal
Serum urea nitrogen, normal
Hepatic function, normal
Cortisol (8 AM) = 13.3 μg/dL (5-25 μg/dL) (SI: 366.9 nmol/L [137.9-689.7 nmol/L])

The emergency department physician calls 2 days later and reports that the patient is being evaluated for severe hypoglycemia. The fingerstick glucose measurement was 42 mg/dL (2.3 mmol/L) in the emergency department, and the patient was treated with an ampule of D50. He has responded well, and the follow-up glucose level is 82 mg/dL (4.6 mmol/L).

The following laboratory tests results are from a sample drawn when the patient redevelops hypoglycemia:
Serum glucose = 44 mg/dL (70-99 mg/dL) (SI: 2.4 mmol/L [3.9-5.5 mmol/L])
Insulin =11.0 μIU/mL (1.4-14.0 μIU/mL) (SI: 76.4 pmol/L [9.7-97.2 pmol/L])
C-peptide = 0.9 ng/mL (0.9-4.3 ng/mL) (SI: 0.30 nmol/L [0.30-1.42 nmol/L])
Proinsulin = 24.7 pg/mL (26.5-176.4 pg/mL) (SI: 2.8 pmol/L [3.0-20.0 pmol/L])
β-Hydroxybutyrate = 1.6 mg/dL (<3.0 mg/dL) (SI: <153.7 μmol/L [<300 μmol/L])

A sulfonylurea serum screen is ordered, but the sample is not collected properly and the test is not run.

Which of the following is the most likely etiology of this patient's hypoglycemia?
A. Use of exogenous insulin
B. Use of an insulin secretogogue
C. Non-insulinoma pancreatogenous hypoglycemia syndrome
D. Insulin-secreting neuroendocrine tumor
E. Non–insulin-mediated hypoglycemia

50 A 53-year-old man attends the outpatient clinic for routine follow-up. Tall-cell variant papillary thyroid cancer with neck node involvement was diagnosed 5 years earlier (American Joint Committee on Cancer stage T2 N1b M0), and he underwent total thyroidectomy and left lateral compartment neck node dissection followed by radioactive iodine remnant ablation with a 158-mCi dose of ^{131}I. He developed low-volume pulmonary metastases 6 months following diagnosis and was given 2 further doses of 150-mCi of ^{131}I. Two years following completion of ^{131}I administration, he developed acute myelogenous leukemia, which was treated with chemotherapy and a stem-cell bone marrow transplant. He is asymptomatic and remains in complete remission from leukemia. He reports that his mother recently died of breast cancer and his brother was diagnosed with colon carcinoma 3 months ago. He remains on treatment with levothyroxine, 150 mcg daily.

On physical examination, his height is 71 in (180.3 cm) and weight is 181 lb (82.3 kg) (BMI = 25.2 kg/m^2). His blood pressure is 134/78 mm Hg, and pulse rate is 76 beats/min. He has a visible thyroidectomy scar but no palpable thyroid enlargement and no palpable cervical lymphadenopathy. Lung fields are clear to auscultation and the rest of his examination findings are normal.

Laboratory test results:

Hemoglobin = 15.8 g/dL (13.8-17.2 g/dL) (SI: 158 g/L [138-172 g/L])

White blood cell count = 8200/μL (4500-11,000/μL) (SI: 8.2 x 10^9/L [4.5-11.0 x 10^9/L])

Platelet count = 203 x 10^3/μL (150-450 x 10^3/μL) (SI: 203 x 10^9/L [150-450 x 10^9/L])

TSH = <0.01 mIU/L (0.5-5.0 mIU/L)

Free T$_4$ = 1.9 ng/dL (0.8-1.8 ng/dL) (SI: 24.5 pmol/L [10.30-23.17 pmol/L])

Thyroglobulin following rhTSH stimulation = <0.1 ng/mL

Neck ultrasonography shows no residual disease in the thyroid bed and no cervical lymphadenopathy. Chest CT shows stable low-volume lung metastases bilaterally and is unchanged from a CT scan performed 18 months ago.

Which of the following factors is most likely to have contributed to the development of acute myeloid leukemia in this patient?

A. Male sex

B. Family history of solid-organ malignancies

C. Cumulative ^{131}I dose of 458 mCi

D. Age >45 years when undergoing ^{131}I administration

E. Tall-cell variant papillary thyroid cancer

51 A 52-year-old man is referred for evaluation of an elevated PTH level. His medical history is notable for morbid obesity, for which he underwent laparoscopic Roux-en-Y gastric bypass at age 42 years. He lost approximately 150 lb (68.2 kg) (~80% of his excess body weight) after surgery, and he has successfully maintained this weight loss. He also had a history of type 2 diabetes mellitus that resolved following bariatric surgery. He has no history of craniocervical irradiation, low-trauma fractures, or nephrolithiasis. His family history is notable for parathyroidectomy in 1 of 8 siblings to treat primary hyperparathyroidism at age 60 years. He takes no prescription medications but does take calcium citrate, 600 mg twice daily, and cholecalciferol, 5000 IU daily. Review of systems is negative for abnormal or frequent stools.

Physical examination findings, including exam of the anterior neck, are unremarkable.

Laboratory test results:

Serum calcium = 9.4 mg/dL (8.2-10.2 mg/dL) (SI: 2.4 mmol/L [2.1-2.6 mmol/L])

Serum phosphate = 3.5 mg/dL (2.3-4.7 mg/dL) (SI: 1.1 mmol/L [0.7-1.5 mmol/L])

Serum creatinine = 0.9 mg/dL (0.6-1.1 mg/dL) (SI: 79.6 μmol/L [53.0-97.2 μmol/L])

Serum albumin = 4.2 mg/dL (3.5-5.0 g/dL) (SI: 42 g/L [35-50 g/L])

Serum intact PTH = 95 pg/mL (10-65 pg/mL) (SI: 95 ng/L [10-65 ng/L])

Serum 25-hydroxyvitamin D = 50 ng/mL (30-80 ng/mL) (SI: 124.8 nmol/L [74.9-199.7 nmol/L])

Urinary calcium = 54 mg/24 h (100-300 mg/24 h) (SI: 1.4 mmol/d [2.5-7.5 mmol/d])

Urinary creatinine = 1.5 g/24 h (1.0-2.0 g/24 h) (SI: 13.3 mmol/d [8.8-17.7 mmol/d])

Which of the following is the best next step in this patient's management?

A. Increase the cholecalciferol dosage to 10,000 IU daily

B. Perform DXA scanning to include measurement of the nondominant, proximal one-third radius

C. Perform parathyroid technetium ^{99m}Tc sestamibi scan

D. Refer to endocrine surgery for consideration of parathyroidectomy

E. Prescribe calcitriol, 0.5 mcg daily

52 A 32-year-old woman is diagnosed with Cushing disease during the workup for 20-lb (9.1-kg) weight gain, hypertension, and menstrual irregularities. A 6-mm pituitary microadenoma is identified, and she undergoes transsphenoidal surgery. Pathology confirms an ACTH-staining adenoma. Thirty-six hours after surgery, her laboratory values are as follows:

Morning cortisol = 1.0 μg/dL (5-25 μg/dL) (SI: 27.6 nmol/L [137.9-689.7 nmol/L])
ACTH = <5.0 pg/mL (10-60 pg/mL) (SI: <1.1 pg/mL [2.2-13.2 pmol/L])

She is discharged from the hospital on a hydrocortisone regimen of 15 mg in the morning and 5 mg in the afternoon.

She misses her follow-up appointment, and you are now seeing her 11 months after surgery. She feels well. She has lost about 15 lb (6.8 kg), and she is normotensive off all blood pressure medication. Her menstrual periods are now regular. She still takes hydrocortisone, which has been renewed by her primary care physician.

Which of the following represents her most likely current early-morning hormonal picture before the hydrocortisone dose?

Answer	Cortisol	ACTH	DHEA-S
A.	↑	↑	↑
B.	↓	normal	↑
C.	↓	↓	↓
D.	normal	normal	↑
E.	↓	normal	↓

53 A 72-year-old man is seen in your clinic for management of type 2 diabetes mellitus, which was diagnosed 7 years ago. He takes metformin and sitagliptin, and his hemoglobin A_{1c} level has been around 8% (64 mmol/mol). He has no known microvascular complications. He was doing well until 3 months ago when he started to have right lower-extremity thigh pain. This has since progressed and he currently has right foot drop requiring a brace. The pain is quite intense and he now needs a wheelchair for mobility. He has also lost 10 lb (4.5 kg). His medical history includes osteoarthritis, hypertension, and dyslipidemia.

On physical examination, he is seated in a wheelchair and appears frail. His height is 69 in (175.3 cm), and weight is 170 lb (77.3 kg) (BMI = 25.1 kg/m^2). His blood pressure is 130/68 mm Hg, and pulse rate is 94 beats/min. Findings on examination of the heart, lungs, and abdomen are normal. Both lower extremities have decreased sensation, and no definitive nerve distribution pattern is evident on examination. Right plantar flexion is weak.

He undergoes nerve conduction studies, and electromyography confirms diabetic amyotrophy.

Which of the following is the best first step in the management of this patient's diabetic amyotrophy?
   A. Methylprednisolone
   B. Intravenous immunoglobulin
   C. Cyclophosphamide
   D. Duloxetine
   E. Tighter glycemic control (hemoglobin A_{1c} <7.5% [<58 mmol/mol])

54 A 57-year-old man is referred for evaluation of recurrent nephrolithiasis. He has had 2 episodes of kidney stones over the past year. His dietary calcium intake is approximately 800 mg daily, and he does not take any calcium or vitamin D supplements. A recent kidney stone analysis revealed that the composition of the stone was 85% calcium oxalate and 15% calcium phosphate. He was advised to take a citrate supplement, but he could not tolerate it due to gastrointestinal adverse effects, namely diarrhea. He takes a vitamin C supplement daily. He has no history of fragility fractures, thyroid disease, or parathyroid disease.

His physical examination findings are unremarkable.

Laboratory test results:
Serum calcium = 9.5 mg/dL (8.2-10.2 mg/dL) (SI: 2.4 mmol/L [2.1-2.6 mmol/L])
Serum phosphate = 3.0 mg/dL (2.3-4.7 mg/dL) (SI: 1.0 mmol/L [0.7-1.5 mmol/L])
Serum creatinine = 1.0 mg/dL (0.7-1.3 mg/dL) (SI: 88.4 μmol/L [61.9-114.9 μmol/L])
Serum intact PTH = 34 pg/mL (10-65 pg/mL) (SI: 34 ng/L [10-65 ng/L])
Serum 25-hydroxyvitamin D = 32 ng/mL (30-80 ng/mL [optimal]) (SI: 79.9 nmol/L [74.9-199.7 nmol/L])
Serum albumin = 3.9 g/dL (3.5-5.0 g/dL) (SI: 39 g/L [35-50 g/L])
Urinary calcium = 330 mg/24 h (100-300 mg/24 h) (SI: 8.3 mmol/d [2.5-7.5 mmol/d])
Urinary sodium = 130 mEq/24 h (40-217 mEq/24 h) (SI: 130 mmol/d [40-217 mmol/d])
Urinary oxalate = 35 mg/24 h (<40 mg/24 h) (SI: 399 mmol/d [<456 mmol/d])
Urinary calcium oxalate saturation ratio = 10.6 (0-6)
Urinary uric acid = 484 mg/24 h (<800 mg/24 h) (SI: 2.9 mmol/d [<4.7 mmol/d])
Urinary citrate = 1076 mg/24 h (320-1240 mg/24 h) (SI: 56.0 mmol/d [16.7-64.5 mmol/d])
Urinary creatinine = 1.5 g/24 h (1.0-2.0 g/24 h) (SI: 13.3 mmol/d [8.8-17.7 mmol/d])
Urine total volume = 1000 mL/24 h

In addition to increasing his fluid intake, which of the following should be recommended now to decrease his future risk of developing kidney stones?
A. Decrease his dietary oxalate intake
B. Decrease his dietary calcium intake
C. Increase his vitamin C intake
D. Increase his salt intake
E. Start hydrochlorothiazide

55 You are asked to evaluate a 32-year-old woman because her surgical team is concerned that she may have adrenal insufficiency. She is currently in the surgical intensive care unit after undergoing a total colectomy for ulcerative colitis 6 days ago. She had not used systemic corticosteroids for her colitis for more than 1 year before surgery. She has no other relevant personal or family medical history.

Her postoperative course has been complicated by a hospital-acquired pneumonia for which she is being treated with intravenous antibiotics.

The patient is weak and tired but claims to be feeling steadily better. Her height is 64 in (162.6 cm), and weight is 100 lb (45.5 kg) (BMI = 17.2 kg/m^2). Her blood pressure is 101/64 mm Hg, and pulse rate is 72 beats/min. She is afebrile. She is pale, but her mucous membranes are moist. On respiratory examination, crackles are detected at the right base.

She is receiving intravenous normal saline at a rate of 125 mL/h and her urine output is 100 mL/h. She is not receiving inotropic support.

Laboratory test results:
Sodium = 132 mEq/L (136-142 mEq/L) (SI: 132 mmol/L [136-142 mmol/L])
Potassium = 4.4 mEq/L (3.5-5.0 mEq/L) (SI: 4.4 mmol/L [3.5-5.0 mmol/L])
Chloride = 103 mEq/L (96-106 mEq/L) (SI: 103 mmol/L [96-106 mmol/L])
Serum urea nitrogen = 6 mg/dL (8-23 mg/dL) (SI: 2.1 mmol/L [2.9-8.2 mmol/L])
Creatinine = 0.52 mg/dL (0.6-1.1 mg/dL) (SI: 46.0 μmol/L [61.9-114.9 μmol/L])
Glucose = 96 mg/dL (70-99 mg/dL) (SI: 5.3 mmol/L [3.9-5.5 mmol/L])
Albumin = 1.8 g/dL (3.5-5.0 g/dL) (SI: 18 g/L [35-50 g/L])
Cortisol (random) = 12.5 μg/dL (5-25 μg/dL) (SI: 345 nmol/L [137.9-689.7 nmol/L])

Which of the following would you recommend to the surgical team responsible for this patient's care?
A. Perform a high-dose (250 mcg) ACTH-stimulation test
B. Perform a low-dose (1 mcg) ACTH-stimulation test
C. Initiate intravenous hydrocortisone, 100 mg every 6 hours
D. Measure cortisol at 8 AM
E. Pursue no further evaluation or treatment

56 A 26-year-old woman with hypothyroidism is referred to you for management of obesity. The patient tells you she has been overweight since age 8 years. She is currently at her highest weight (280 lb [127.3 kg]; BMI = 47 kg/m²), and she reports that her weight gain has been gradual. In the past, she followed self-administered diets and took over-the-counter medications for weight loss, without success. You recommend a comprehensive lifestyle program and refer her to your colleagues in the bariatric surgery clinic. The patient agrees to undergo Roux-en-Y gastric bypass.

At a follow-up visit 3 months after her operation, she has lost 62 lb (28.2 kg). She says that she feels better overall. Her current medications include levothyroxine, multivitamin with minerals, iron with vitamin C, and a calcium supplement. She does not smoke cigarettes.

On physical examination, her height is 63.5 in (161.3 cm) and weight is 218 lb (99.1 kg) (BMI = 38 kg/m²). Her blood pressure is 120/65 mm Hg, and pulse rate is 68 beats/min. She has thyromegaly but no palpable nodules. Her lungs are clear to auscultation bilaterally, her heart sounds are regular, and she has no peripheral edema. Her abdomen is soft and nontender.

Laboratory test result:
    TSH = 1.2 mIU/L (0.5-5.0 mIU/L)

You congratulate her on her weight-loss efforts and encourage her to continue following a meal plan and an exercise program. The patient shares that she has started dating and you discuss birth control.

Which of the following would be your first-choice recommendation for birth control in this patient?
   A. Intrauterine device
   B. Drospirenone/ethinyl estradiol
   C. Desogestrel/ethinyl estradiol
   D. Norethindrone
   E. Norethindrone/ethinyl estradiol

57 A 63-year-old woman returns for follow-up consultation regarding type 2 diabetes mellitus complicated only by nonproliferative diabetic retinopathy. Her current regimen includes metformin, 1000 mg twice daily; insulin glargine (100 units/mL), 70 units once nightly; and insulin lispro, 15 units before each meal. She has no specific concerns except that she experiences hypoglycemia in the late afternoons, with glucose values ranging between 50 and 60 mg/dL (2.8-3.3 mmol/L) that are associated with symptoms; this occurs about once weekly. Her hemoglobin A₁c level is 7.2% (55 mmol/mol), and she has been reluctant to make changes to her regimen, which she thinks works very well. She is adherent to dietary recommendations and is reasonably active, doing water aerobics twice weekly and yoga once weekly. Review of glucometer data is notable for a 30-day mean glucose value of 172 mg/dL (9.5 mmol/L).

She checks her glucose twice daily, and the glucometer download shows the following:
    Fasting glucose values = 82-256 mg/dL (4.6-14.2 mmol/L); average = 186 mg/dL (10.3 mmol/L)
    Prelunch values = 97-148 mg/dL (5.4-8.2 mmol/L); average = 118 mg/dL (6.5 mmol/L)
    Predinner values = 88-212 mg/dL (4.9-11.8 mmol/L); average = 152 mg/dL (8.5 mmol/L)
    Bedtime values = 111-178 mg/dL (6.2-9.9 mmol/L); average = 150 mg/dL (8.3 mmol/L)

On physical examination, her height is 65 in (165 cm) and weight is 175 lb (79.5 kg) (BMI = 29.1 kg/m²). Her blood pressure is 132/84 mm Hg, and pulse rate is 84 beats/min. Examination findings are otherwise unremarkable.

Laboratory test results:
    Serum urea nitrogen, normal
    Creatinine, normal
    Liver enzymes, normal

Which of the following is the best next step in this patient's management?
- A. Change basal insulin to U300 glargine, 70 units once daily
- B. Change basal insulin to U100 degludec, 70 units once daily
- C. Order a continuous glucose monitor
- D. Reduce the prandial insulin lispro dose to 10 units
- E. Discontinue prandial insulin and add a GLP-1 receptor agonist once weekly

58 A 45-year-old woman is referred for evaluation and treatment of hypercalcemia. Elevated serum calcium was first noted 4 years ago (10.8 mg/dL [2.7 mmol/L]) on routine testing and has remained stable since then. She has no history of craniocervical irradiation, confounding medication use (calcium, thiazides, lithium), nephrolithiasis, or fractures. Her medical history is unremarkable. She is premenopausal and does not take calcium or vitamin D supplements. Her family history is negative for renal stones or fractures. Review of systems is notable for fatigue and some short-term memory issues, but negative for bone pain or anxiety/depression.

On physical examination, she appears well. She has normal spinal curvature, no palpable neck masses, and no flank tenderness.

Laboratory test results:
  Serum calcium = 10.8 mg/dL (8.2-10.2 mg/dL) (SI: 2.7 mmol/L [2.1-2.6 mmol/L])
  Serum phosphate = 3.8 mg/dL (2.3-4.7 mg/dL) (SI: 1.2 mmol/L [0.7-1.5 mmol/L])
  Serum creatinine = 0.9 mg/dL (0.6-1.1 mg/dL) (SI: 79.6 µmol/L [53.0-97.2 µmol/L])
  Serum albumin = 4.2 mg/dL (3.5-5.0 g/dL) (SI: 42 g/L [35-50 g/L])
  Serum magnesium = 1.7 mg/dL (1.5-2.3 mg/dL) (SI: 0.70 [0.6-0.9 mmol/L])
  Serum intact PTH = 85 pg/mL (10-65 pg/mL) (SI: 85 ng/L [10-65 ng/L])
  Plasma ionized calcium = 5.6 mg/dL (4.60-5.08 mg/dL) (SI: 1.4 mmol/L [1.2-1.3 mmol/L])
  Serum 25-hydroxyvitamin D = 8 ng/mL (30-80 ng/mL) (SI: 20.0 nmol/L [74.9-199.7 nmol/L])
  Urinary calcium = 45 mg/24 h (100-300 mg/24 h) (SI: 1.1 mmol/d [2.5-7.5 mmol/d])
  Urinary creatinine = 1.0 g/24 h (1.0-2.0 g/24 h) (SI: 8.8 mmol/d [8.8-17.7 mmol/d])

DXA shows normal bone mineral density for age at the anteroposterior lumbar spine, right femoral neck, right total hip, and left proximal one-third radius.

Which of the following is the best next step in this patient's management?
- A. Measure serum calcium levels of all local first-degree family members
- B. Reassure the patient that she does not meet the criteria for referral for surgical management of hyperparathyroidism
- C. Measure serum PTHrP
- D. Start cinacalcet, 30 mg daily, and follow-up in 4 weeks
- E. Start cholecalciferol, 2000 IU daily, and follow-up in 8 weeks

59 A 65-year-old woman with a 50-year history of type 1 diabetes mellitus is admitted to the hospital with pain and swelling of the lateral aspect of her right thigh. The onset was abrupt and was not precipitated by vigorous exercise or trauma. She does not use her right thigh for insulin injection.

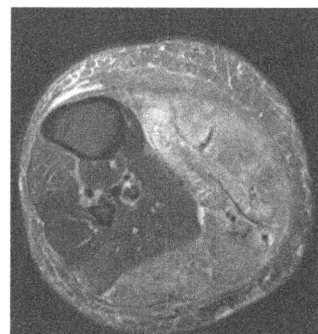

Laboratory test results:
  Erythrocyte sedimentation rate, elevated
  Creatine kinase, normal
  Serum glucose = 400 mg/dL (70-99 mg/dL) (SI: 22.2 mmol/L [3.9-5.5 mmol/L])
  Urinalysis, positive for protein but negative for ketones
  Serum creatinine = 3.5 mg/dL (0.6-1.1 mg/dL) (SI: 309.4 µmol/L [53.0-97.2 µmol/L])

Doppler ultrasonography of the lower extremities is negative for abnormalities. MRI of her right thigh is shown (*see image*). There is soft-tissue swelling on the anterior thigh and increased signal on the T2-weighted image of the lateral muscle groups.

Which of the following is the most likely diagnosis?
  A. Acute deep venous thrombosis
  B. Muscle abscess
  C. Polymyositis
  D. Osteomyelitis
  E. Muscle infarction

60 A 60-year-old man is referred for management of hyperlipidemia that was initially detected many years ago. Statin therapy has been attempted multiple times, but he developed myalgias on each of the medications he tried. Symptoms resolved when each drug was discontinued. He has longstanding type 2 diabetes mellitus, hypertension, gout, and stage 3 chronic kidney disease. He currently takes furosemide, chlorthalidone, candesartan, cholecalciferol, and oxycodone. His diabetes is managed with insulin glargine and insulin lispro. He quit smoking cigarettes 15 years ago and drinks 2 alcoholic beverages nightly. His parents are deceased and his family history is unremarkable for any form of cardiovascular disease.

On physical examination, his blood pressure is 159/81 mm Hg. His height is 68.5 in (174 cm), and weight is 202 lb (91.8 kg) (BMI = 30.3 kg/m^2). There are dark pigmented areas on both shins, a 3/6 ejection systolic murmur along the left sternal border, and bilateral 1+ pitting pedal edema.

Laboratory test results (sample drawn while fasting):
  Total cholesterol = 329 mg/dL (<200 mg/dL [optimal]) (SI: 8.52 mmol/L [<5.18 mmol/L])
  Triglycerides = 326 mg/dL (<150 mg/dL [optimal]) (SI: 3.68 mmol/L [<1.70 mmol/L])
  HDL cholesterol = 42 mg/dL (>60 mg/dL [optimal]) (SI: 1.09 mmol/L [>1.55 mmol/L])
  LDL cholesterol = 222 mg/dL (<100 mg/dL [optimal]) (SI: 5.75 mmol/L [<2.59 mmol/L])
  Non-HDL cholesterol = 287 mg/dL (<130 mg/dL [optimal]) (SI: 7.43 mmol/L [<3.37 mmol/L])
  Apolipoprotein B = 183 mg/dL (50-110 mg/dL) (SI: 1.8 g/L [0.5-1.1 g/L])
  Creatinine = 2.3 mg/dL (0.7-1.3 mg/dL) (SI: 203.3 μmol/L [61.9-114.9 μmol/L])
  Estimated glomerular filtration rate = 31 mL/min per 1.73 m^2 (>60 mL/min per 1.73 m^2)
  Hemoglobin A$_{1c}$ = 9.4% (4.0%-5.6%) (79 mmol/mol [20-38 mmol/mol])
  TSH = 4.23 mIU/L (0.5-5.0 mIU/L)

Which of the following is the best next step in this patient's management?
  A. Colesevelam
  B. Fish oil
  C. Evolocumab
  D. Fenofibrate
  E. Ezetimibe

61 A 42-year-old man presents with a 3-month history of palpitations, nervousness, heat intolerance, frequent bowel movements, intermittent blurred vision, increased eye prominence, and weight loss. He also reports erectile dysfunction.

Initial laboratory test results ordered by his primary care physician:
  TSH = <0.01 mIU/L (0.5-5.0 mIU/L)
  Free T$_4$ = 7.2 ng/dL (0.8-1.8 ng/dL) (SI: 92.7 pmol/L [10.30-23.17 pmol/L])
  Total testosterone = 2691 ng/dL (300-900 ng/dL) (SI: 93.4 nmol/L [10.4-31.2 nmol/L])

On physical examination, his blood pressure is 110/70 mm Hg, pulse rate is 100 beats/min, and BMI is 21 kg/m^2. He has classic stigmata of severe Graves disease, including a diffusely enlarged thyroid gland, bilateral severe exophthalmos, and prominent lid lag. The rest of his examination findings are unremarkable except for a bruit heard over the thyroid gland, warm, moist skin, and a fine hand tremor. Examination of the external genitalia reveals a normal phallus and a testicular volume of 18 mL bilaterally.

Repeated laboratory test results:

TSH = <0.01 mIU/L (0.5-5.0 mIU/L)

Free T_4 = 7.5 ng/dL (0.8-1.8 ng/dL) (SI: 96.5 pmol/L [10.30-23.17 pmol/L])

Total T_3 = 923 ng/dL (70-200 ng/dL) (SI: 14.2 nmol/L [1.08-3.08 nmol/L])

Total testosterone = 2570 ng/dL (300-900 ng/dL) (SI: 89.2 nmol/L [10.4-31.2 nmol/L])

Thyroid-stimulating immunoglobulin = 323% (≤120% of basal activity)

Which of the following diagnostic tests is the best next step to investigate this patient's elevated testosterone?

A. Adrenal CT

B. Pituitary MRI

C. Measurement of FSH and LH

D. Measurement of hCG

E. Measurement of SHBG

62 A 51-year-old woman is referred for evaluation of low bone density. She reports multiple fractures sustained as a child and adolescent due to falls (toes, fingers, arms, and legs), and she recently sustained a fracture of her right wrist after a fall. She underwent surgical menopause at age 44 years. She has excellent dietary calcium intake (~1500 mg daily) and takes a vitamin D supplement. She has no family history of osteoporosis or other bone disorders.

On physical examination, her height is 60 in (152.4 cm), and she has scoliosis. She has mild bowing of her lower extremities.

DXA scan documents a T-score of –2.7 in the right total hip.

A pathogenic variant in which of the following genes most likely explains her clinical presentation?

A. *COL1A1* or *COL1A2* (collagen alpha-1 chain or collagen alpha-2 chain)

B. *LRP5* (LDL receptor-related protein 5)

C. *GNAS* (α subunit of the stimulatory guanine nucleotide-binding protein [G protein])

D. *PHEX* (phosphate-regulating endopeptidase on the X chromosome)

E. *DMP1* (dentin matrix acidic phosphoprotein 1)

63 A 32-year-old woman seeks evaluation for hirsutism. After menarche at age 12 years, the patient had regular menses until she started combined oral contraceptives in high school. Three years ago, she discontinued oral contraceptives to try for pregnancy and conceived without difficulty. She stopped breastfeeding early due to the development of frequent migraine headaches with aura and the need for preventative and abortive medications. Three months after she stopped breastfeeding, she developed acne and hair growth on her face, abdomen, arms, and legs. Her menses have not returned over the past year since she stopped breastfeeding. She has a family history of venous thromboembolic disease. Her mother developed lower-extremity deep venous thrombosis after gall bladder surgery, and her sister recently had pulmonary embolism after starting oral contraceptives.

On physical examination, she has significant terminal hair growth with a Ferriman-Gallwey score of 15. Acne lesions are not cystic and are clustered along the jawline without evidence of scarring. She has no acanthosis.

Her testosterone concentration is mildly elevated. Her prolactin level and thyroid function tests are normal and a pregnancy test is negative. With 10 days of micronized progesterone, she has a withdrawal bleed. Currently, she does not plan to try conceiving again and is most concerned about her poor self-image due to the acne and hair growth.

Which of the following is the best next step?
- A. Metformin
- B. Spironolactone and levonorgestrel-releasing intrauterine device
- C. Combined oral contraceptives
- D. Progestin-only oral contraceptives
- E. Topical retinoid, clindamycin, and eflornithine

64 A 67-year-old man presents to the emergency department with severe headache, vomiting, and left third nerve palsy. Brain MRI shows a large heterogeneous sellar mass with chiasmatic compression and invasion of the left cavernous sinus. An obvious visual field defect is detected, and pituitary apoplexy is diagnosed. A random cortisol concentration is less than 1.0 µg/dL (<27.6 nmol/L). He receives intravenous glucocorticoids and undergoes emergency transsphenoidal surgery. Pathology documents a hemorrhagic pituitary macroadenoma, with negative stains for ACTH, GH, and prolactin. Postoperative MRI shows no obvious residual adenoma.

You see him 3 days after surgery. He remains on hydrocortisone. He tells you that a couple years ago he had complained of erectile dysfunction, and his primary care physician documented low testosterone. He was prescribed testosterone replacement but had discontinued it a few months later because his wife was undergoing chemotherapy for breast cancer and was not interested in sex.

Current laboratory test results:
Free T$_4$ = 0.6 ng/dL (0.8-1.8 ng/dL) (SI: 7.7 pmol/L [10.30-23.17 pmol/L])
Testosterone, undetectable
Prolactin, undetectable

You prescribe levothyroxine, 75 mcg daily, and testosterone replacement and continue the hydrocortisone, 15 mg in the morning and 5 mg in the afternoon.

You see him 6 weeks later. He is feeling well. The third nerve palsy has resolved. He is adhering to his regimen of hydrocortisone, levothyroxine, and testosterone.

Laboratory test results:
Free T$_4$ = 1.2 ng/dL (0.8-1.8 ng/dL) (SI: 15.4 pmol/L [10.30-23.17 pmol/L])
Testosterone = 360 ng/dL (300-900 ng/dL) (SI: 12.5 mol/L [10.4-31.2 nmol/L])
Prolactin = 1.0 ng/dL (4-23 ng/dL) (SI: 0.04 nmol/L [0.17-1.00 nmol/L])

Which of the following is the best next step in this patient's management?
- A. Continue the same therapies
- B. Stop testosterone therapy and measure testosterone in 3 weeks
- C. Stop levothyroxine and measure free T$_4$ in 2 weeks
- D. Stop hydrocortisone and measure cortisol at 8 AM the next day
- E. Prescribe liothyronine

65 A 58-year-old man with a 7-year history of diabetes mellitus is seen in the endocrinology clinic for follow-up. He is being treated with metformin, 2000 mg daily; pioglitazone, 45 mg daily; and dulaglutide, 1.5 mg weekly via subcutaneous injection. He has had acceptable glucose control recently, and his current hemoglobin A$_{1c}$ measurement is 7.4% (57 mmol/mol). He has no retinopathy. He has long-lasting symptoms of numbness and tingling in both feet and lancinating-type pain in his feet that is bothersome. The symptoms are worse at rest and at night. He does not have calf pain with walking. He asks for something to treat the neuropathic pain.

His urinary albumin excretion is elevated, and his hypertension is being treated with losartan, amlodipine, spironolactone, and furosemide. He takes fenofibrate and atorvastatin to treat combined dyslipidemia. He has a history of a silent myocardial infarction. A stress echocardiogram done 6 months ago demonstrated a fixed area of hypokinesia in the inferolateral left ventricle, and there was evidence of diastolic dysfunction.

He smokes one-half pack of cigarettes per day and has smoked for 32 years. He has 2 to 3 servings of alcohol per week.

On physical examination, his height is 71 in (180 cm) and weight is 228 lb (103.6 kg) (BMI = 31.8 kg/m²). His blood pressure is 141/82 mm Hg, and pulse rate is 82 beats/min. He has central weight distribution. Findings on cardiac examination reveal a grade II/VI systolic ejection murmur and an S_4. Findings on lung and abdominal examinations are unremarkable. He has grade 1 pedal edema. The distal pulses are moderately reduced. There are hammer toe deformities of the second through fourth toes of each foot, and hyperkeratosis is evident on the corresponding metatarsal head areas and distal interphalangeal joints of the second through fourth toes of each foot. He has reduced sensation to 10-g monofilament testing and vibrational sense in each foot. The ankle reflexes are blunted.

Laboratory test results:
    Creatinine = 1.3 mg/dL (0.7-1.3 mg/dL) (SI: 114.9 µmol/L [61.9-114.9 µmol/L])
    Estimated glomerular filtration rate = 59 mL/min per 1.73 m² (>60 mL/min per 1.73 m²)
    Electrolytes, normal
    Serum urea nitrogen, normal
    TSH = 2.73 mIU/L (0.5-5.0 mIU/L)
    Vitamin B_{12} = 560 pg/mL (180-914 pg/mL) (SI: 560 ng/L [180-914 ng/L])
    Serum protein electrophoresis, normal

Which of the following is the best treatment for this patient's diabetic neuropathy pain?
    A. Fluoxetine
    B. Oxycodone
    C. Insulin
    D. Amitriptyline
    E. Pregabalin

66 A 58-year-old man with hypertension, hyperlipidemia, and obesity presents for a follow-up visit to manage testosterone therapy. Ten months ago, he was documented to have 2 low testosterone measurements when he presented with symptoms of fatigue, poor sleep, worsening erectile function, and mild lower urinary symptoms. Secondary hypogonadism was diagnosed, and he was prescribed a topical testosterone gel. While on the testosterone therapy, he has noticed a significant increase in his energy and a mild increase in his urinary symptoms. He is uncertain whether the therapy has improved his sexual function, so a phosphodiesterase 5 inhibitor has been prescribed. Current medications include testosterone gel, lisinopril, atorvastatin, and vardenafil as needed.

On physical examination, his height is 67 in (170 cm) and weight is 210 lb (96 kg) (BMI = 33 kg/m²). His blood pressure is 144/87 mm Hg, and pulse rate is 71 beats/min. Testicular volume is 12 to 15 mL bilaterally. The prostate is mildly enlarged without nodules. The rest of the examination findings are normal.

Laboratory and radiology test results:

Measurement	Baseline	12 Months on Testosterone	Reference Range
Total testosterone	238 and 261 ng/dL (SI: 8.3 and 9.1 nmol/L)	672 ng/dL (SI: 23.3 nmol/L)	300-900 ng/dL (SI: 10.4-31.2 nmol/L)
PSA	1.2 ng/mL (SI: 1.2 µg/L)	2.9 ng/mL (SI: 2.9 µg/L)	<3.8 ng/mL (SI: <3.8 µg/L)
Hematocrit	47% (SI: 0.47)	51% (SI: 0.51)	41%-50% (SI: 0.41-0.50)
Chemistry panel	Normal	Normal	...
DXA scan	Hip T-score, −1.2 Spine T-score, −1.0	Hip T-score, −1.2 Spine T-score, −1.1	...

Which of the following is the best next step in this patient's management?
    A. Continue testosterone therapy at the current dosage
    B. Decrease the testosterone dosage due to elevated hematocrit
    C. Decrease the testosterone dosage to target testosterone <500 ng/dL (<17.4 nmol/L) given his age
    D. Increase the testosterone dosage due to lack of increase in T-scores
    E. Refer for urologic evaluation

67 A 52-year-old woman is referred to you for evaluation of an abnormal bone density study. A recent DXA scan documented osteopenia in the lumbar spine (T-score, –1.6). She was osteoporotic in the hip, with right femoral neck and total hip T-scores of –3.5 and –3.0, respectively. She was prescribed risedronate, 150 mg monthly, but she elected to hold off on therapy until her consultation with you.

She has a history of recurrent metatarsal stress fractures without significant trauma. She underwent natural menopause 1 year ago and has not taken hormone therapy. She takes calcium, 600 mg twice daily, and cholecalciferol, 2000 IU daily, but no multivitamin or additional supplements. Review of systems is notable for multiple previous tooth extractions due to poor dentition and ongoing mild but vague right upper thigh pain. On review of her family history, her mother had a femoral fracture in her 50s, although she was not diagnosed with osteoporosis nor treated specifically for this condition.

On physical examination, she has no significant height loss. She has multiple missing teeth. She has mild tenderness to palpation over the right anterolateral upper femur. There is no evident thoracic kyphosis.

Laboratory test results:
Serum calcium = 9.5 mg/dL (8.2-10.2 mg/dL) (SI: 2.4 mmol/L [2.1-2.6 mmol/L])
Serum phosphate = 4.0 mg/dL (2.3-4.7 mg/dL) (SI: 1.3 mmol/L [0.7-1.5 mmol/L])
Serum alkaline phosphatase = 30 U/L (50-120 U/L) (SI: 0.5 μkat/L [0.84-2.00 μkat/L])
Serum ALT = 35 U/L (10-40 U/L) (SI: 0.58 μkat/L [0.17-0.67 μkat/L])
Serum AST = 42 IU/L (20-48 U/L) (SI: 0.70 μkat/L [0.33-0.80 μkat/L])
Serum albumin = 4.0 mg/dL (3.5-5.0 g/dL) (SI: 40 g/L [35-50 g/L])
Serum creatinine = 1.0 mg/dL (0.6-1.1 mg/dL) (SI: 88.4 μmol/L [53.0-97.2 μmol/L])
Serum intact PTH = 45 pg/mL (10-65 pg/mL) (SI: 45 ng/L [10-65 ng/L])
Serum 25-hydroxyvitamin D = 48 ng/mL (30-80 ng/mL) (SI: 119.8 nmol/L [74.9-199.7 nmol/L])
Urinary calcium = 200 mg/24 h (100-300 mg/24 h) (SI: 5.0 mmol/d [2.5-7.5 mmol/d])
Urinary creatinine = 1.2 g/24 h (1.0-2.0 g/24 h) (SI: 10.6 mmol/d [8.8-17.7 mmol/d])

Which of the following is this patient's most likely diagnosis?
A. Osteogenesis imperfecta type 1
B. Paget disease of bone
C. Hypophosphatasia
D. Hypophosphatemic rickets
E. Celiac disease

68 A colleague in primary care refers a 32-year-old woman who is 2 months postpartum following the birth of her second child. Graves disease was diagnosed 2 years earlier and this was initially treated with methimazole. Her antithyroid drug regimen was changed to propylthiouracil 3 months before she became pregnant, and antithyroid drug treatment was discontinued at 16 weeks' gestation. She reports that she felt nauseated while taking propylthiouracil. The patient remained euthyroid during pregnancy but has now presented with a 4-week history of palpitation, weight loss of 11 lb (5 kg), heat intolerance, and tremulousness. She reports that she is breastfeeding her baby and she is keen to continue this.

On physical examination, her height is 68 in (172.7 cm) and weight is 150 lb (68.2 kg) (BMI = 22.8 kg/m^2). Her blood pressure is 124/62 mm Hg, and pulse rate is 110 beats/min. There is a tremor of the outstretched hands, and her hands are moist. She has mild periorbital and conjunctival swelling. A small, soft, diffusely enlarged thyroid gland is palpable in her neck.

Laboratory test results:
TSH = <0.01 mIU/L (0.5-5.0 mIU/L)
Free T$_4$ = 3.1 ng/dL (0.8-1.8 ng/dL) (SI: 39.9 pmol/L [10.30-23.17 pmol/L])
TRAb = 23.0 IU/L (≤1.75 IU/L)

Which of the following is the best next step in this patient's management?
A. Start methimazole and continue breastfeeding
B. Start propylthiouracil and continue breastfeeding
C. Start propranolol and continue breastfeeding
D. Recommend total thyroidectomy and continue breastfeeding
E. Stop breastfeeding due to risk of hyperthyroidism in infant

69 A 24-year-old woman with an 8-year history of type 1 diabetes mellitus is admitted to the hospital for management of a hyperglycemic crisis. She usually has good glycemic control. Her most recent hemoglobin A_{1c} value was 6.8% (51 mmol/mol) 8 weeks ago. The night before admission, her insulin pump malfunctioned overnight and she was not able to keep up with her fluid needs or her insulin with subcutaneous injections. She had nausea, vomiting, and abdominal pain. Urine ketones were strongly positive. She has no other notable medical history.

On physical examination, she is awake and able to answer questions, but she appears fatigued and pauses between sentences. She is afebrile, blood pressure is 96/68 mm Hg, pulse rate is 112 beats/min, and respiratory rate is 24 breaths/min. Her height is 64 in (162.5 cm), and weight is 121 lb (55 kg) (BMI = 20.8 kg/m^2). Oral examination reveals dry mucous membranes. Lungs are clear to auscultation. She is tachypneic, and Kussmaul respiration is noted. Cardiac examination is notable for tachycardia. There is diffuse abdominal tenderness but no rebound, guarding, or focal pain. The rest of her examination findings are normal.

Laboratory test results:
    pH = 6.9 (7.35-7.45)
    Anion gap = 17
    Bicarbonate = 10 mEq/L (21-28 mEq/L) (SI: 10 mmol/L [21-28 mmol/L])
    Blood glucose = 268 mg/dL (70-99 mg/dL) (SI: 14.9 mmol/L [3.9-5.5 mmol/L])
    Serum urea nitrogen = 56 mg/dL (8-23 mg/dL) (SI: 20.0 mg/dL [2.9-8.2 mmol/L])
    Creatinine = 2.6 mg/dL (0.6-1.1 mg/dL) (SI: 229.8 μmol/L [53.0-97.2 μmol/L])
    Sodium = 135 mEq/L (136-142 mEq/L) (SI: 135 mmol/L [136-142 mmol/L])
    Potassium = 3.2 mEq/L (3.5-5.0 mEq/L) (SI: 3.2 mmol/L [3.5-5.0 mmol/L])
    Magnesium = 1.7 mg/dL (1.5-2.3 mg/dL) (SI: 0.7 mmol/L [0.6-0.9 mmol/L])
    Phosphate = 3.6 mg/dL (2.3-4.7 mg/dL) (SI: 1.2 mmol/L [0.7-1.5 mmol/L])

Which of the following is the best initial step in this patient's management?
A. Infuse 1000 mL 0.9% NaCl with 40 mEq of KCl over 1 hour
B. Give 6 units regular insulin intravenously and infuse 1000 mL 0.9% NaCl with 40 mEq KCl over 1 hour
C. Infuse 1000 mL 0.45% NaCl with 40 mEq KCl over 1 hour
D. Give 6 units regular insulin intravenously and infuse 0.45% NaCl at 100 cc/h with 20 mEq KCl per L
E. Infuse 0.45% NaCl at 100 cc/h with 40 mEq of KCl per L

70 A 41-year-old woman with hypothyroidism presents for ongoing management. She has a history of depression and nonadherence to her prescribed medical therapy of levothyroxine, 150 mcg daily.

At today's visit, she appears dispirited. Her main concerns are feeling tired and gaining weight. Her blood pressure is 136/80 mm Hg, pulse rate is 60 beats/min, and BMI is 30 kg/m^2.

Laboratory test results:
    TSH = 26 mIU/L (0.5-5.0 mIU/L)
    Total cholesterol = 220 mg/dL ([optimal] <200 mg/dL) (SI: 5.70 mmol/L [<5.18 mmol/L])

She admits to not taking her levothyroxine on a regular basis, but she thinks she takes it 4 to 5 days a week. You begin a trial of observed daily therapy for 6 weeks and also repeat vital signs assessment and biochemical evaluation.

Her pulse rate is now 75 beats/min. Laboratory test results:

TSH = 3.2 mIU/L (0.5-5.0 mIU/L)

Total cholesterol = 190 mg/dL (<200 mg/dL [optimal]) (SI: 4.92 mmol/L [<5.18 mmol/L])

She states that she feels slightly less fatigued, but that she cannot continue daily therapy because it is too inconvenient. You decide to administer 7 times the patient's daily levothyroxine dose given as an observed once-weekly oral dose. After 6 weeks of weekly therapy, you perform an assessment before administering the next weekly dose. The assessment includes measurement of TSH, free T_4, total cholesterol, and heart rate, as well as an evaluation for hyperthyroid symptoms.

Which of the following best represents the patient's most likely response to the change from once-daily to once-weekly therapy?

Answer	Free T_4	TSH	Total Cholesterol	Hyperthyroid Symptoms	Heart Rate
A.	↑	↓	↔	↑	↑
B.	↓	↑	↑	↓	↓
C.	↓	↑	↑	↔	↔
D.	↑	↓	↓	↑	↑
E.	↑	↓	↓	↔	↔

↑ or ↓ indicates direction of the change in the parameter during once-weekly therapy compared with once-daily therapy. ↔ indicates no change in the parameter during once-weekly therapy compared with once-daily therapy.

71 A 52-year-old man comes for consultation regarding resistant hypertension. He reports being diagnosed with hypertension at age 33 years. Over the subsequent 19 years, he has been treated with numerous antihypertensive medications, although he does not recall all of their names. Four years ago, he was noted to have hypokalemia with a serum potassium value of 2.9 mEq/L (2.9 mmol/L) and he was started on potassium supplements.

Currently, he presents with a blood pressure of 142/88 mm Hg. A biochemical evaluation for primary aldosteronism is performed while the patient is in the seated position. He is currently taking the following medications: hydrochlorothiazide, 25 mg daily; verapamil, 120 mg twice daily; enalapril, 20 mg daily; amiloride, 10 mg twice daily; hydralazine, 25 mg 3 times daily; and potassium chloride, 20 mEq daily.

Laboratory test results:

Serum aldosterone = 39 ng/dL (4-21 ng/dL) (SI: 1082 pmol/L [111.0-582.5 pmol/L])

Plasma renin activity = 1.7 ng/mL per h (0.6-4.3 ng/mL per h)

Aldosterone-to-renin ratio (ng/dL per ng/mL per h) = 23

Serum potassium = 3.8 mEq/L (3.5-5.0 mEq/L) (SI: 3.8 mmol/L [3.5-5.0 mmol/L])

Plasma metanephrines, normal

Cortisol following 1-mg dexamethasone suppression test = 0.8 µg/dL (22.1 nmol/L)

Which of the following is the most appropriate interpretation of the test results?
  A. "Positive screen" for primary aldosteronism
  B. "Negative screen" for primary aldosteronism
  C. Results cannot be interpreted; stop amiloride for a few weeks and repeat testing
  D. Results cannot be interpreted; stop hydrochlorothiazide for a few weeks and repeat testing
  E. Results cannot be interpreted; stop enalapril for a few weeks and repeat testing

72 A 28-year-old woman presents to the clinic with a 6-week history of weight loss of 6.5 lb (3 kg) in addition to palpitation, tremor, and heat intolerance. She gave birth to her firstborn baby 8 months ago and continues to breastfeed. She reports no notable medical history, and she is not taking any regular medication. Her mother has celiac disease, but there is no other family history of note.

On physical examination, her height is 65 in (165.1 cm) and weight is 123 lb (55.8 kg) (BMI = 20.5 kg/m^2). Her blood pressure is 132/68 mm Hg, and pulse rate is 110 beats/min. There is a tremor of the outstretched hands, and her hands are moist. There are no signs of thyroid ophthalmopathy or dermopathy. Her thyroid gland is palpable in her neck, and there is no palpable cervical lymphadenopathy. Findings on systems examination are otherwise unremarkable.

Laboratory test results:
    TSH = <0.01 mIU/L (0.5-5.0 mIU/L)
    Free T$_4$ = 3.1 ng/dL (0.8-1.8 ng/dL) (SI: 39.9 pmol/L [10.30-23.17 pmol/L])

Which of the following is the most appropriate next investigation?
    A. Thyroid ultrasonography
    B. ^{131}I isotope scan
    C. Measurement of TPO antibodies
    D. Measurement of serum free T$_3$
    E. Measurement of TRAb

73 A 48-year-old man presents with a 4-month history of flushing (mainly affecting his face and upper chest), as well as profuse, watery diarrhea and abdominal cramps. He has no relevant medical history. He takes no medications.

On physical examination, he appears well. His height is 71 in (180 cm), and weight is 165 lb (75 kg) (BMI = 23 kg/m^2). His blood pressure is 144/92 mm Hg, and pulse rate is 74 beats/min. Findings on abdominal examination suggest hepatomegaly; the liver is palpable to 1 inch below the costal margin.

Laboratory test results:
    Chromogranin A = 280 ng/mL (<93 ng/mL) (SI: 280 ng/mL [<93 µg/L])
    ALT = 185 U/L (10-40 U/L) (SI: 3.09 µkat/L [0.17-0.67 µkat/L])
    AST = 210 U/L (20-48 U/L) (SI: 3.51 µkat/L [0.33-0.80 µkat/L])
    Albumin = 3.4 g/dL (3.5-5.0 g/dL) (SI: 34 g/L [35-50 g/L])
    Bilirubin (total) = 5 mg/dL (0.3-1.2 mg/dL) (SI: 85.5 µmol/L [5.1-20.5 µmol/L])
    Urinary 5-hydroxyindole acetic acid = 17 mg/24 h (2-9 mg/24 h) (SI: 88.9 µmol/d [10.5-47.1 µmol/d])

Abdominal CT is shown (*see images*). Several small heterogeneous lesions within the liver are suspicious for malignancy. In addition, a hyperdense lesion suspicious for malignancy is seen within the terminal ileum, as well as neoplastic-type nodal masses that are noted within the mesentery along the ileocolic vessels and adherent to the terminal ileum (*arrows*).

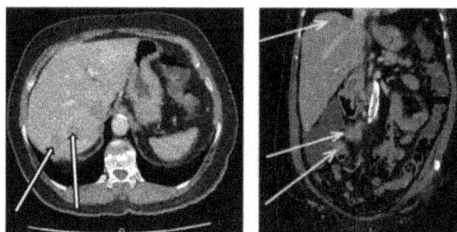

Biopsy of the liver lesions documents metastatic neuroendocrine carcinoma (grade 2; Ki67 index, 5%). Octreotide LAR, 30 mg monthly, is initiated.

In addition to somatostatin analogue therapy, which of the following is the most appropriate management option?
    A. Observation with regular imaging and assessment of biomarkers
    B. Surgery to remove the primary tumor and debulk liver metastases
    C. Ablation therapy of liver metastases
    D. Peptide receptor radionuclide therapy with ^{177}Lu-DOTATATE
    E. Everolimus

74 A 65-year-old woman with type 2 diabetes mellitus, hypercholesterolemia, class III obesity, severe arthritis, and depression presents for a follow-up visit. Her medications include metformin, liraglutide, atorvastatin, and naproxen. During the visit, the patient reports that she has had chest pain for the past 2 months. The patient describes the pain as dull and being associated with pressure on her chest. The pain is substernal, radiates to her left shoulder, and only occurs when she is more active than usual. After resting for 5 to 10 minutes, the pain resolves. Both her father and paternal grandmother had type 2 diabetes and they both had a myocardial infarction at age 65 years. She mentions that her arthritis is worsening and that she is having more difficulty with ambulation.

On physical examination, her blood pressure is 146/88 mm Hg and pulse rate is 68 beats/min. Her height is 61 in (154.9 cm), and weight is 256 lb (116.4 kg) (BMI = 48.4 kg/m^2). The patient is in no distress, she breathes normally on room air, and her lungs are clear to auscultation bilaterally. On cardiac examination, she has distant heart sounds, normal rate and regular rhythm, no murmur, and no abnormal heart sounds. She has no peripheral edema. On knee examination, she has reduced range of motion and crepitus bilaterally. Her abdomen is soft and nontender.

Laboratory test results:
Hemoglobin A$_{1c}$ = 6.6% (4.0%-5.6%) (49 mmol/mol [20-38 mmol/mol])
Creatinine = 0.9 mg/dL (0.6-1.1 mg/dL) (SI: 79.6 µmol/L [53.0-97.2 µmol/L])
Total cholesterol = 202 mg/dL (<200 mg/dL [optimal]) (SI: 5.23 mmol/L [<5.18 mmol/L])
Triglycerides = 287 mg/dL (<150 mg/dL [optimal]) (SI: 3.24 mmol/L [<1.70 mmol/L])
HDL cholesterol = 35 mg/dL (>60 mg/dL [optimal]) (SI: 0.91 mmol/L [>1.55 mmol/L])
LDL cholesterol = 109 mg/dL (<100 mg/dL [optimal]) (SI: 2.82 mmol/L [<2.59 mmol/L])

You order electrocardiography, which shows low QRS voltage on all the precordial leads and nonspecific T-wave flattening.

Which of the following cardiac tests is the best next step in this patient's workup?
- A. Transthoracic dobutamine stress echocardiography
- B. Stress radionuclide myocardial perfusion imaging with positron emission tomography
- C. CT coronary artery calcium scoring
- D. Exercise stress testing with electrocardiography
- E. Exercise stress testing with echocardiography

75 A 45-year-old man is referred to you for evaluation of hypoglycemia. For the past 6 months, he has noticed that any time he eats a carbohydrate-heavy meal, he becomes lightheaded within 40 minutes and must stop what he is doing. Using his wife's glucometer, he documented a glucose value of 50 mg/dL (2.8 mmol/L) during one of these episodes. Once, while driving, he was forced to stop his car on the shoulder of the road because of these symptoms. When he has such an episode, he eats a hard candy or consumes a nondiet soft drink and he feels better. These episodes have made working difficult, as he must stop his activities to treat his symptoms. He has tried to modify his diet by reducing starch and sweets, but he still occasionally has these episodes. He has no history of diabetes. His wife has type 2 diabetes. His weight has been stable. He has not traveled recently or had gastric banding or bariatric surgery. He exercises by walking, jogging, or using cardio equipment 30 minutes daily.

His current medications are lisinopril, 10 mg daily, and atorvastatin, 10 mg daily. He takes no over-the-counter products.

Findings on physical examination are normal. His height is 69.5 in (176.5 cm), and weight is 165 lb (75 kg) (BMI = 24 kg/m^2).

In addition to testing his blood for oral hypoglycemic agents, which of the following should be the next step in this patient's evaluation?
- A. 5-Hour mixed-meal test
- B. Oral glucose tolerance test
- C. Admit for a 48-hour fast
- D. Selective arterial calcium stimulation test
- E. Insulin antibody assessment

76 A 39-year-old woman was recently started on an immune checkpoint inhibitor for recurrence of melanoma with skeletal metastases. A melanoma had been resected from her thigh 5 years ago and further therapy was not recommended at that time. The recurrence was found after she presented with shoulder pain and was found to have a destructive lesion in her humeral head. She was started on combination therapy with ipilimumab and nivolumab, and after the third dose she felt unwell.

When she presents for her fourth dose today, she describes feeling weak, fatigued, dizzy, and nauseated, and she has a poor appetite. Her blood pressure is 105/65 mm Hg, pulse rate is 85 beats/min, and BMI is 20 kg/m^2. On examination, she appears sick. Findings are notable for absence of hyperpigmentation, an unremarkable neck examination, and diffuse mild abdominal tenderness.

Laboratory test results:
  Serum sodium = 134 mEq/L (136-142 mEq/L) (SI: 134 mmol/d [136-142 mmol/d])
  Serum potassium = 4.1 mEq/L (3.5-5.0 mEq/L) (SI: 4.1 mmol/L [3.5-5.0 mmol/L])
  Serum urea nitrogen = 25 mg/dL (8-23 mg/dL) (SI: 8.9 mmol/L [2.9-8.2 mmol/L])
  ACTH = 5 pg/mL (10-60 pg/mL) (SI: 1.1 pmol/L [2.2-13.2 pmol/L])
  Cortisol (8 AM) = 3 µg/dL (5-25 µg/dL) (SI: 82.8 nmol/L [137.9-689.7 nmol/L])
  Serum TSH = 1.0 mIU/L (0.5-5.0 mIU/L)

A pituitary-directed MRI shows diffuse enlargement of the pituitary gland consistent with hypophysitis. The patient is initially started on high-dosage glucocorticoids and later transitioned to a body surface area–based dose of hydrocortisone. She feels better with less weakness and no further dizziness, but continues to have malaise and fatigue. Her appetite has improved and she has no polydipsia or polyuria.

Which of the following is the most likely explanation for the patient's current symptoms?
  A. Secondary hypothyroidism
  B. Primary hypogonadism
  C. Primary adrenal insufficiency
  D. Diabetes insipidus
  E. Type 1 diabetes mellitus

77 A 78-year-old woman presents for evaluation of hypercalcemia. She has had mild hypercalcemia for the past 3 years. She had been on hydrochlorothiazide for hypertension; this was discontinued a few months ago and her hypercalcemia persisted. She takes no calcium or vitamin D supplements. She has no history of fragility fractures, kidney stones, or thyroid disease. She reports progressive fatigue and a 20-lb (9.1-kg) weight loss in the past few months.

On physical examination, her vital signs are normal. Cervical adenopathy is appreciated on neck examination. She had a recent unremarkable chest radiograph.

Laboratory test results:
  Serum calcium = 11.6 mg/dL (8.2-10.2 mg/dL) (SI: 2.9 mmol/L [2.1-2.6 mmol/L])
  Serum phosphate = 3.1 mg/dL (2.3-4.7 mg/dL) (SI: 1.0 mmol/L [0.7-1.5 mmol/L])
  Serum creatinine = 1.1 mg/dL (0.6-1.1 mg/dL) (SI: 97.2 µmol/L [53.0-97.2 µmol/L])
  Serum intact PTH = 20 pg/mL (10-65 pg/mL) (SI: 20 ng/L [10-65 ng/L])
  Serum 25-hydroxyvitamin D = 30 ng/mL (30-80 ng/mL [optimal]) (SI: 74.9 nmol/L [74.9-199.7 nmol/L])
  Serum 1,25-dihydroxyvitamin D = 70 pg/mL (16-65 pg/mL) (SI: 182 pmol/L [41.6-169.0 pmol/L])
  Serum albumin = 3.7 g/dL (3.5-5.0 g/dL) (SI: 37 g/L [35-50 g/L])

Which of the following is the best next step in the evaluation of this patient's hypercalcemia?
  A. Tuberculin skin test
  B. Measurement of PTHrP
  C. Serum protein electrophoresis
  D. Bone scan
  E. CT of the chest, abdomen, and pelvis

78 A 19-year-old man returns for follow-up of type 1 diabetes mellitus of 16 years' duration and is accompanied by his mother. He has no specific concerns and reports no hospitalizations or emergency department visits. He has had no episodes of severe hypoglycemia. He uses an insulin pump. In the past, he has been extremely diligent about checking his blood glucose and correcting when necessary, but today you note that there are several days when he did not check his blood glucose at all. His point-of-care hemoglobin A_{1c} level today is 8.5% (69 mmol/mol), whereas in the last few years his hemoglobin A_{1c} has typically been less than 7.0% (<53 mmol/mol). There have been no changes in his medical or family history. He has previously denied use tobacco, alcohol, or illicit drugs. Although he was in community college, he has since left, expressing dissatisfaction with schoolwork. However, he is interested in studying either business or computers. He continues to live with his family and notes several conflicts that have been causing stress.

On physical examination, he is a thin, well-developed man in no distress. His height is 70 in (177.8 cm), and weight is 126 lb (57.3 kg) (BMI = 18.1 kg/m^2) (notably 6 lb [2.7 kg] less than at his last visit). His blood pressure is 146/81 mm Hg, and pulse rate is 81 beats/min. Findings on heart, lung, and abdominal examinations are unremarkable. Skin is notable for hypertrophy at one of his pump insertion sites in the buttocks.

Which of the following is the best next step in this patient's management?

- A. Prescribe a continuous glucose monitor
- B. Request a nutritional consultation to ensure adequate caloric intake
- C. Request consultation with a mental health care provider
- D. Arrange for him to attend a diabetes education class
- E. Advise rotation of his insulin insertion sites and avoidance of hypertrophied sites

79 A 54-year-old woman is referred for evaluation of primary aldosteronism. She has a 10-year history of resistant hypertension, as well as hypokalemia with a documented potassium level as low as 2.8 mEq/L (2.8 mmol/L). Her blood pressure is 160/100 mm Hg while being treated with diltiazem and doxazosin. A diagnosis of primary aldosteronism is confirmed when her serum aldosterone level is found to be 44 ng/dL (1221 pmol/L) in the context of a plasma renin activity less than 0.6 ng/mL per h (aldosterone-to-renin ratio >73).

Abdominal CT reveals a 1.9 x 1.3-cm left-sided adrenal adenoma. Adrenal venous sampling performed with simultaneous sampling of the inferior vena cava and each adrenal vein reveals the following results, which are interpreted to suggest a left-sided aldosterone-producing adenoma:

Inferior Vena Cava		Right Adrenal Vein		Left Adrenal Vein	
Aldosterone	**Cortisol**	**Aldosterone**	**Cortisol**	**Aldosterone**	**Cortisol**
15.0 ng/dL (416 pmol/L)	9.6 µg/dL (265 nmol/L)	6.5 ng/dL (180 pmol/L)	24.2 µg/dL (668 nmol/L)	220 ng/dL (6103 pmol/L)	31.2 µg/dL (861 nmol/L)
A/C ratio = 1.56		A/C ratio = 0.27		A/C ratio = 7.05	

Values are presented in conventional units with SI units in parentheses. Results following ACTH stimulation were also obtained; however, only the baseline values are presented here for simplicity.

The patient undergoes a successful left-sided laparoscopic adrenalectomy. On the second postoperative day, her blood pressure is 133/75 mm Hg off all of antihypertensive medications. On the seventh postoperative day, her blood pressure is 98/55 mm Hg off all of antihypertensive medications, and her potassium level is 6.1 mEq/L (6.1 mmol/L), with a rise in creatinine to 1.8 mg/dL (159.1 µmol/L) (increased from 1.0 mg/dL [88.4 µmol/L] before surgery).

Which of the following sets of laboratory results is most likely to be observed in this patient now?

	Plasma Renin Activity (ng/mL per h)[a]	Serum Aldosterone (ng/dL)[b]
A.	<0.6	25
B.	<0.6	44
C.	<0.6	<4
D.	5.5	25
E.	5.5	<4

[a]The lower limit of the reference range for the plasma renin activity is 0.6 ng/mL per h.
[b]The lower limit of the reference range for the serum aldosterone assay is 4 ng/dL.

80 A 27-year-old man presents to discuss the potential effects of exercise on testosterone levels. His medical history is unremarkable except for a diagnosis of generalized anxiety disorder. The patient has never been overweight and reports having a "fast metabolism." As part of a New Year's resolution, he intends to begin a regular exercise regimen to improve his fitness and overall health. He does not currently exercise regularly but used to play recreational tennis and lift weights in high school and college. Recently, he has been spending several hours each week on Internet forums related to sports and exercise. He has encountered conflicting information regarding whether certain exercise regimens or sports can alter testosterone levels. He is anxious about choosing an exercise program that will not lower his testosterone level. At his routine annual physical, he requested measurement of his baseline testosterone level. He currently takes no medications.

On physical examination, his height is 69 in (175 cm) and weight is 152 lb (69 kg) (BMI = 22 kg/m^2). His blood pressure is 125/72 mm Hg, and pulse rate is 75 beats/min. Examination findings are unremarkable. Testicular volume is 15 mL bilaterally.

Laboratory test results:

Total testosterone = 481 ng/dL (300-900 ng/dL) (SI: 16.7 nmol/L [10.4-31.2 nmol/L])

Complete blood cell count, normal

Chemistry panel, normal

Extended participation in which of the following activities should be avoided given the patient's concerns?
A. Cycling
B. Playing soccer
C. Powerlifting
D. Swimming
E. Wrestling

81 You are asked for advice regarding a 38-year-old woman who is 7 weeks pregnant. She has previously had 3 early first-trimester miscarriages. She underwent in vitro fertilization treatment to achieve this pregnancy. She reports increasing tiredness over the past 2 months, as well as mild nausea. She has no notable medical history. She is currently taking a pregnancy-specific multivitamin preparation containing folic acid and iodine. She reports a family history of autoimmune hypothyroidism in her mother and aunt.

On physical examination, her height is 66 in (167.6 cm) and weight is 154 lb (70 kg) (BMI = 24.9 kg/m^2). Her blood pressure is 128/64 mm Hg, and pulse rate is 68 beats/min. Her thyroid gland is not palpable. Physical examination findings are otherwise unremarkable. A pregnancy test done in the clinic is positive.

Laboratory test results:

TSH = 3.8 mIU/L (0.5-5.0 mIU/L)

Free T$_4$ = 1.0 ng/dL (0.8-1.8 ng/dL) (SI: 12.9 pmol/L [10.30-23.17 pmol/L])

Which of the following is most appropriate next step in this patient's management?
A. Measurement of TSH in 4 weeks
B. Measurement of TPO antibody titer
C. Measurement of thyrotropin receptor–blocking antibodies
D. Measurement of free T$_3$
E. Thyroid ultrasonography

82 A 24-year-old man with type 1 diabetes mellitus is concerned about the frequency of hypoglycemia he is experiencing. The patient is an avid cyclist and often bikes on mountain trails for 2 to 3 hours at a time. He starts to ride anytime between 8 and 9 AM and does so 4 to 5 days a week. He does not check his blood glucose nor adjust insulin consistently before activity. His hemoglobin A$_{1c}$ level is 6.4% (46 mmol/mol), and he has no diabetes-related complications. He has awareness of hypoglycemia when his blood glucose level reaches 65 mg/dL (3.6 mmol/L).

His insulin regimen consists of insulin glargine, 8 units daily; insulin aspart, 1 unit for every 16 g of carbohydrate; and correction with insulin aspart of 1 unit for every 50 mg/dL that glucose rises above 150 mg/dL (>8.3 mmol/L).

On physical examination, he is afebrile. His blood pressure is 92/68 mm Hg, and pulse rate is 58 beats/min. His height is 71 in (180.3 cm), and weight is 147 lb (66.8 kg) (BMI = 20.5 kg/m^2). The rest of the examination findings are normal.

Blood glucose levels for the last 6 days are shown (*see table*). He cycled on days 1, 2, 4, and 5 (marked in the table with *).

Day	8-9 AM	10-11 AM	11 AM-12 PM	12-1 PM	1-2 PM	2-3 PM	3-4 PM	4-5 PM	5-6 PM	6-7 PM	7-8 PM	8-9 PM	9-10 PM
1*	231 (12.8)	...	68 (3.8)	...	...	173 (9.6)	...	...	...	40 (2.2)	...	...	294 (16.3)
2*	57 (3.2)	...	...	...	23 (1.3)	...	103 (5.7)	66 (3.7)	...	...	127 (7.0)	...	123 (6.8)
3	224 (12.4)	...	...	87 (4.8)	...	124 (6.9)	184 (10.2)	...	251 (13.9)	...	206 (11.4)	...	156 (8.7)
4*	214 (11.9)	33 (1.8)	...	82 (4.6)	...	38 (2.1)	62 (3.4)	...	...	...	...	...	157 (8.7)
5*	100 (5.6)	116 (6.4)	...	82 (4.6)	...	62 (3.4)	...	146 (8.1)	192 (10.7)	...		133 (7.4)	152 (8.4)
6	233 (12.9)	...	43 (2.4)	...	...	...	203 (11.3)	...	...	113 (6.3)	...	...	116 (6.4)

Values are shown in mg/dL with SI units (mmol/L) in parentheses.

After reviewing the blood glucose values, which of the following is the first change you would you recommend?

A. Start continuous glucose monitoring
B. Change the meal ratio for all meals to 1 unit per 20 g carbohydrate on the days he exercises
C. Lower insulin glargine to 6 units on the days that he plans to exercise
D. Change meal ratio for breakfast and lunch to 1 unit per 20 g carbohydrate
E. Start insulin pump therapy

83 A 36-year-old man is referred for evaluation of an abnormal left humerus x-ray. He describes a 2- to 3-year history of constant aching in his left mid-upper arm that has gradually worsened over time. He recalls no antecedent trauma. He has no history of fractures. He describes frequent headaches involving both parietal regions, which are poorly responsive to ibuprofen. He takes no medications or supplements. The rest of his medical history and accompanying family history are unremarkable. Review of systems is notable for an unintentional 10-lb (4.5-kg) weight loss.

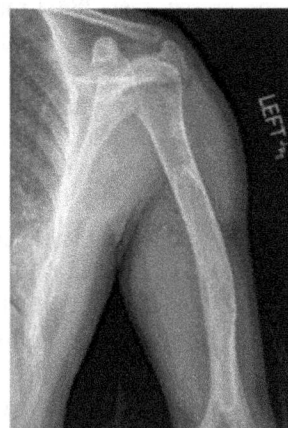

On physical examination, he has mild, diffuse tenderness over the left mid-humerus without an apparent mass or deformity. There is a hyperpigmented, irregular macular lesion over his upper back and neck that extends from the midline laterally. The thyroid is palpably enlarged and nodular without a dominant lesion. Deep tendon reflexes are brisk with a shortened recovery phase. The rest of his examination findings, including exam of the cranium, are normal.

Anteroposterior radiograph of the left humerus is shown (*see image*).

Laboratory test results:
    Complete blood cell count, normal
    Creatinine, normal
    AST, normal
    ALT, normal
    Total bilirubin, normal
    Calcium, normal
    Phosphate, normal
    Intact PTH, normal
    TSH = 0.03 mIU/L (0.5-5.0 mIU/L)
    Free T$_4$ = 2.5 ng/dL (0.8-1.8 ng/dL) (SI: 32.2 ng/dL [10.30-23.17 pmol/L])
    25-Hydroxyvitamin D, normal
    Alkaline phosphatase = 310 U/L (50-120 U/L) (SI: 5.18 μkat/L [0.84-2.00 μkat/L])

Which of the following is this patient's most likely diagnosis?
    A. Celiac disease
    B. Fibrous dysplasia
    C. Graves disease
    D. Paget disease of bone
    E. Tumor-induced osteomalacia

84 An obstetrician refers a 36-year-old woman for management of lipids. She is currently 27 weeks' gestation with her first child. The pregnancy has been uneventful and she has no chest pain or angina but reports occasional palpitations, shortness of breath, and fatigue. After she noticed the recent development of lumps in the dorsal aspect of her hands, her obstetrician ordered a lipid panel. She has a known history of hypercholesterolemia treated sporadically with atorvastatin, but she had been off therapy for 2 years before her current pregnancy. On review of her family history, her father died of a myocardial infarction at age 42 years, her 28-year-old brother has untreated hypercholesterolemia, and a paternal uncle had a myocardial infarction at age 45 years.

On physical examination, her blood pressure is 100/60 mm Hg and pulse rate is 95 beats/min. Tendon xanthomas are noted on the dorsal aspect of both hands.

Laboratory test results (sample drawn while fasting):
    Total cholesterol = 359 mg/dL (<200 mg/dL [optimal]) (SI: 9.30 mmol/L [<5.18 mmol/L])
    Triglycerides = 116 mg/dL (<150 mg/dL [optimal]) (SI: 1.31 mmol/L [<1.70 mmol/L])
    HDL cholesterol = 42 mg/dL (>60 mg/dL [optimal]) (SI: 1.09 mmol/L [>1.55 mmol/L])
    LDL cholesterol = 294 mg/dL (<100 mg/dL [optimal]) (SI: 7.61 mmol/L [<2.59 mmol/L])
    Non-HDL cholesterol = 317 mg/dL (<130 mg/dL [optimal]) (SI: 3.37 mmol/L [<3.37 mmol/L])

Which of the following is the best next step in this patient's management?
    A. Start a statin
    B. Start ezetimibe
    C. Start niacin
    D. Start LDL apheresis
    E. Defer treatment until after the baby is delivered

85 A 72-year-old man is noted to have a repeatedly low serum TSH level of less than 0.01 mIU/L. Thyroid hormone levels are normal. The patient's only other medical problem is hypertension that is well controlled on a single agent.

When seen by his primary care physician, the patient states that he feels well and has no complaints. His vital signs are normal. His physical examination findings are notable for a left-sided nodule that is about 3 cm in dimension and feels firm to palpation. The rest of the physical examination fails to show any features suggestive of hyperthyroidism.

A radioactive iodine scan is performed and there is homogeneously increased iodine uptake throughout the thyroid gland, but with a cold defect corresponding to the patient's palpable left thyroid nodule. FNA biopsy of the nodule is performed under ultrasound guidance and the cytology is read as atypia of undetermined significance. No right lobe nodules are identified. After surgical consultation, the patient elects to undergo a left lobectomy, and the left-sided nodule is found to be a benign hyperplastic nodule. A 7-mm papillary thyroid cancer is also identified. Cancer cells are identified abutting, but not penetrating, the inked posterior surgical margins.

Which of the following is the best next step in this patient's management?
- A. Completion thyroidectomy
- B. Levothyroxine therapy to achieve a TSH level between 0.1 and 0.3 mIU/L
- C. Radioactive iodine therapy
- D. Initiation of methimazole
- E. Monitoring the patient's TSH without further therapy now

86 A 56-year-old woman is referred to you by a general surgeon for endocrine workup before elective adrenalectomy. Abdominal CT performed to evaluate left iliac fossa discomfort demonstrated an incidental 5.8-cm right-sided adrenal mass (*see image, white arrow*). The precontrast density is −44 Hounsfield units.

The patient's only current medication is oral hormone therapy (estradiol and norethindrone preparation). She underwent a right upper lobectomy for a T2 N0 M0 non–small cell lung cancer 6 years ago, and she sees her oncologist annually. She reports no recent changes in weight.

On physical examination, she does not appear cushingoid. Her height is 67 in (170.2 cm), and weight is 172 lb (78.2 kg) (BMI = 26.9 kg/m^2). Her blood pressure is 138/74 mm Hg. Findings on abdominal examination are normal.

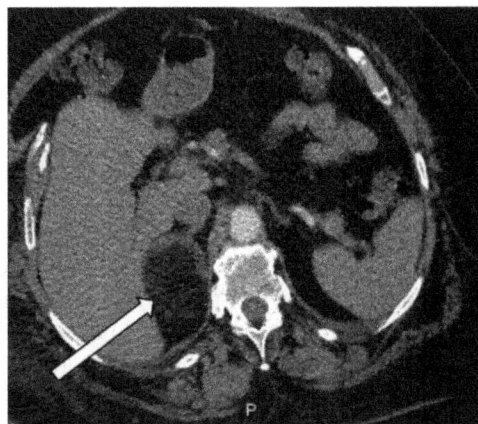

Laboratory test results:
Urinary cortisol = 28 µg/24 h (4-50 µg/24 h) (SI: 77.3 nmol/d [11-138 nmol/d])
Urinary metanephrine = 356 µg/24 h (<400 µg/24 h) (SI: 1804 nmol/d [<2028 nmol/d])
Urinary normetanephrine= 763 µg/24 h (<900 µg/24 h) (SI: 4166 nmol/d [<4914 nmol/d])
Plasma cortisol (8 AM; after 1 mg dexamethasone the night before) = 5.5 µg/dL (<2.0 µg/dL) (SI: 151.7 nmol/L [<50 nmol/L])
Plasma aldosterone = 4 ng/dL (1-21 ng/dL) (SI: 111.0 pmol/L [27.7-582.5 pmol/L])
Plasma renin activity = 4.0 ng/mL per h (0.6-4.3 ng/mL per h)

Which of the following would you advise?
- A. Cancel surgery, no further routine imaging required
- B. Cancel surgery, arrange regular follow-up CT every 6 months
- C. Perform adrenal biopsy
- D. Perform PET-CT
- E. Prescribe perioperative hydrocortisone

87 A 45-year-old man with type 1 diabetes mellitus requests to see a physician for sudden fatigue while mowing his lawn today. He reports that he initially felt well, but after 30 minutes of pushing the lawnmower, he was extremely fatigued and had to shut down the mower and sit in the shade. He stated that the grass was quite high and required more effort than usual to mow. After resting, he felt somewhat better, but he did not feel well enough to resume mowing. His wife noticed him sitting in the shade and she drove him to your office. The patient reports that he typically has no problems with exercise and states that most days he walks 30 minutes. He uses an insulin pump and continuous glucose sensor and reports his blood glucose values typically range from 80 to 220 mg/dL (4.4-12.2 mmol/L). When he measured his glucose while sitting in the shade, it was 220 mg/dL (12.2 mmol/L). He does not recall his most recent hemoglobin A_{1c} measurement. He has no diabetes-related complications. His only other medication in addition to insulin is lisinopril, 10 mg daily.

On physical examination, his blood pressure is 110/80 mm Hg and pulse rate is 60 beats/min and regular. His height is 70.5 in (179 cm), and weight is 165 lb (75 kg) (BMI = 23.3 kg/m^2). The patient has sweaty clothes, but examination findings are normal.

The weather report shows the outdoor temperature to be 90°F (32.2°C).

In addition to measuring his glucose and obtaining routine laboratory tests, which of the following is the best next step?
  A. Check core body temperature
  B. Measure TSH and free T_4
  C. Perform electrocardiography
  D. Check urine for ketones
  E. Perform an ACTH-stimulation test

88 A 38-year-old woman presents with a 6-month history of palpitation, tremor, anxiety, weight loss of 15 lb (6.8 kg), tiredness, heat intolerance, and increased frequency of bowel movements. She also reports increasing neck swelling but has no symptoms of choking or dysphagia. She has no eye symptoms. There is no notable medical history, and she is not taking any regular medication. Her sister underwent treatment of Graves disease with a prolonged course of antithyroid drugs 5 years earlier.

On physical examination, her height is 66 in (167.6 cm) and weight is 172 lb (78.2 kg) (BMI = 27.8 kg/m^2). Her blood pressure is 126/68 mm Hg, and pulse rate is 104 beats/min in a regular rhythm. She has a fine tremor of the outstretched hands but no signs of thyroid eye disease. A large, firm, diffuse goiter is palpable in her neck and there is no retrosternal extension or tracheal deviation. Physical examination findings are otherwise unremarkable.

Laboratory test results:
  TSH = 2.2 mIU/L (0.5-5.0 mIU/L)
  Free T_4 = 4.8 ng/dL (0.8-1.8 ng/dL) (SI: 61.8 pmol/L [10.30-23.17 pmol/L])
  Free T_3 = 12.3 pg/mL (0.8-1.8 ng/dL) (SI: 18.9 pmol/L [3.53-6.45 pmol/L])
  TPO antibodies = 10 IU/mL (<2.0 IU/mL) (SI: 10 kIU/L [<2.0 kIU/L])
  LH = 4.0 mIU/mL (1.0-18.0 mIU/mL) (SI: 4.0 IU/L [1.0-18.0 IU/L])
  FSH = 2.8 mIU/mL (2.0-12.0 mIU/mL) (SI: 2.8 IU/L [2.0-12.0 IU/L])
  IGF-1 = 134.4 ng/mL (106-277 ng/mL (SI: 17.6 nmol/L [13.9-36.3 nmol/L])
  SHBG = 24.9 µg/mL (2.2-14.6 µg/mL) (SI: 221.5 nmol/L [20-130 nmol/L])
  α-Subunit of pituitary glycoprotein hormones = 1.74 ng/mL (<1.2 ng/mL) (SI: 1.74 µg/L [<1.2 µg/L])

Which of the following is the most likely diagnosis?
  A. Graves disease
  B. Resistance to thyroid hormone
  C. Hashimoto thyroiditis
  D. Pituitary TSH-producing adenoma
  E. Artifact in laboratory TSH assay

89 A 33-year-old man is self-referred for consultation regarding fertility evaluation. The patient has been married for 2 years and his 37-year-old wife has been unable to conceive for the past 14 months despite regular unprotected intercourse 1 to 3 times a week. His wife reports regular menses and has a 6-year-old daughter from a previous relationship. Before marriage, the patient did not father or attempt to father a child. His medical history is notable for hyperlipidemia. His only current medication is atorvastatin.

On physical examination, his height is 70 in (178 cm) and weight is 156 lb (71 kg) (BMI = 22 kg/m²). His blood pressure is 120/76 mm Hg, and pulse rate is 78 beats/min. Examination findings are unremarkable. Testicular volume is 20 mL bilaterally.

Laboratory test result:

Total testosterone = 673 ng/dL (300-900 ng/dL) (SI: 23.4 nmol/L [10.4-31.2 nmol/L])

You recommend obtaining a semen analysis.

To obtain an optimal sample, what should you advise the patient regarding the timing and location for collection?

A. At an andrology laboratory 2 to 3 days after abstinence with or without an isotonic lubricant

B. At an andrology laboratory 7 to 8 days after abstinence with or without an isotonic lubricant

C. At home 2 to 3 days after abstinence without an isotonic lubricant

D. At home 7 to 8 days after abstinence without an isotonic lubricant

E. The timing and location are not important, as long as the sample is brought to the andrology lab within 6 hours

90 A 55-year-old woman is referred for evaluation of osteoporosis, which was diagnosed based on a screening bone density test done 2 years ago (lowest T-score of –2.5 in the lumbar spine; Z-score, –1.5). She was started on weekly alendronate, which she has been taking correctly and is tolerating well. She recently sustained a right foot fracture after falling, and a repeated DXA scan revealed a 6% decline in her lumbar spine bone mineral density. She takes a multivitamin daily. She had surgical menopause at age 40 years and has since been on estradiol therapy for hot flashes. She underwent lithotripsy for a kidney stone 1 year ago. She has no family history of osteoporosis.

Her physical examination findings are unremarkable.

Laboratory test results:

Serum calcium = 9.6 mg/dL (8.2-10.2 mg/dL) (SI: 2.4 mmol/L [2.1-2.6 mmol/L])

Serum phosphate = 4.4 mg/dL (2.3-4.7 mg/dL) (SI: 1.4 mmol/L [0.7-1.5 mmol/L])

Serum creatinine = 0.7 mg/dL (0.6-1.1 mg/dL) (SI: 61.9 µmol/L [53.0-97.2 µmol/L])

Serum 25-hydroxyvitamin D = 35 ng/mL (30-80 ng/mL [optimal]) (SI: 87.4 nmol/L [74.9-199.7 nmol/L])

Serum albumin = 4.0 g/dL (3.5-5.0 g/dL) (SI: 40 g/L [35-50 g/L])

Urinary calcium = 350 mg/24 h (100-300 mg/24 h) (SI: 8.8 mmol/d [2.5-7.5 mmol/d])

Urinary sodium = 96 mEq/24 h (40-217 mEq/24 h) (SI: 96 mmol/d [40-217 mmol/d])

Urinary creatinine = 1.0 g/24 h (1.0-2.0 g/24 h) (SI: 8.8 mmol/d [8.8-17.7 mmol/d])

Complete blood cell count, normal

TSH, normal

Liver panel, normal

In addition to dietary counseling, which of the following recommendations should you make regarding this patient's management?

A. Discontinue alendronate and start zoledronic acid

B. Discontinue alendronate and start denosumab

C. Discontinue alendronate and start an anabolic agent

D. Start hydrochlorothiazide

E. No change is needed at this time; repeat DXA in 1 to 2 years

91 A 64-year-old woman with type 2 diabetes mellitus seeks help to improve her glucose control. Her medical history is notable for hypertension, hyperlipidemia, and obesity. All of her siblings have diabetes. Diabetes was diagnosed 4 years ago, and the patient was initially treated with oral agents, but insulin was started within 6 months of diagnosis because of hyperglycemia. Two years ago, her regimen was transitioned from premixed insulin to multiple daily injections. She has no acute concerns other than polyuria. Specifically, she has no easy bruising, unusual stretch marks, bone fractures, or hirsutism. She has had no episodes of hypoglycemia.

Her current treatment regimen consists of U100 insulin glargine, 74 units 2 times daily; insulin aspart, 54 units before meals; liraglutide, 1.8 mg once daily; and metformin, 1000 mg twice daily. Her hemoglobin A_{1c} level is 10.5% (91 mmol/mol), and it has decreased from 12.1% (109 mmol/mol) documented 5 months ago. She checks her blood glucose via fingerstick only once daily in the morning, and her meter shows a range from 106 to 182 mg/dL (5.9-10.1 mmol/L), with an average fasting glucose level of 132 mg/dL (7.3 mmol/L). Other relevant medications include hydrochlorothiazide, pravastatin, and lisinopril.

On physical examination, her height is 62 in (157.5 cm) and weight is 230 lb (104.5 kg) (BMI = 42.1 kg/m^2). Her blood pressure is 137/74 mm Hg, and pulse rate is 92 beats/min.

Laboratory test results:
Total cholesterol = 179 mg/dL (<200 mg/dL [optimal]) (SI: 4.63 mmol/L [<5.18 mmol/L])
Triglycerides = 403 mg/dL (<150 mg/dL [optimal]) (SI: 4.55 mmol/L [<1.70 mmol/L])
HDL cholesterol = 28 mg/dL (>60 mg/dL [optimal]) (SI: 0.73 mmol/L [>1.55 mmol/L])

Which of the following is the best next step in this patient's management?
A. Start insulin pump therapy
B. Increase U100 glargine to 100 units twice daily
C. Switch insulin regimen to U500 insulin only, 120 units twice daily
D. Switch insulin regimen to U500 insulin only, 160 units twice daily
E. Switch basal insulin only, from insulin glargine to U200 degludec

92 A 54-year-old woman with a history of HIV infection and asthma presents with polyuria, polydipsia, and a blood glucose value of 317 mg/dL (17.6 mmol/L). She has no history of hyperglycemia or diabetes mellitus. HIV was diagnosed 20 years ago and is well controlled, with a recent CD_4 cell count greater than 500 and an undetectable viral load. Her medications include a ritonavir-based (protease inhibitor) antiretroviral regimen, inhaled fluticasone (250 mcg twice daily), salmeterol (50 mcg twice daily), atorvastatin, and lisinopril.

On physical examination, she has several features of Cushing syndrome, including moon facies, dorsocervical fat pad, central adiposity, lipoatrophy of the arms and legs, and violaceous striae.

Her primary care physician had measured morning cortisol, which returned surprisingly low at 1.7 μg/dL (46.9 nmol/L) and prompted further testing (ACTH-stimulation test):

Measurement	8 AM	→→→→→	9 AM
Cortisol	1.3 μg/dL (SI: 35.7 nmol/L)	Administration of intravenous cosyntropin, 250 mcg	8.4 μg/dL (SI: 231.7 nmol/L)
ACTH	<5 pg/mL (SI: 1.1 pmol/L)		...
Aldosterone	4.3 ng/dL (SI: 119.3 pmol/L)		8.9 ng/dL (SI: 246.9 pmol/L)
Plasma renin activity	1.1 ng/mL per h		...

Which of the following is the most likely diagnosis?
A. Primary adrenal insufficiency
B. Cushing syndrome with fluticasone-induced secondary adrenal insufficiency
C. Hyperglycemia-induced secondary adrenal insufficiency
D. Cushing syndrome due to ectopic ACTH secretion
E. Cushing syndrome due to an ACTH-secreting pituitary adenoma

93 A 51-year-old man with type 2 diabetes mellitus, hypertension, gastroesophageal reflux disease, depression, and a seizure disorder seeks help for weight loss. He has gradually gained weight over the last 10 years, with his highest weight of 270 lb (122.7 kg) recorded 2 months ago. Under the guidance of his primary care physician, he has been able to lose 4 lb (1.8 kg) in 2 months. His current meal plan includes 1 meal replacement each day (at lunch time). He started an exercise program, and he plans to walk a 5K in the coming months. He questions whether he can continue to adhere to this meal plan, as he is getting bored of eating the same lunch food every day. He reports being very hungry late in the day, and he regularly eats snacks just before bedtime. He is familiar with counting carbohydrates and calories. He consumes only sugar-free drinks. His medications include metformin, canagliflozin, pantoprazole, amlodipine, lisinopril, sertraline, and topiramate. His diabetes control has been suboptimal, and his last 2 hemoglobin A_{1c} measurements were greater than 8.0% (>64 mmol/mol).

On physical examination, his blood pressure is 157/82 mm Hg and pulse rate is 72 beats/min. His height is 67 in (170.2 cm), and weight is 266.2 lb (121 kg) (BMI = 41.7 kg/m²). He has acanthosis nigricans on his neck, his lungs are clear to auscultation, his heart sounds are regular, his abdomen is soft, and he has trace lower-extremity edema bilaterally.

You discuss weight-loss treatment options. You suggest that he visit your colleagues in the bariatric surgery clinic, but he declines the referral. You recommend a new meal plan (without the meal replacement) and encourage him to continue his exercise program. You also discuss the possibility of starting a weight-loss medication.

Which of the following medications is the best recommendation for this patient?
   A. Lorcaserin
   B. Orlistat
   C. Liraglutide
   D. Naltrexone/bupropion
   E. Phentermine

94 A 55-year-old woman is referred for evaluation of foot pain and fatigue. She reports gradual onset of fatigue over 5 years, accompanied by more frequent bilateral midfoot pain that is worse with ambulation. She has been menopausal since age 45 years and has not taken hormone therapy. She did have a bone density assessment 1 year ago, which revealed osteopenia with lumbar spine and femoral neck T-scores of –1.8 and –2.3. She was prescribed alendronate, but she stopped after 1 month due to severe worsening of her foot pain. She has no known history of fractures. She takes supplemental calcium, 600 mg twice daily, and cholecalciferol, 800 IU daily, but no other medications. Her family history is notable for osteoporosis in her mother with vertebral fractures in her 70s. Review of systems is otherwise unremarkable. She has had no significant height loss since young adulthood.

On physical examination, she has mild tibial and midfoot tenderness to palpation and squeezing. She has to use her arms to rise from a sitting position. Otherwise, her examination findings are unrevealing.

Laboratory test results:
   Serum calcium = 9.2 mg/dL (8.2-10.2 mg/dL) (SI: 2.3 mmol/L [2.1-2.6 mmol/L])
   Serum phosphate = 1.5 mg/dL (2.3-4.7 mg/dL) (SI: 0.5 mmol/L [0.7-1.5 mmol/L])
   Serum creatinine = 0.9 mg/dL (0.6-1.1 mg/dL) (SI: 79.6 µmol/L [53.0-97.2 µmol/L])
   Serum albumin = 3.7 mg/dL (3.5-5.0 g/dL) (SI: 37 g/L [35-50 g/L])
   Serum intact PTH = 60 pg/mL (10-65 pg/mL) (SI: 60 ng/L [10-65 ng/L])
   Serum 25-hydroxyvitamin D = 32 ng/mL (30-80 ng/mL) (SI: 79.9 nmol/L [74.9-199.7 nmol/L])
   Serum 1,25-dihydroxyvitamin D = 14 pg/mL (16-65 pg/mL) (SI: 36.4 pmol/L [41.6-169.0 pmol/L])
   Alkaline phosphatase = 165 U/L (50-120 U/L) (SI: 2.76 µkat/L [0.84-2.00 µkat/L])
   ALT = 28 U/L (10-40 U/L) (SI: 0.47 µkat/L [0.17-0.67 µkat/L])
   AST = 37 U/L (20-48 U/L) (SI: 0.62 µkat/L [0.33-0.80 µkat/L])

Which of the following is this patient's most likely diagnosis?
   A. Primary hyperparathyroidism
   B. Pseudogout
   C. Hypophosphatasia
   D. Postmenopausal osteoporosis
   E. Tumor-induced osteomalacia

95 A 45-year-old man with a history of end-stage renal disease due to polycystic kidney disease had a cadaveric kidney transplant 1 week ago. He was transfused with 2 units of packed red blood cells perioperatively. Induction immunosuppressive therapy was started, which included immunosuppressive antibody therapy (rabbit antithymocyte globulin); prednisone, 20 mg daily; mycophenolate mofetil, 1 g twice daily; and tacrolimus, 8 mg twice daily. During hospitalization, his fasting blood glucose measurements were in the range of 130 to 160 mg/dL (7.2-8.9 mmol/L), and postprandial measurements were in the range of 160 to 250 mg/dL (8.9-13.9 mmol/L).

In addition to his kidney problems, his medical history includes hypertension for which he takes lisinopril, 20 mg daily. He has no known history of type 2 diabetes.

On physical examination, his height is 71 in (180.3 cm) and weight is 182 lb (82.7 kg) (BMI = 25.4 kg/m^2). His blood pressure is 132/76 mm Hg, and pulse rate is 88 beats/min. Examination findings are unremarkable except for a surgical scar on left side of his abdomen. The scar appears to be healing well.

Which of the following is the best next step at this office visit to confirm whether this patient has posttransplant diabetes mellitus?
   A. Use blood glucose values measured during the hospital stay
   B. Measure fasting blood glucose
   C. Perform an oral glucose tolerance test
   D. Measure hemoglobin A$_{1c}$
   E. Defer testing

96 You are asked to evaluate a 32-year-old woman who presents with an unplanned pregnancy of approximately 18 weeks' gestation. She has a history of acromegaly treated by debulking pituitary surgery 3 years ago. A small tumor remnant remains in the cavernous sinus. As a result, IGF-1 and GH levels failed to normalize after surgery and she required management with intramuscular lanreotide with the subsequent addition of pegvisomant. She feels well and has no concerns.

On physical examination, she has mild acromegalic facies. Her blood pressure is 112/78 mm Hg, and pulse rate is 100 beats/min. Visual fields are normal.

Laboratory test results 2 months before pregnancy:
   GH = 1.8 ng/mL (0.01-3.61 ng/mL) (SI: 1.8 µg/L [0.01-3.61 µg/L])
   IGF-1 = 195 ng/mL (113-297 ng/mL) (SI: 25.5 nmol/L [14.8-38.9 nmol/L])
   Prolactin = 19 ng/mL (4-30 ng/mL) (SI: 0.83 nmol/L [0.17-1.30 nmol/L])

Current laboratory test results:
   GH = 4.0 ng/mL (SI: 4.0 µg/L)
   IGF-1 = 320 ng/mL (SI: 41.9 nmol/L)
   Prolactin = 220 ng/mL (SI: 9.6 nmol/L)

Pituitary-directed MRI performed 3 months previously is shown (*see image*). Residual tumor is visible in the left side of the pituitary (*white arrow*), extending into cavernous sinus (stable compared with MRI 1 year ago).

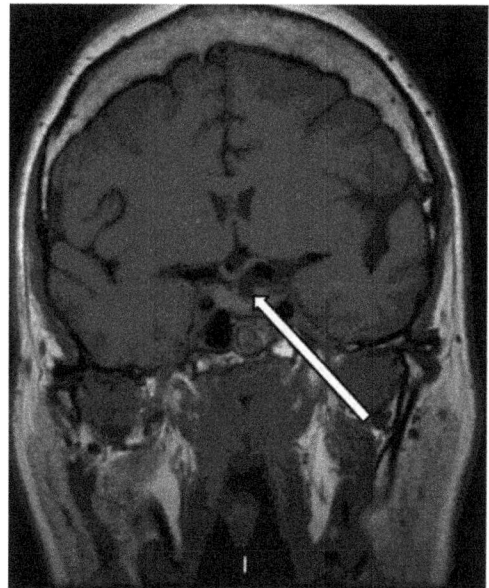

Which of the following should you recommend as the best next management step for this patient?
   A. Continue current therapy
   B. Stop pegvisomant and continue lanreotide
   C. Stop pegvisomant and lanreotide; start cabergoline
   D. Stop current therapy; restart if IGF-1 continues to rise
   E. Stop current therapy; do not routinely monitor IGF-1 during pregnancy

97 A 22-year-old woman was diagnosed with Graves disease approximately 1 year ago. Her treatment with methimazole has been notable for periods of both overtreatment and undertreatment. The patient now elects to undergo treatment with radioactive iodine. Her methimazole is discontinued 5 days before her planned treatment. Three days before radioactive iodine therapy, the following laboratory results are obtained:

TSH = 0.12 mIU/L (0.5-5.0 mIU/L)
Free T_4 = 1.9 ng/dL (0.8-1.8 ng/dL) (SI: 24.5 pmol/L [10.30-23.17 pmol/L])
Total T_3 = 220 ng/dL (70-200 ng/dL) (SI: 3.4 nmol/L [1.08-3.08 nmol/L])
β-hCG = <6.0 mIU/mL (<6.0 mIU/mL) (SI: <6.0 IU/L [<6.0 IU/L])

A thyroid uptake with ^{123}I shows 95% uptake at 24 hours, and the patient is treated with a 10 mCi dose of ^{131}I.

Two months later at a follow-up endocrinology visit, the patient states that she is pregnant and thinks that her last menstrual period was approximately 3 weeks before her radioiodine therapy. Her vital signs are normal. Her thyroid exam reveals a slightly firm thyroid gland. Her deep tendon reflexes are normal and she has no tremor of her outstretched hands.

Laboratory test results:
TSH = 15.0 mIU/L (0.5-5.0 mIU/L)
Free T_4 = 0.8 ng/dL (0.8-1.8 ng/dL) (SI: 10.30 pmol/L [10.30-23.17 pmol/L])
β-hCG = 75,000 mIU/mL (<6.0 mIU/mL) (SI: 75,000 IU/L [<6.0 IU/L])

An obstetrics evaluation confirms a viable pregnancy, and the estimated gestational age is 11 weeks.

Which of the following is the most likely fetal consequence of the patient's radioactive iodine therapy?
A. Fetal goiter
B. Whole-body radiation exposure to the fetus
C. Fetal hypothyroidism
D. Fetal hyperthyroidism
E. Fetal death

98 You are asked to consult on a 41-year-old woman 17 months after kidney-pancreas transplant. She has had type 1 diabetes mellitus since age 8 years. She has advanced microvascular complications from diabetes, including proliferative retinopathy for which she has had laser photocoagulative treatment in both eyes. She has peripheral neuropathy and neuropathic pain. She developed end-stage kidney disease, which led to the transplant. In the 3 years before transplant, she had multiple episodes of severe hypoglycemia requiring frequent paramedic calls and emergency department treatment due to hypoglycemia unawareness. Her husband has administered glucagon multiple times in the past.

Before surgery, she was treated with an insulin pump and used a continuous glucose sensor for 3 years. Her glycemic control was suboptimal, in part to avoid severe hypoglycemia. Since surgery, she has been treated with prednisone and the dosage was tapered to 5 mg daily 6 months after the transplant. She is also treated with tacrolimus and mycophenolate. There was a single episode of acute kidney rejection that occurred 6 weeks after surgery. Renal function has improved steadily since then. She has been off insulin since 7 days after undergoing the transplant. Her hemoglobin A_{1c} level was 6.0% (42 mmol/mol) 6 months after transplant and 6.3% (45 mmol/mol) 12 months after transplant.

Her current home medication list includes pregabalin, fosinopril, metoprolol, fluoxetine, and atorvastatin. She completed a 14-day course of levofloxacin for treatment of a sinus infection 3 weeks ago. She is asymptomatic now. She does not smoke cigarettes or drink alcohol.

On physical examination, her height is 67 in (170 cm) and weight is 153 lb (69.5 kg), (BMI = 24.0 kg/m²). Her blood pressure is 128/79 mm Hg, and pulse rate is 74 beats/min. On eye examination, laser scars are evident. On cardiac examination, there is a regular rate, S_1, S_2, and a grade I-II/VI systolic ejection murmur along the base and aortic interspaces. Findings on lung and abdominal examinations are unremarkable. The distal pulses are normal, but she has reduced sensation to 10-g monofilament testing and reduced vibrational sense in each foot. The ankle and patellar reflexes are blunted.

Laboratory test results:

Hemoglobin A_{1c} = 7.3% (4.0%-5.6%) (56 mmol/mol [20-38 mmol/mol])
Fasting glucose = 139 mg/dL (<70-99 mg/dL) (SI: 7.7 mmol/L [3.9-5.5 mmol/L])
C-peptide = 1.9 ng/mL (0.9-4.3 ng/mL) (SI: 0.6 nmol/L [0.30-1.42 nmol/L])
Electrolytes, normal
Creatinine = 1.5 mg/dL (0.6-1.1 mg/dL) (SI: 132.6 μmol/L [53.0-97.2 μmol/L])
Estimated glomerular filtration rate = 53 mL/min per 1.73 m^2 (>60 mL/min per 1.73 m^2)
Amylase = 56 U/L (26-102 U/L) (SI: 0.9 μkat/L [0.43-1.70 μkat/L])

Which of the following is the most likely explanation for her elevated fasting glucose and hemoglobin A_{1c}?
- A. Pancreas rejection
- B. Transient hyperglycemia after transplant
- C. Posttransplant diabetes mellitus
- D. Autoimmune β-cell destruction (recurrence of type 1 diabetes)
- E. Sinus infection

99 A 56-year-old man comes to see you for management of panhypopituitarism due to surgery and radiation therapy for a large pituitary macroadenoma 15 years ago. He does not have his old medical records. For several years, he has taken hydrocortisone, 15 mg in the morning and 5 mg in the afternoon; levothyroxine, 100 mcg daily; and testosterone gel, 1.62%, 2 pump presses daily. About 6 months ago, GH replacement therapy was added (0.2 mg daily). He describes several months of tiredness and sleepiness. His weight has been stable, and he has no joint pain.

On physical examination, his blood pressure is 125/85 mm Hg and pulse rate is 72 beats/min. His height is 70 in (178 cm), and weight is 198 lb (90 kg) (BMI = 28.4 kg/m^2). His abdomen is mildly prominent. He has small testes. There is no hand or pedal edema.

Laboratory test results:

Free T_4 = 0.9 ng/dL (0.8-1.8 ng/dL) (SI: 11.6 pmol/L [10.30-23.17 pmol/L])
Total testosterone = 425 ng/dL (300-900 ng/dL) (SI: 14.7 nmol/L [10.4-31.2 nmol/L])
IGF-1 = 198 ng/mL (78-220 ng/mL) (SI: 25.9 nmol/L [10.2-28.8 nmol/L])
Basic metabolic panel, normal

Which of the following is the best next step in this patient's management?
- A. Increase the testosterone dosage
- B. Decrease the hydrocortisone dosage
- C. Decrease the GH dosage
- D. Increase the levothyroxine dosage
- E. Recommend no change in therapy

100 A 50-year-old woman is referred for recommendations on treatment of osteoporosis that was recently identified by DXA scan. She has no history of low-trauma fractures as an adult. Her medical history is notable only for hypertension treated with lisinopril. She underwent natural menopause at age 46 years and did not take hormone therapy. She does not take calcium or vitamin D supplements, but she does consume 4 servings of dairy products per day. Her family history is notable for osteoporosis in her father who suffered a hip fracture in his 70s. Review of systems is notable for vague bilateral lower leg pain that is longstanding and worse with ambulation. She has no significant height loss.

On physical examination, she has no evident thoracic kyphosis. There is moderate anterior tibial tenderness to direct palpation. The rest of her examination findings are noncontributory.

Laboratory test results:
    Serum calcium = 8.3 mg/dL (8.2-10.2 mg/dL) (SI: 2.2 mmol/L [2.1-2.6 mmol/L])
    Serum phosphate = 2.3 mg/dL (2.3-4.7 mg/dL) (SI: 0.7 mmol/L [0.7-1.5 mmol/L])
    Serum creatinine = 0.9 mg/dL (0.6-1.1 mg/dL) (SI: 79.6 μmol/L [53.0-97.2 μmol/L])
    Serum albumin = 4.4 mg/dL (3.5-5.0 g/dL) (SI: 44 g/L [35-50 g/L])
    Serum intact PTH = 90 pg/mL (10-65 pg/mL) (SI: 90 ng/L [10-65 ng/L])
    Serum 25-hydroxyvitamin D = 9 ng/dL (30-80 ng/mL) (SI: 22.5 nmol/L [74.9-199.7 nmol/L])
    Serum 1,25-dihydroxyvitamin D = 68 pg/mL (16-65 pg/mL) (SI: 176.8 pmol/L [41.6-169.0 pmol/L])
    Alkaline phosphatase = 145 U/L (50-120 U/L) (SI: 2.42 μkat/L [0.84-2.00 μkat/L])
    AST = 25 U/L (20-48 U/L) (SI: 0.42 μkat/L [0.33-0.80 μkat/L])
    ALT = 30 U/L (10-40 U/L) (SI: 0.50 μkat/L [0.17-0.67 μkat/L])

DXA results are shown (*see images and tables*):

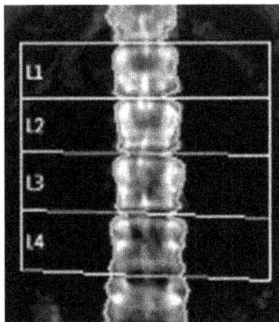

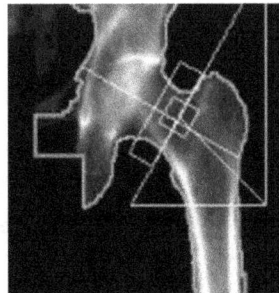

Region	BMD, g/cm^2	T-Score
L1	0.642	−4.3
L2	0.703	−4.5
L3	0.698	−4.5
L4	0.618	−5.2
Total	0.662	−4.6

Region	BMD, g/cm^2	T-Score
Neck	0.682	−3.0
Total	0.788	−2.2

Which of the following is the most appropriate treatment in the management of this woman's bone disorder?
    A. Ergocalciferol
    B. Alendronate
    C. Denosumab
    D. Calcium citrate
    E. Elemental phosphorus and calcitriol

101 A 25-year-old woman is referred by her gynecologist for evaluation of hyperprolactinemia. For the past 3 years, she has been using oral contraceptives to treat cystic acne. She developed arm and leg numbness on a different generic form of her oral contraceptive and decided to stop therapy 6 months ago, which resolved paresthesias. Her periods were regular for 3 months and then stopped 3 months before her current presentation.

Laboratory test results (ordered by her gynecologist):
 TSH = 0.5 mIU/L (0.5-5.0 mIU/L)
 FSH = 6.2 mIU/mL (2.0-12.0 mIU/mL [follicular]) (SI: 6.2 IU/L [2.0-12.0 IU/L])
 LH = 27.5 mIU/mL (1.0-18.0 mIU/mL [follicular]) (SI: 27.5 IU/L [1.0-18.0 IU/L])
 Prolactin = 42 ng/mL (4-30 ng/mL) (SI: 1.83 nmol/L [0.17-1.30 nmol/L])
 hCG, negative

Menarche occurred at age 12 years, and she experienced regular menses until she started oral contraceptives. She has had no galactorrhea.

On physical examination, her Ferriman-Gallwey score is 8 based on terminal hair growth on the upper lip, upper and lower abdomen, and inner thighs. Acne is visible along her jaw. She has no acanthosis.

Which of the following is the best next step to determine whether she has clinically significant hyperprolactinemia?
 A. Perform pelvic ultrasonography
 B. Perform pituitary MRI
 C. Prescribe progesterone treatment for 10 days
 D. Measure random progesterone concentration
 E. Measure estradiol concentration

102 A 58-year-old man with hypertension, type 2 diabetes mellitus, hypercholesterolemia, hypothyroidism, and severe osteoarthritis is referred to your weight-loss clinic by his orthopedic surgeon. The patient must lose 20 to 25 lb (9.1-11.4 kg) to be a surgical candidate for left knee replacement. The patient tells you he has never participated in a weight-loss program and he is motivated to follow your advice, as his knee pain is severe. He no longer can walk without a cane. Current medications include metformin, atorvastatin, amlodipine, hydrochlorothiazide, meloxicam, and levothyroxine.

On physical examination, his blood pressure is 155/91 mm Hg and pulse rate is 61 beats/min. His height is 67 in (170.2 cm), and weight is 275 lb (125 kg) (BMI = 43.1 kg/m^2). He is in distress due to knee pain, his lungs are clear to auscultation, and his heart sounds are regular. His left knee is swollen and has decreased range of motion.

You discuss medical weight-loss options. He does not think he can exercise because of his knee pain. He is willing to follow the meal plan you recommend. After a long discussion, you start him on a full replacement meal plan (using protein shakes) that will provide him with 800 calories daily.

Laboratory test result:
 TSH = 1.7 mIU/L (0.5-5.0 mIU/L)

Which of the following medications should this patient stop the first day he starts his new meal plan?
 A. Hydrochlorothiazide
 B. Atorvastatin
 C. Metformin
 D. Amlodipine
 E. Levothyroxine

103 A 56-year-old man is referred to you by his primary care physician for possible diabetes mellitus. His medical history is notable for HIV, treated with antiretroviral therapy. His viral load is zero, and he has no history of opportunistic infections. He also has hypertension and dyslipidemia. On review of systems, he notes the inability to lose weight, with a steady weight gain of 50 lb (22.7 kg) over the past 10 years. Current medications include a once-daily combination pill for antiretroviral therapy and atorvastatin, 10 mg daily. His antiretroviral therapy regimen was recently changed.

On physical examination, his blood pressure is 130/80 mm Hg and pulse rate is 80 beats/min. His height is 66.5 in (169 cm), and weight is 220 lb (100 kg) (BMI = 35 kg/m^2). He has moderate truncal obesity and no lipoatrophy.

Laboratory test result:
Glucose = 95 mg/dL (70-99 mg/dL) (SI: 5.3 mmol/L [3.9-5.5 mmol/L])

Which of the following is the best next step to monitor for possible diabetes?
A. Perform an oral glucose tolerance test
B. Measure hemoglobin A$_{1c}$
C. Measure random glucose every 3 months
D. Measure fasting glucose every 3 months
E. Prescribe a glucometer to test fasting glucose monthly

104 A 23-year-old woman is referred for additional evaluation of weight gain and difficulty sleeping. She has just graduated from college and is having trouble finding a job. She reports a 15.5-lb (7-kg) weight gain over the past 3 months even though she thinks her caloric intake has been low and physical activity has been high. Her current weight is 145 lb (66 kg). At night, she has had difficulty falling asleep and staying asleep. She takes norgestimate-ethinyl estradiol daily for contraception.

On physical examination, her blood pressure is 131/92 mm Hg. She has a small dorsocervical fat pad, but no obvious moon facies, supraclavicular fat pads, striae, lipoatrophy, or lipodystrophy.

Her primary care physician had performed an evaluation for Cushing syndrome (testing performed at 8 AM following 1-mg of dexamethasone taken at 11 PM the night before):

Cortisol = 15 µg/dL (SI: 413.8 nmol/L)
ACTH = 28 pg/mL (10-65 pg/mL) (SI: 6.2 pmol/L [2.2-14.3 pmol/L])

On the basis of these lab values, her primary care physician performed both pituitary and adrenal imaging. Pituitary MRI showed a possible 5-mm pituitary adenoma; however, the finding was small enough that confidence for an abnormality was low. Abdominal CT was also performed and demonstrated a 1.1-cm left adrenal adenoma.

Which of the following is the most appropriate next step?
A. Inferior petrosal sinus sampling
B. Transsphenoidal pituitary adenoma resection
C. Laparoscopic left-sided adrenalectomy
D. Late-night salivary cortisol testing
E. CT imaging of the chest

105 A 35-year-old woman with no relevant medical history is admitted to the hospital for evaluation and management of hypocalcemia. She reports a 2-week history of paresthesias in her extremities, as well as muscle cramping. She had a recent illness with nausea, vomiting, and diarrhea. Despite treatment with intravenous and oral calcium and vitamin D supplements, she remains hypocalcemic. She is currently receiving calcium, 750 mg by mouth 3 times daily, and calcitriol, 0.25 mcg 3 times daily. She has no family history of calcium disorders.

On physical examination, her blood pressure is 120/70 mm Hg and pulse rate is 80 beats/min. Her height is 64 in (162.6 cm), and weight is 106 lb (48.2 kg) (BMI = 18.2 kg/m^2). The Chvostek sign is elicited on examination.

Laboratory test results:
Serum calcium = 6.5 mg/dL (8.2-10.2 mg/dL) (SI: 1.6 mmol/L [2.1-2.6 mmol/L])
Serum phosphate = 3.5 mg/dL (2.3-4.7 mg/dL) (SI: 1.1 mmol/L [0.7-1.5 mmol/L])
Serum creatinine = 0.8 mg/dL (0.6-1.1 mg/dL) (SI: 70.7 µmol/L [53.0-97.2 µmol/L])
Serum intact PTH = 17 pg/mL (10-65 pg/mL) (SI: 17 ng/L [10-65 ng/L])
Serum 25-hydroxyvitamin D = 30 ng/mL (30-80 ng/mL [optimal]) (SI: 74.9 nmol/L [74.9-199.7 nmol/L])
Serum albumin = 4.0 g/dL (3.5-5.0 g/dL) (SI: 40 g/L [35-50 g/L])

Which of the following should be measured as the best next step in the evaluation of this patient's hypocalcemia?
A. 24-Hour urinary calcium
B. Serum magnesium
C. 1,25-Dihydroxyvitamin D
D. Tissue transglutaminase antibodies
E. PTH antibodies

106 A 72-year-old man presents with a 6-month history of an enlarging neck swelling. He describes a feeling of choking at night and increasing dysphagia when eating solid foods. He has mild shortness of breath on exertion and reports "3-pillow" orthopnea. He has no symptoms of thyroid dysfunction, and his weight has remained stable over the last 12 months. He underwent quadruple-vessel bypass surgery for ischemic heart disease 11 months ago. His current medications are aspirin, lisinopril, and atorvastatin. There is no notable family history.

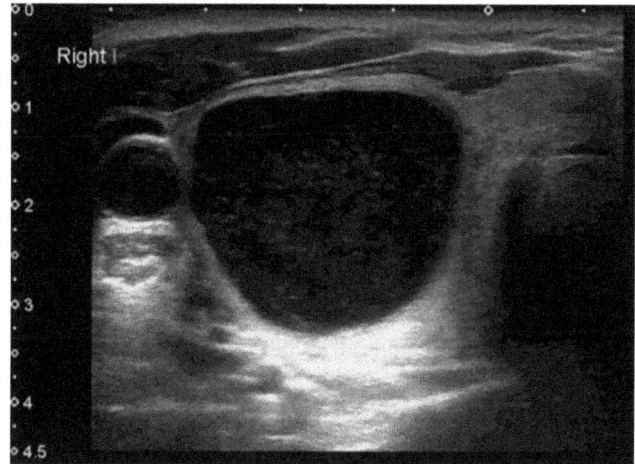

On physical examination, his height is 68 in (172.7 cm) and weight is 143 lb (65 kg) (BMI = 21.7 kg/m^2). His blood pressure is 143/82 mm Hg, and pulse rate is 76 beats/min in a regular rhythm. His trachea is deviated to the left, and his lung fields are clear. His heart sounds are normal, and findings on abdominal examination are unremarkable. A right-sided goiter is visible in his neck, and palpation reveals a smooth, 4 x 5-cm, right-sided thyroid swelling that moves with swallowing. There is no palpable cervical lymphadenopathy. The Pemberton sign is negative, and there is no clinical evidence of retrosternal extension.

Laboratory test results:
    TSH = 3.7 mIU/L (0.5-5.0 mIU/L)
    Free T$_4$ = 1.3 ng/dL (0.8-1.8 ng/dL) (SI: 16.7 pmol/L [10.30-23.17 pmol/L])

Thyroid ultrasonography is shown (*see image*).

Which of the following is the most likely diagnosis?
A. Anaplastic thyroid cancer
B. Differentiated thyroid malignancy with cystic degeneration
C. Benign thyroid cyst
D. Multinodular goiter
E. Thyroglossal duct cyst

107 A 35-year-old previously healthy man was recently diagnosed with type 2 diabetes mellitus. He now presents to the endocrine clinic for further management.

Laboratory test results at diagnosis:
    Blood glucose = 350 mg/dL (70-99 mg/dL) (SI: 19.4 mmol/L [3.9-5.5 mmol/L])
    Hemoglobin A$_{1c}$ = 10.2% (4.0%-5.6%) (88 mmol/mol [20-38 mmol/mol])
    LDL cholesterol = 162 mg/dL (<100 mg/dL [optimal]) (SI: 4.20 mmol/L [<2.59 mmol/L])
    Triglycerides = 240 mg/dL (<150 mg/dL [optimal]) (SI: 2.71 mmol/L [<1.70 mmol/L])

The following treatment regimen was prescribed: insulin glargine, 15 units once daily; metformin, 1000 mg twice daily; atorvastatin, 40 mg daily; and supplemental insulin at mealtimes as needed. At today's visit, he reports that his blood glucose is now under control (most values are in the range of 100-150 mg/dL [5.6-8.3 mmol/L]). He has started to eat better and exercise regularly, and he has lost an additional 5 lb (2.3 kg) since diabetes was diagnosed.

On physical examination, his height is 71 in (180 cm) and weight is 230 lb (104 kg) (BMI = 32.1 kg/m^2). His blood pressure is 146/77 mm Hg, and pulse rate is 88 beats/min. Skin examination reveals skin tags and acanthosis nigricans. The rest of the examination findings are normal.

He is very concerned about retinopathy and loss of vision due to diabetes.

Which of the following would you recommend to reduce this patient's risk of diabetic retinopathy?
 A. Stop insulin and add pioglitazone
 B. Stop insulin and add a GLP-1 receptor agonist
 C. Add lisinopril
 D. Add a fibrate
 E. Reassure the patient that he does not need any change in management now

108 A 62-year-old transgender woman is referred to the endocrine clinic by her primary care physician for management of gender dysphoria. The patient reports being in denial of her gender identity for much of her life. At age 53 years, she established care with both a psychologist and psychiatrist after suffering an emotional breakdown. At that time, she came out as transgender to these mental health professionals. She then came out to family and friends 2 years later. She has presented as female in public on several occasions but is fearful of offending others. At age 56, she began cross-sex hormone therapy with estrogen and antiandrogens. She has been on numerous estrogen formulations, including oral, sublingual, transdermal, and intramuscular. Despite attempts with different doses and formulations of estrogen, her testosterone and estradiol levels have never reached target. She was advised to discontinue hormone therapy for 3 weeks to reassess baseline testosterone.

On physical examination, her height is 69 in (175 cm) and weight is 185 lb (84 kg) (BMI = 27 kg/m^2). Her blood pressure is 145/88 mm Hg, and pulse rate is 85 beats/min. Her physical examination findings are notable for a testicular volume of 15 mL bilaterally and sparse body hair.

Laboratory test results:

	Treatment Regimen			
Measurement	None	Spironolactone: 100 mg twice daily	Estradiol: 2 mg daily Spironolactone: 200 mg twice daily	Estradiol: 4 mg daily Spironolactone: 100 mg twice daily
Serum estradiol	Not measured	Not measured	37 pg/mL (SI: 135.8 pmol/L)	35 pg/mL (SI: 128.5 pmol/L)
Serum testosterone	877 ng/dL (SI: 30.4 nmol/L)	677 ng/dL (SI: 23.5 nmol/L)	506 ng/dL (SI: 17.6 nmol/L)	580 ng/dL (SI: 20.1 nmol/L)

Reference ranges (female): estradiol: 10-180 pg/mL (SI: 36.7-660.8 pmol/L); testosterone: 8-60 ng/dL (SI: 0.3-2.1 nmol/L).

Which of the following is the best next step to lower her androgen levels?
 A. Increase the estradiol dosage
 B. Increase the estradiol and spironolactone dosages
 C. Switch the mode of estradiol delivery from oral to sublingual
 D. Recommend the addition of progesterone
 E. Recommend elective orchiectomy

109 A 21-year-old man is referred to you by his former pediatric endocrinologist. GH deficiency was diagnosed at age 4 years when he presented with growth failure. At that time, MRI showed anterior pituitary hypoplasia and ectopic posterior pituitary (*see image*) and he failed a GH stimulation test. Hypothyroidism was diagnosed at age 6 years. He continued GH replacement until age 16, when he decided to stop. He underwent spontaneous puberty. He currently takes levothyroxine, 100 mcg daily. He reports low energy but works 30 hours a week while attending school full time. His weight has been stable, and he has had no nausea or reduced appetite.

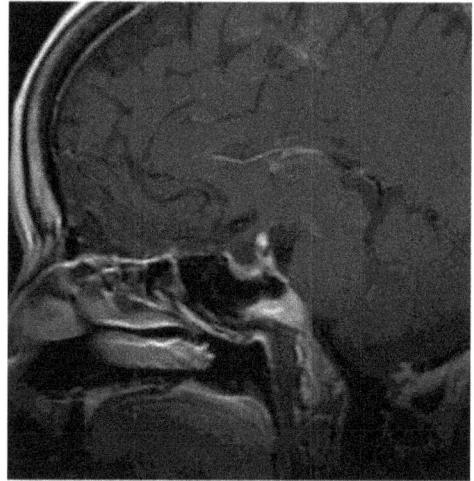

On physical examination, he looks healthy. His blood pressure is 118/75 mm Hg, and pulse rate is 74 beats/min. His height is 70 in (178 cm) (close to his midparental target height), and weight is 157.5 lb (72 kg) (BMI = 22.7 kg/m^2). He is fully androgenized. His testes are 12 mL bilaterally.

Laboratory test results:

Free T$_4$ = 1.3 ng/dL (0.8-1.8 ng/dL) (SI: 16.7 pmol/L [10.30-23.17 pmol/L])

TSH = 1.45 mIU/L (0.5-5.0 mIU/L)

Total testosterone = 423 ng/dL (300-900 ng/dL) (SI: 14.7 nmol/L [10.4-31.2 nmol/L])

IGF-1 = 83 ng/mL (116-341 ng/mL) (SI: 10.9 ng/mL [15.2-44.7 nmol/L])

Which of the following is the best next step in this patient's management?

A. Increase the levothyroxine dosage

B. Perform an ACTH-stimulation test

C. Reinitiate GH therapy

D. Initiate testosterone therapy

E. Measure prolactin

110 A 24-year-old woman is being seen in follow-up for treatment of diabetes mellitus. She is 24 weeks' gestation with her first pregnancy and she is feeling well. She met with a dietician twice in the last 10 weeks and continues to adhere to a diabetic meal plan. Fetal ultrasonography done at 7 weeks' gestation showed a viable fetus without abnormalities. The patient has gained 12 lb (5.5 kg) with the pregnancy. She exercises regularly.

A monogenic form of diabetes was diagnosed at age 15 years after she presented with elevated random urinary glucose levels. She has always been on dietary treatment. She does not have any diabetes-related microvascular complications, nor does she have a history of hypertension or dyslipidemia. Her only medication is a prenatal vitamin.

Her older brother was diagnosed with diabetes at age 17 years. He was found to have a pathogenic variant in the hepatocyte nuclear factor 1α gene (*HNF1A*) (MODY 3) and is treated with a sulfonylurea and basal insulin. The patient's mother, 2 maternal uncles, and maternal grandmother all have diabetes.

On physical examination, her height is 66.5 in (169 cm) and weight is 153 lb (69.5 kg) (BMI = 24.3 kg/m^2). Her blood pressure is 107/64 mm Hg, and pulse rate is 62 beats/min. Examination findings are normal.

Laboratory test results:

Hemoglobin A$_{1c}$ = 5.2% (4.0%-5.6%) (33 mmol/mol [20-38 mmol/mol])

TSH = 1.2 mIU/mL (0.5-5.0 mIU/L)

Recent fingerstick glucose values are as follows:

Date	Fasting	2-Hour Post Breakfast	2-Hour Post Lunch	2-Hour Post Evening Meal
Day 1	111 mg/dL (SI: 6.2 mmol/L)	...	115 mg/dL (SI: 6.4 mmol/L)	133 mg/dL (SI: 7.4 mmol/L)
Day 2	106 mg/dL (SI: 5.9 mmol/L)	96 mg/dL (SI: 5.3 mmol/L)	109 mg/dL (SI: 6.0 mmol/L)	121 mg/dL (SI: 6.7 mmol/L)
Day 3	98 mg/dL (SI: 5.4 mmol/L)	104 mg/dL (SI: 5.8 mmol/L)	101 mg/dL (SI: 5.6 mmol/L)	142 mg/dL (SI: 7.9 mmol/L)
Day 4	101 mg/dL (SI: 5.6 mmol/L)	99 mg/dL (SI: 5.5 mmol/L)	112 mg/dL (SI: 6.2 mmol/L)	...
Day 5	89 mg/dL (SI: 4.9 mmol/L)	105 mg/dL (SI: 5.8 mmol/L)	117 mg/dL (SI: 6.5 mmol/L)	145 mg/dL (SI: 8.0 mmol/L)
Day 6	104 mg/dL (SI: 5.8 mmol/L)	100 mg/dL (SI: 5.6 mmol/L)	...	138 mg/dL (SI: 7.7 mmol/L)

Which of the following is the best treatment option?
A. Start NPH insulin at bedtime
B. Start insulin degludec at bedtime
C. Start insulin aspart before the evening meal
D. Start NPH insulin at bedtime and insulin aspart before the evening meal
E. Continue dietary treatment alone

111 A 45-year-old woman is referred for management of very high triglyceride levels. She reports that she was found to have elevated triglycerides 8 years ago on a routine physical, but no therapy was offered. She has gained 25 lb (11.4 kg) over the past 5 years since the birth of her son, and she works a sedentary job. She has no other medical problems and takes no medications. She does not smoke cigarettes or drink alcohol. She is originally from China and her family history is unrevealing except for type 2 diabetes mellitus in her 79-year-old father.

On physical examination, her blood pressure is 133/77 mm Hg. Her height is 60.5 in (153.5 cm), and weight is 145.5 lb (kg) (BMI = 27.9 kg/m^2). There is some abdominal adiposity, but examination findings are otherwise unremarkable.

Laboratory test results (sample drawn while fasting):

Measurement	7 Months Ago	Today's Visit	Reference Ranges
Total cholesterol	202 mg/dL (SI: 5.23 mmol/L)	300 mg/dL (SI: 7.77 mmol/L)	<200 mg/dL (SI: <5.18 mmol/L)
Triglycerides	282 mg/dL (SI: 3.19 mmol/L)	495 mg/dL (SI: 5.59 mmol/L)	<150 mg/dL (SI: <1.70 mmol/L)
LDL cholesterol	107 mg/dL (SI: 2.77 mmol/L)	...	<100 mg/dL (SI: <2.59 mmol/L)
HDL cholesterol	37 mg/dL (SI: 0.96 mmol/L)	25 mg/dL (SI: 0.65 mmol/L)	>60 mg/dL (SI: >1.55 mmol/L)
Non-HDL cholesterol	165 mg/dL (SI: 4.27 mmol/L)	275 mg/dL (SI: 7.12 mmol/L)	<130 mg/dL (SI: <3.37 mmol/L)
TSH	1.3 mIU/L	5.1 mIU/L	0.5-5.0 mIU/L
Creatinine	0.6 mg/dL (SI: 53.0 µmol/L)	0.6 mg/dL (SI: 53.0 µmol/L)	0.6-1.1 mg/dL (SI: 53.0-97.2 µmol/L)
Hemoglobin A$_{1c}$	5.4% (36 mmol/mol)	5.7% (39 mmol/mol)	4.0%-5.6% (20-38 mmol/mol)
Glucose	98 mg/dL (SI: 5.4 mmol/L)	113 mg/dL (SI: 6.3 mmol/L)	70-99 mg/dL (SI: 3.9-5.55 mmol/L)

Which of the following is the best next step in managing this patient's lipids?
A. Refer for medical nutrition therapy
B. Start a statin
C. Start fish oil
D. Start levothyroxine
E. Start fenofibrate

112 A 75-year-old woman is noted to have a thyroid mass when hospitalized to receive intravenous antibiotics for pneumonia. Upon discharge from the hospital, she is advised to follow-up with an endocrinologist. At the time of her evaluation, the patient describes hoarseness and a sensation of pressure when turning her head. Her only other medical problem is type 2 diabetes mellitus that is well controlled with sitagliptin monotherapy.

On physical examination, her blood pressure is 135/80 mm Hg and pulse rate is 75 beats/min. Her height is 62 in (157.5 cm), and weight is 137 lb (62.3 kg) (BMI = 25.1 kg/m^2). Neck examination reveals a firm 4.5-cm mass occupying most of the right lobe of the thyroid gland.

FNA biopsy yields cells with features of papillary thyroid cancer. The patient undergoes a total thyroidectomy, and pathologic examination shows anaplastic thyroid cancer with a mixed spindle-cell and giant-cell pattern. Small areas of papillary thyroid cancer are also identified. Genomic testing reveals the presence of *TP53* and *BRAF* pathogenic variants in various areas of the tumor. The patient is referred to a comprehensive cancer center for ongoing therapy, and external beam radiation with radiosensitizing chemotherapy is initiated.

Which of the following factors best predicts a more favorable prognosis for this patient?
A. Complete tumor resection
B. Coexistence of papillary and anaplastic thyroid cancer within her thyroid gland
C. Spindle-cell growth pattern
D. Presence of a *BRAF* pathogenic variant
E. Tumor size <5 cm

113
A 25-year-old Hispanic woman is referred by her gynecologist for evaluation of hirsutism and abnormal test results. Menarche was at age 14 years. She has always had irregular menses—fewer than 6 per year. Excessive hair growth began in her teens and has progressively worsened into her 20s. Initially, the hair growth began on her face, but it is now notable on her back and chest. Both of her parents have type 2 diabetes mellitus. Her primary care physician has been treating her with oral contraceptives for polycystic ovary syndrome and atorvastatin for hyperlipidemia.

On physical examination, her height is 63 in (160 cm) and weight is 195 lb (88.6 kg) (BMI = 34.5 kg/m^2). She has terminal hair growth on her upper lip, chin, neck, chest, abdomen, upper arms, thighs, and upper and lower back with a Ferriman-Gallwey score of 26. Acanthosis nigricans is present on the back of her neck.

Laboratory test results:
Total testosterone = 27 ng/dL (8-60 ng/dL) (SI: 0.9 nmol/L [0.3-2.1 nmol/L])
17-Hydroxyprogesterone = 433 ng/dL (<80 ng/dL [follicular]) (SI: 13.1 nmol/L [<2.42 nmol/L])
Fasting glucose = 112 mg/dL (70-99 mg/dL) (SI: 6.2 mmol/L [3.9-5.5 mmol/L])
Total cholesterol = 194 mg/dL (<200 mg/dL [optimal]) (SI: 5.02 mmol/L [<5.18 mmol/L])
Triglycerides = 398 mg/dL (<150 mg/dL [optimal]) (SI: 4.50 mmol/L [<1.70 mmol/L])
HDL cholesterol = 43 mg/dL (>60 mg/dL [optimal]) (SI: 1.11 mmol/L [>1.55 mmol/L])
LDL cholesterol = 71 mg/dL (<100 mg/dL [optimal]) (SI: 1.84 mmol/L [<2.59 mmol/L])

You proceed with an ACTH-stimulation test (250 mcg cosyntropin) and obtain the following results:

Time point	Cortisol	17-Hydroxyprogesterone
Baseline	17 µg/dL (SI: 469.0 nmol/L)	1460 ng/dL (SI: 44.2 nmol/L)
30 min	20 µg/dL (SI: 551.8 nmol/L)	3100 ng/dL (SI: 93.9 nmol/L)
60 min	26 µg/dL (SI: 579.3 nmol/L)	3290 ng/dL (SI: 99.7 nmol/L)

The patient is not currently trying to conceive. She wants to primarily address the hair growth, which causes her significant distress.

In addition to continuing oral contraceptives, which of the following is the best treatment plan to address her hirsutism?
A. Spironolactone
B. Hydrocortisone dosed with a reverse diurnal rhythm
C. Flutamide
D. Dexamethasone at bedtime
E. Metformin

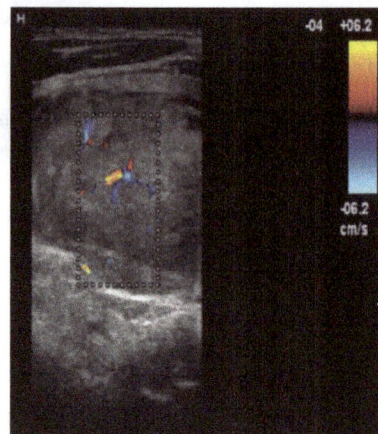

114 A 62-year-old woman presents with a 5-month history of an enlarging neck swelling. She has no feeling of choking and no dysphagia with solids or liquids. She is asymptomatic and, in particular, she does not report symptoms of thyroid dysfunction. She has a history of hypertension that is controlled with an ACE inhibitor. Her father has type 2 diabetes mellitus.

On physical examination, her height is 69 in (175.3 cm) and weight is 154 lb (70 kg) (BMI = 22.7 kg/m^2). Her blood pressure is 132/78 mm Hg, and pulse rate is 72 beats/min in a regular rhythm. Examination of her neck reveals a right-sided thyroid swelling measuring 5 x 6 cm that moves with swallowing. There is no palpable cervical lymphadenopathy. Findings on systems examination are otherwise unremarkable.

Laboratory test results:
  TSH = 2.1 mIU/L
  Free T$_4$ = 1.4 ng/dL (0.8-1.8 ng/dL) (SI: 18.0 pmol/L [10.30-23.17 pmol/L])

Neck ultrasonography reveals a right-sided, 6 x 5 x 3.5-cm, slightly hyperechoic nodule with a regular margin and some internal vascularity (*see image*).

FNA biopsy is undertaken and cytologic analysis reveals a moderately cellular specimen in which the thyroid epithelial cells show a considerable degree of nuclear polymorphism, nuclear crowding, and overlap. Occasional nuclear grooves and intranuclear pseudo-inclusions are also noted. The specimen is considered suspicious for malignancy (Bethesda Category 5).

The patient undergoes a right hemithyroidectomy, and the histopathologic evaluation indicates the presence of a noninvasive follicular thyroid neoplasm with papillary-like nuclear features (NIFTP).

Which of the following is the best next step?
  A. Completion thyroidectomy
  B. Completion thyroidectomy followed by remnant ablation with ^{131}I
  C. Administration of an ablative dose of ^{131}I now
  D. High-dosage levothyroxine therapy to suppress serum TSH to <0.1 mIU/L
  E. Observation with occasional monitoring of serum thyroglobulin and neck ultrasonography

115 A 48-year-old man is referred to you for new-onset type 2 diabetes mellitus. He describes increased thirst and polyuria for the past 3 months. His weight has been unchanged. The patient has been taking metformin, 1000 mg twice daily, for the past 2 years. He has no diabetes-related complications.

On physical examination, his blood pressure is 130/90 mm Hg and pulse rate is 100 beats/min. His height is 70 in (178 cm), and weight is 195 lb (109 kg) (BMI = 28 kg/m^2). He has acanthosis nigricans at the base of the neck. Examination findings are otherwise normal.

Laboratory test result:
  Hemoglobin A$_{1c}$ = 7.4% (4.0%-5.6%) (57 mmol/mol [20-38 mmol/mol])

Which of the following is the most important target when considering the addition of a second diabetes medication?
  A. Postprandial glucose
  B. Fasting glucose
  C. Both fasting and postprandial glucose
  D. Insulin resistance
  E. Body weight

116 A 58-year-old woman is referred for a newly developed sellar mass. Scalp melanoma was diagnosed 4 months ago. She had wide resection and was found to have positive neck lymph nodes. Ipilimumab was prescribed, 3 mg/kg intravenously every 3 weeks. Two weeks after the third dose, she developed headaches, and a noncontrast brain MRI showed a diffusely enlarged pituitary gland (*see image*). She was feeling tired and had noticed reduction of appetite. She has had no polyuria or polydipsia.

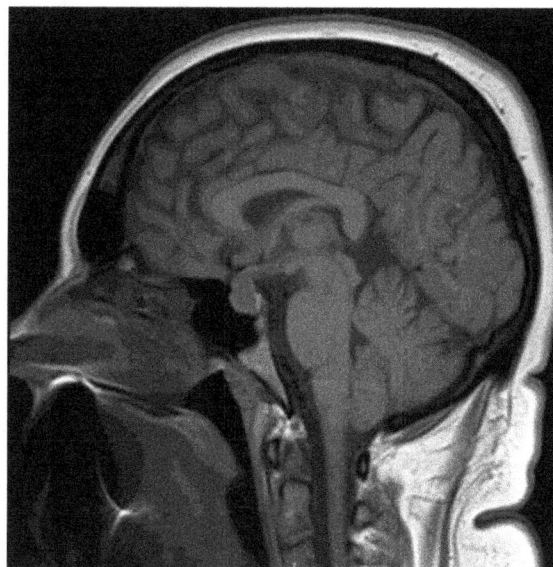

Laboratory test results obtained by her oncologist:

Free T_4 = 0.6 ng/dL (0.8-1.8 ng/dL) (SI: 7.7 pmol/L [10.30-23.17 pmol/L])

TSH = 1.45 mIU/L (0.5-5.0 mIU/L)

Cortisol (8 AM) = 2.0 µg/dL (5-25 µg/dL) (SI: 55.2 nmol/L [137.9-689.7 nmol/L])

ACTH (8 AM) = 6.0 pg/mL (10-60 pg/mL) (SI: 1.3 pmol/L [2.2-13.2 pmol/L])

Her oncologist already initiated hydrocortisone and levothyroxine therapy 1 week ago, and her symptoms have improved. Her headaches have also improved, and they are controlled by acetaminophen.

On physical examination, her blood pressure is 115/76 mm Hg and pulse rate is 72 beats/min. Her height is 64 in (162.5 cm), and weight is 158 lb (71.8 kg) (BMI = 27.1 kg/m^2). Her examination findings are normal, including visual fields by confrontation.

Which of the following is the best next step in this patient's management?
A. Refer to neuro-ophthalmology
B. Refer to neurosurgery for biopsy to rule out pituitary metastasis
C. Start rituximab
D. Start high-dosage prednisone (1 mg/kg per day)
E. Start intravenous immunoglobulins

117 A 26-year-old woman has an 8-year history of type 1 diabetes mellitus. Her glycemic control was poor for the first 3 years, but over the past 5 years she has been able to maintain her hemoglobin A_{1c} level in the range of 6.3% to 7.5% (45-58 mmol/mol). She lives in a small town with limited availability of medical care. She has never had a retinal examination. A diabetes management center with specialized ophthalmopathy care is a 5-hour drive. She has access to retinal photography and CT imaging in a town 1 hour away.

Which of the following is the best next step to screen for proliferative retinopathy in this patient?
A. Fluorescein angiography
B. Nonmydriatic digital stereoscopic photography
C. Automated digital retinal imaging
D. Optical coherence CT
E. Ophthalmoscopy and fundus examination by an eye specialist

118 A 47-year-old woman presents for management of cardiovascular risk. Two years ago, coronary angiography revealed significant 3-vessel disease, and a 3-vessel bypass was performed. Atorvastatin, 40 mg daily (her maximum tolerated dosage), and fenofibrate were started at that time. Type 2 diabetes mellitus diagnosed 1 year ago is treated with metformin. She also takes aspirin, lisinopril, and hydrochlorothiazide. Five months ago, she developed chest tightness and 1 bypass graft was found to be occluded and successfully stented. She now returns for further management.

She is sedentary and has multiple dietary indiscretions. She has a remote history of 20 pack-years of cigarette smoking. She does not drink alcohol. Her family history is remarkable for a father with coronary artery disease at age 50 years requiring 3-vessel coronary bypass and a 41-year-old brother with coronary artery disease and stent placement.

On physical examination, her blood pressure is 144/83 mm Hg. Her height is 66.5 in (169 cm), and weight is 264 lb (120 kg) (BMI = 42 kg/m^2). There are no xanthomas. She has central adiposity.

Laboratory test results (sample drawn when fasting):

Measurement	Time of Assessment		Reference Ranges
	16 Months Ago	Today's Visit (on simvastatin and fenofibrate)	
Total cholesterol	232 mg/dL (SI: 6.01 mmol/L)	205 mg/dL (SI: 5.31 mmol/L)	<200 mg/dL (SI: <5.18 mmol/L)
Triglycerides	381 mg/dL (SI: 4.31 mmol/L)	375 mg/dL (SI: 4.24 mmol/L)	<150 mg/dL (SI: <1.70 mmol/L)
LDL cholesterol	116 mg/dL (SI: 3.00 mmol/L)	96 mg/dL (SI: 2.49 mmol/L)	<100 mg/dL (SI: <2.59 mmol/L)
HDL cholesterol	40 mg/dL (SI: 1.04 mmol/L)	34 mg/dL (SI: 0.88 mmol/L)	>60 mg/dL (SI: >1.55 mmol/L)
Non-HDL cholesterol	192 mg/dL (SI: 4.97 mmol/L)	171 mg/dL (SI: 4.43 mmol/L)	<130 mg/dL (SI: <3.37 mmol/L)
TSH	3.2 mIU/L	3.6 mIU/L	0.5-5.0 mIU/L
Creatinine	0.95 mg/dL (SI: 84.0 µmol/L)	0.95 mg/dL (SI: 84.0 µmol/L)	0.6-1.1 mg/dL (SI: 53.0-97.2 µmol/L)
Hemoglobin A$_{1c}$	6.6% (49 mmol/mol)	6.3% (45 mmol/mol)	4.0%-5.6% (20-38 mmol/mol)

In addition to emphasizing aggressive lifestyle management efforts, which of the following is the best next step in this patient's management?
A. No change in therapy
B. Increase atorvastatin dosage to 80 mg daily
C. Add ezetimibe
D. Add niacin
E. Add alirocumab

119 A 28-year-old woman presents with concerns about hirsutism and seeks help interpreting an extensive laboratory workup performed elsewhere. She describes having a normal birth, normal childhood development and growth, and no known genital malformations. Menarche was at age 12 years and thereafter she had regular menses occurring every 27 to 28 days until age 25. Between ages 25 and 28, she had irregular menses described as occurring every 32 to 35 days, and occasionally occurring after more than 40 days. At age 22, she started noting the development of terminal hairs on her chin and above her upper lip, as well as below her umbilicus. She would tweeze these unwanted hairs daily. She has had no acne on her face or chest, alopecia, or deepening of her voice. She is mainly concerned about the hirsutism.

On physical examination, her blood pressure is 112/60 mm Hg. Her height is 64 in (162.5 cm), and weight is 169 lb (76.8 kg) (BMI = 29 kg/m^2). She has evidence of tweezed terminal hairs on her chin, upper lip, and abdomen below the umbilicus. There is no evidence of terminal hairs on her back, chest, or upper arms. There is no acne or alopecia. She has no overt signs of Cushing syndrome. External genitalia are normal without clitoromegaly.

The samples for the laboratory tests were drawn in the morning on the third day following a menses. An elevated DHEA-S level was documented, which prompted a dynamic ACTH-stimulation study.

Measurement	8 AM	Reference Range
DHEA-S	398 µg/dL (SI: 10.8 µmol/L)	44-332 µg/dL (1.19-9.00 µmol/L)
Total testosterone	35 ng/dL (SI: 1.2 nmol/L)	8-60 ng/dL (SI: 0.3-2.1 nmol/L)
Prolactin	11 ng/mL (SI: 0.5 nmol/L)	4-30 ng/mL (SI: 0.17-1.30 nmol/L)
FSH	3.5 mIU/mL (SI: 3.5 IU/L)	2.0-12.5 mIU/mL (SI: 2.0-12.0 IU/L)
LH	7.6 mIU/mL (SI: 7.6 IU/L)	1.0-18.0 mIU/mL (SI: 1.0-18.0 IU/L)

Measurement	8 AM	→→→→→	9 AM
Cortisol	12.7 µg/dL (SI: 350.4 nmol/L)		23.0 µg/dL (SI: 634.5 nmol/L)
17-Hydroxyprogesterone	211 ng/dL (SI: 6.4 nmol/L)		278 ng/dL (SI: 8.4 nmol/L)
17-Pregnenalone	41 ng/dL (SI: 1.2 nmol/L)	Administration of intravenous cosyntropin, 250 mcg	1050 ng/dL (SI: 31.6 nmol/L)
11-Deoxycorticosterone	7.8 ng/dL (SI: 0.23 nmol/L)		17.0 ng/dL (SI: 0.51 nmol/L)
Aldosterone	12 ng/dL (SI: 332.9 pmol/L)		19 ng/dL (SI: 527.1 pmol/L)

Which of the following is the most likely diagnosis?
A. Polycystic ovary syndrome
B. Nonclassic 21-hydroxylase deficiency
C. 11β-Hydroxylase deficiency
D. 17α-Hydroxylase deficiency
E. Nonclassic 3β-hydroxysteroid dehydrogenase deficiency

120 A 59-year-old woman comes to your clinic for initial consultation regarding type 2 diabetes mellitus of more than 5 years' duration. She has peripheral neuropathy, and she notes numbness in both legs extending from her feet to her upper calves, as well as ongoing discomfort in her knees and hips, which are more chronic problems.

Upon directed questioning, you learn she has experienced polyuria and unintentional weight loss of 10 lb (4.5 kg) over the last 3 months. She currently takes metformin, 2000 mg once daily. Her medical history is otherwise notable for hypercholesterolemia, pyelonephritis, and cholecystectomy. Data from her glucometer show a mean blood glucose value of 186 mg/dL (10.3 mmol/L), and she checks blood glucose once daily. She has poor adherence to recommendations for lifestyle modifications. She consumes sweets daily, although she is open to improving her diet. Exercise is difficult because of her joint discomfort. She also reports recently starting vitamin B_{12} injections.

On physical examination, her blood pressure is 148/92 mm Hg and pulse rate is 98 beats/min. Her height is 64 in (162.6 cm), and weight is 188 lb (85.5 kg) (BMI = 32.3 kg/m^2). Notably, there is no acanthosis nigricans, facial plethora, moon facies, dorsocervical fat pad fullness, or wide violaceous striae. Foot exam shows no worrisome wounds, and peripheral pulses are normal. There is loss of Achilles tendon reflexes. Vibratory sensation and monofilament sensation are both impaired.

Her current hemoglobin A_{1c} level is 9.2% (77 mmol/mol).

In addition to referral to a nutritionist to aid with lifestyle modifications, which of the following should be added as the best next step in managing this patient's hyperglycemia?
A. Glimepiride
B. Insulin detemir
C. Empagliflozin
D. Liraglutide
E. Liraglutide and empagliflozin

ENDOCRINE SELF-ASSESSMENT PROGRAM 2019

Part II

ANSWER: D) Add spironolactone to the current regimen

This patient has a definite biochemical diagnosis of primary aldosteronism. The recently updated Endocrine Society Clinical Practice Guideline on this topic continues to recommend use of the aldosterone-to-renin ratio (ARR) as an initial screening test to identify individuals at risk for primary aldosteronism. A value greater than 30 (when plasma aldosterone and plasma renin activity are in conventional units) merits investigation. Ordinarily, an elevated ARR alone is insufficient to diagnose primary aldosteronism and a further confirmatory test is required. There are 4 potential tests to confirm primary aldosteronism as outlined in the guideline: (1) oral sodium-loading test and measurement of 24-hour urinary sodium; (2) saline suppression test; (3) fludrocortisone suppression test; and (4) captopril challenge test. The guideline does not recommend any single test as the gold standard. Moreover, the guideline suggests that confirmatory testing is not required in clear-cut cases of primary aldosteronism with spontaneous hypokalemia, undetectable plasma renin levels, and a plasma aldosterone concentration greater than 20 ng/dL (>550 pmol/L), which was the case in this vignette.

Occasionally, confirmation testing is not required when a clear case of primary aldosteronism has been identified on initial screening. The required criteria are an elevated ARR, plasma aldosterone concentration greater than 20 ng/dL (>554.8 pmol/L), and spontaneous hypokalemia. All 3 criteria are met in this vignette. Moreover, this patient also demonstrates elevated urinary aldosterone excretion in a salt-replete condition, which fulfills the criteria for a diagnostic oral sodium-loading test. Therefore, the diagnosis of primary aldosteronism has been made, and no further confirmatory testing, such as a saline suppression test (Answer C), is required.

Ideally, the ARR should be assessed while the patient is on no treatment or, if that is not possible, while taking antihypertensive therapy that has minimal effects on its individual constituents (for example, α-adrenergic blockers and nondihydropyridine calcium channel blockers). In practice, this is often very difficult and carries a risk of worsening blood pressure control. Therefore, with the exception of potassium-sparing diuretics, the ARR can be measured while the patient is on any antihypertensive agent as long as the effect of that agent on aldosterone and renin is recognized and taken into account. Thus, repeating laboratory testing after discontinuing enalapril (Answer E) is unnecessary. Enalapril usually reduces plasma aldosterone levels and increases plasma renin activity. Therefore, the elevated plasma aldosterone and low plasma renin activity in this patient are particularly suspicious.

Given that primary aldosteronism has already been confirmed, the next question relates to further management. Adrenal venous sampling (Answer B) is usually required in patients older than 35 years to confirm unilateral aldosterone excess before surgery due to the increased risk of adrenal incidentalomas in this age group. This is an invasive procedure that carries clinical risk (albeit small) and therefore should be performed only in individuals who would choose adrenalectomy if their aldosterone excess can be lateralized. It is not appropriate in this patient who has clearly stated that she would rather avoid surgery if possible.

This patient's blood pressure is well controlled according to the Eighth Joint National Committee Guideline for the Management of High Blood Pressure in Adults (JNC VIII), which recommends a target blood pressure less than 140/90 mm Hg for adults younger than 60 years. However, the recently published SPRINT trial demonstrated that in patients at high risk for cardiovascular disease but who did not have a history of diabetes, intensive blood pressure control (target systolic blood pressure <120 mm Hg) improved cardiovascular outcomes and overall survival compared with standard therapy (target systolic blood pressure 135-139 mm Hg). Moreover (and in reaction to the SPRINT trial), the recently published Guideline for the Prevention, Detection, Evaluation, and Management of High Blood Pressure in Adults issued by the American College of Cardiology and the American Heart Association redefines "hypertension" as systolic blood pressure between 130 and 139 mm Hg and diastolic blood pressure between 80 and 89 mm Hg. Therefore, in this patient who has a high cardiovascular risk, the target systolic blood pressure should be lower than the value documented in the vignette. Thus, simply continuing current therapy (Answer A) is incorrect.

Finally, there is a plethora of evidence that patients with primary aldosteronism are at considerably higher risk of stroke, atrial fibrillation, and other cardiovascular events than those with primary hypertension of similar severity and duration. Therefore, in proven cases of aldosterone excess, simply lowering the blood pressure to target using conventional antihypertensive agents is not enough, and amelioration of the effects of aldosterone excess is required. This can be achieved by surgery or by the use of mineralocorticoid-receptor antagonists such as spironolactone (Answer D), which should achieve the dual goal of a lower target blood pressure and protection from the deleterious effects of aldosterone excess. Prescribing spironolactone is the best next management step in this case.

Educational Objective
Manage aldosterone excess, as well as control blood pressure, in primary aldosteronism.

UpToDate Topic Review(s)
Diagnosis of primary aldosteronism
Treatment of primary aldosteronism

Reference(s)

Funder JW, Carey RM, Mantero F, et al. The management of primary aldosteronism: case detection, diagnosis, and treatment: an Endocrine Society Clinical Practice Guideline. *J Clin Endocrinol Metab.* 2016;101(5):1889-1916. PMID: 26934393

Whelton PK, Carey RM, Aronow WS, et al. 2017 ACC/AHA/AAPA/ABC/ACPM/AGS/APhA/ASH/ASPC/NMA/PCNA guideline for the prevention, detection, evaluation, and management of high blood pressure in adults: a report of the American College of Cardiology/American Heart Association Task Force on Clinical Practice Guidelines. *Hypertension.* 2018;71(6):e13-e115. PMID: 29133356

Berlowitz DR, Foy CG, Kazis LE, et al; SPRINT Research Group. Effect of intensive blood-pressure treatment on patient-reported outcomes. *N Engl J Med.* 2017;377(8):733-744. PMID: 28834483

Savard S, Amar L, Plouin PF, Steichen O. Cardiovascular complications associated with primary aldosteronism: a controlled cross-sectional study. *Hypertension.* 2013;62(2):331-336. PMID: 23753408

2 ANSWER: C) Denosumab

This patient has osteoporosis in the setting of multiple comorbidities and she has already sustained a right hip fragility fracture. She is at high risk for future fracture and should be counseled on fall prevention, as well as treated with pharmacologic therapy for osteoporosis. With her history of esophageal carcinoma and esophagogastrectomy, an oral bisphosphonate such as alendronate (Answer A) should be avoided. An intravenous bisphosphonate such as zoledronic acid (Answer B) would be a good option if her renal function were better, but it is not recommended to use this agent in the setting of chronic kidney disease with an estimated glomerular filtration rate less than 35 mL/min per 1.73 m^2.

Teriparatide (PTH 1-34) (Answer D) and abaloparatide (Answer E), both of which are anabolic agents used in the treatment of osteoporosis, are contraindicated in this patient with a history of radiation therapy to the skeleton due to their black box warning of osteosarcoma. Abaloparatide is an analogue of PTHrP that was approved by the US FDA in April 2017 for the treatment of postmenopausal osteoporosis. In a phase III trial of postmenopausal women with osteoporosis randomly assigned to abaloparatide (80 mcg daily by subcutaneous injection), placebo, or open-label teriparatide (20 mcg daily by subcutaneous injection), abaloparatide significantly reduced the risk of new vertebral and nonvertebral fractures compared with placebo, similar to the reduction in fracture rates in the teriparatide group at 18 months. However, the incidence of hypercalcemia was lower with abaloparatide than with teriparatide.

Denosumab (Answer C) would be the most appropriate agent to treat her osteoporosis. Denosumab is a fully human monoclonal antibody to the receptor activator of nuclear factor kappaB ligand (RANKL). By blocking the binding of RANKL to RANK, it reduces the formation, function, and survival of osteoclasts, which results in decreased bone resorption and increased bone density. Denosumab is administered by subcutaneous injection once every 6 months. It is not excreted by the kidneys; therefore, it can be used in patients with reduced kidney function without the need for a dosage change. In order to avoid hypocalcemia with denosumab use, it is important to ensure that patients maintain an adequate amount of calcium and vitamin D supplementation, especially with conditions that predispose to hypocalcemia, such as chronic kidney disease or malabsorption syndromes. Denosumab should not be given to patients with preexisting hypocalcemia until it is corrected. Because of emerging concerns about an increased risk of vertebral fracture after discontinuation of denosumab, the need for indefinite administration of denosumab or switching to an alternative therapy if possible should be discussed with patients before its initiation.

Educational Objective
Recommend the most appropriate therapeutic agent to treat osteoporosis in the presence of other comorbidities.

UpToDate Topic Review(s)
Overview of the management of osteoporosis in postmenopausal women
Denosumab for osteoporosis

Reference(s)

Silverman S, Christiansen C. Individualizing osteoporosis therapy. *Osteoporos Int.* 2012;23(3):797-809. PMID: 22218417

Miller PD, Hattersley G, Riis BJ, et al; ACTIVE Study Investigators. Effect of abaloparatide vs placebo on new vertebral fractures in postmenopausal women with osteoporosis: a randomized clinical trial. *JAMA*. 2016;316(7):722-733. PMID: 27533157

Lamy O, Gonzalez-Rodriguez E, Stoll D, Hans D, Aubry-Rozier B. Severe rebound-associated vertebral fractures after denosumab discontinuation: 9 clinical cases report. *J Clin Endocrinol Metab*. 2017;102(2):354-358. PMID: 27732330

3 ANSWER: D) Hybrid closed-loop insulin pump and continuous glucose monitoring system

This patient with type 1 diabetes is not meeting reasonable glycemic targets despite adherence to recommendations for self-monitoring and lifestyle. His main issue is the variability of his lifestyle and physical activity. Exploration of technologic solutions is indicated.

Real-time continuous glucose monitors (CGMs) (Answer B) have been studied extensively. Most studies are of relatively short duration, between 12 weeks and 6 months, but they generally show modest reductions in hemoglobin A_{1c} and less time spent in hypoglycemia, although not all studies demonstrate both these effects. It is notable that hypoglycemia unawareness is not a reported problem for this patient. While the use of a CGM would certainly provide this patient with some benefit, there may be better options for him. Flash CGM (Answer E) allows the patient to obtain glucose values by waving the reader close to the CGM, which is inserted into the upper arm. Although it is an attractive option to replace frequent fingerstick blood glucose measurements, flash CGM does not have the option to alert patients if hypoglycemia occurs. While this patient retains hypoglycemia awareness, flash CGM would not be the best choice because he reports frequent hypoglycemia.

Recently, the US FDA approved an insulin pump and CGM to operate in so-called hybrid closed-loop mode (Answer D). This insulin pump has an "auto mode" whereby the pump receives glucose data from the CGM and continuously adjusts the basal rates based on an algorithm. Also, it calculates the insulin sensitivity (or correction) factor based on machine learning algorithms. The patient must enter the number of carbohydrates being consumed, and the physician must set the insulin-to-carbohydrate ratio. This latter point is important—the hybrid closed-loop requires patient adherence to dietary recommendations and patient input at meal times. The pump can operate in a "manual mode" where the algorithm is inactive. Studies comparing the hybrid closed-loop system used in auto mode vs manual mode have been shown to increase time in the target glycemic range, to lower hemoglobin A_{1c}, and to decrease both hyperglycemia and hypoglycemia. Although the largest of such studies was a single-arm, nonrandomized study, the balance of evidence suggests that in this patient with an erratic lifestyle and frequent hypoglycemia, hybrid close-loop technology would be the best option to optimize glucose control.

Continuous subcutaneous insulin injection (CSII) or insulin pump therapy alone (Answer A) may improve glycemic control, although the bulk of this evidence is from studies comparing CSII with the use of intermediate-acting recombinant insulin. Studies comparing CSII alone with a regimen of multiple daily injections with a modern insulin analogue suggest that CSII results in reduced glycemic variability and lower hemoglobin A_{1c} values in patients who have higher hemoglobin A_{1c} values to start. CSII with integrated CGM with the threshold suspend feature (Answer C) most likely improves rates of hypoglycemia and may represent a better option than CSII alone. However, the patient retains hypoglycemia awareness and it would not address his variable lifestyle. As studies with hybrid closed-loop systems have been compared with the same pump operating in auto mode vs manual mode, the hybrid closed-loop system is most likely the best choice for this patient.

CSII/CGM type	Adjusts Basal Rate Continuously	Temporarily Stops Insulin Delivery at a Given Glucose Threshold	Requires Patient to Announce Meal and Enter Carbs	Requires Insulin Sensitivity Factor to be Determined by Provider
CSII + CGM	No	No	Yes	Yes
CSII + CGM + Threshold Suspend	No	Yes	Yes	Yes
CSII + CGM + Hybrid Closed Loop	Yes	Yes	Yes	No

Educational Objective

Optimize glycemic control in a patient with type 1 diabetes and hypoglycemia who has a variable schedule.

UpToDate Topic Review(s)
Management of blood glucose in adults with type 1 diabetes mellitus

Reference(s)

Garg SK, Weinzimer SA, Tamborlane WV, et al. Glucose outcomes with the in-home use of a hybrid closed-loop insulin delivery system in adolescents and adults with type 1 diabetes. *Diabetes Technol Ther.* 2017;19(3):155-163. PMID: 28134564

Beck RW, Riddlesworth T, Ruedy K, et al; DIAMOND Study Group. Effect of continuous glucose monitoring on glycemic control in adults with type 1 diabetes using insulin injections: The DIAMOND Randomized Clinical Trial. *JAMA.* 2017;317(4):371-378. PMID: 28118453

4 ANSWER: A) Clomiphene

This woman has classic polycystic ovary syndrome with symptoms since menarche, fewer than 9 periods per year, and clinical signs of androgen excess with a Ferriman-Gallwey score greater than or equal to 8 even though her total testosterone level is normal. While obesity is strongly associated with polycystic ovary syndrome, the lean phenotype is present in at least 30% (and up to 70%) of women with polycystic ovary syndrome varying by population and race/ethnicity. Although the lean phenotype of polycystic ovary syndrome may be less frequently associated with metabolic complications, metformin (Answer C) has been demonstrated to improve ovulation rates/frequency even in normal-weight women and in women without prediabetes or diabetes. However, in randomized controlled trials of metformin vs clomiphene (Answer A), and even compared with the combination of metformin and clomiphene, clomiphene treatment alone is superior to metformin in increasing pregnancy rates. Although a subsequent randomized controlled trial found that letrozole was superior to clomiphene, letrozole was not a choice in this vignette. There was no increase in teratogenicity reported in a randomized controlled trial of 750 participants, but letrozole is not FDA approved specifically for fertility.

Laparoscopic ovarian drilling (Answer D) (laparoscopic ovarian diathermy or electrocoagulation) is a surgical approach to improve ovulatory function in polycystic ovary syndrome that replaced wedge resection, offering a less invasive surgical approach that reduces the risk for postoperative adhesions. The exact mechanism for why laparoscopic ovarian drilling works is not known, but it most likely involves reduction in local and circulating androgens by destroying/reducing the volume of androgen-producing ovarian stroma thecal cells. Laparoscopic ovarian drilling does not increase pregnancy rates more effectively than any pharmacologic ovulation induction therapy. However, it might be considered in women with polycystic ovary syndrome who are clomiphene-resistant and/or for women with polycystic ovary syndrome who would be at higher risk with multiple pregnancies. Gonadotropins (Answer B) are also considered second-line therapy due to the risk for multiple pregnancies and ovarian hyperstimulation syndrome.

In women with polycystic ovary syndrome who are overweight, weight loss achieved from diet and lifestyle modification (Answer E) has been shown to improve ovulatory frequency. However, there are no randomized controlled trials demonstrating that weight loss improves pregnancy rates. Overweight and obese women with polycystic ovary syndrome who are trying to conceive are encouraged to lose weight with healthful diet and lifestyle approaches for the metabolic benefit, to prevent complications during pregnancy, and to improve the response to medications used for ovarian stimulation.

Age-related changes in fertility and evidence of anovulatory cycles are important considerations that can affect timing of evaluations and treatment decisions for infertility. In women with polycystic ovary syndrome and anovulation or in women older than 35 years, evaluation and treatment for infertility is encouraged after 6 months of unprotected intercourse as opposed to the otherwise recommended 12 months. Especially for this woman who is approaching the age of 32, when female fertility significantly declines, it would be important to consider clomiphene and monitored ovulation induction at this earlier time point of 6 months after trying to conceive. If this woman were younger, metformin could be a reasonable option to increase ovulatory frequency and likelihood of conceiving.

Educational Objective

Provide tailored recommendations to a woman with polycystic ovary syndrome to improve future fertility.

UpToDate Topic Review(s)
Ovulation induction with clomiphene citrate

Reference(s)

Legro RS, Arslanian SA, Ehrmann DA, et al. Diagnosis and treatment of polycystic ovary syndrome: an Endocrine Society Clinical Practice Guideline. *J Clin Endocrinol Metab.* 2013;98(12):4565-4592. PMID: 24151290

Balen AH, Morley LC, Misso M, et al. The management of anovulatory infertility in women with polycystic ovary syndrome: an analysis of the evidence to support the development of global WHO guidance. *Hum Reprod Update.* 2016;22(6):687-708. PMID: 27511809

Committee on Gynecologic Practice of American College of Obstetricians and Gynecologists; Practice Committee of American Society for Reproductive Medicine. Age-related fertility decline: a committee opinion. *Fertil Steril.* 2008;90(3):486-487. PMID: 18847603

5   ANSWER: E) Reduce his insulin glargine and prandial insulin dosages by 50%

Left ventricular assist devices (LVADs) are increasingly used to prolong life in patients with advanced chronic heart failure. An LVAD may be recommended as a bridge to heart transplant or as "destination" therapy. Patients with chronic heart failure have markedly increased insulin resistance compared with that observed in age- and BMI-matched persons without heart failure. The mechanism of insulin resistance in this setting is speculated to be higher catecholamine levels. The elevated sympathetic activity may also reduce endogenous insulin secretion. As heart failure worsens, reduced cardiac output can further impair insulin production. This combination of events frequently causes deterioration in diabetes control, leading to treatment with higher dosages of diabetes medications.

If the LVAD implantation is successful, cardiac output is restored and diabetes control improves. Uriel et al presented data on 15 patients with type 2 diabetes who underwent LVAD implantation. The authors demonstrated that after LVAD implantation, diabetes control greatly improved (hemoglobin A_{1c} 7.7% → 6.0% [61 → 42 mmol/mol]) and patients required 50% less insulin compared with preimplantation dosages. Guglin et al reported similar reductions in hemoglobin A_{1c} and insulin dosages after 3 months in 50 patients who underwent LVAD implantation. The authors described that the timing of improved diabetes control is similar to the timing of recovery of other hemodynamic parameters.

In this vignette, the patient required high dosages of both basal and prandial insulins. He became profoundly hypoglycemic after hospital discharge. In light of the known improvement in insulin resistance after LVAD implantation, an immediate reduction in the dosages of both prandial and basal insulin is the best choice (Answer E).

The incidence of adrenal insufficiency is rare after uncomplicated heart surgery. Thus, an ACTH stimulation test (Answer A) is not the best next step. Changing his basal insulin (Answer B) will not correct the problem, as degludec at the wrong dosage will also cause hypoglycemia. Starting continuous glucose monitoring (Answer C) is certainly appropriate, but this step should not preclude reducing his insulin dosage. Sepsis is certainly possible and is a worrisome complication after LVAD placement. However, the patient would most likely have other systemic signs of sepsis, so measuring lactate and drawing blood cultures (Answer D) is not the most important next step.

Educational Objective

Anticipate the decreased insulin requirement after implantation of a left ventricular assist device in a patient with diabetes mellitus and chronic heart failure.

UpToDate Topic Review(s)

Heart failure in diabetes mellitus

Reference(s)

Uriel N, Naka Y, Colombo PC, et al. Improved diabetic control in advanced heart failure patients treated with left ventricular assist devices. *Eur J Heart Fail.* 2011; 13(2):195-199. PMID: 21098576

Swan JW, Anker SD, Walton C, et al. Insulin resistance chronic heart failure: relation to severity and etiology of heart failure. *J Am Coll Cardiol.* 1997;30(2): 527-532. PMID: 9247528

Guglin M, Maguire K, Missimer T, Faber C, Caldeira C. Improvement in blood glucose control in patients with diabetes after implantation of left ventricular assist devices. *ASAIO J.* 2014;60(3):290-293. PMID: 24614357

6   ANSWER: E) Pheochromocytoma

Pheochromocytomas (Answer E) are chromaffin-cell tumors that originate in the adrenal medulla. The diagnosis of pheochromocytoma should involve evaluation of clinical symptoms, evidence of hormonal activity, and radiographic appearance.

Pheochromocytomas may secrete catecholamines (such as norepinephrine, epinephrine, and, less frequently, dopamine) that induce adrenergic symptoms and signs, such as palpitations, anxiety, sweating, pallor, and elevations in blood pressure and heart rate. However, some pheochromocytomas do not secrete high concentrations of catecholamines, and in some instances, even when high catecholamine concentrations are detected, some patients do not exhibit the classic symptoms. Typically, pheochromocytomas that induce clinical symptoms are associated with metanephrine and/or normetanephrine levels that are substantially higher than the upper limit of the reference range—usually 4 times or more (less commonly 2 or 3 times higher). Importantly, mild elevations above the upper limit of the metanephrines reference range (<2 times) are common and are usually attributed to enhanced sympathoadrenergic tone (eg, in a state of anxiety or stress) and/or the use of norepinephrine reuptake inhibitors (eg, some antidepressant medications and cocaine). In this regard, these milder elevations are frequent causes of false-positive values. Metanephrines are inactive metabolites of catecholamines and elevations either suggest the secretion of high circulating concentrations of catecholamines, or that catecholamines are being metabolized in a tumor to inactive metanephrines before secretion. The absence of classic adrenergic symptoms in this patient does not exclude a pheochromocytoma; however, the marked elevation in normetanephrine levels (approximately 7.5 times the upper limit of the reference range) strongly suggests that this adrenal tumor is a pheochromocytoma.

Once the clinical and/or biochemical characteristics either confirm or strongly suggest a pheochromocytoma, attention should be paid to the radiographic features. Pheochromocytomas are typically 2 cm or larger when a clinical syndrome of adrenergic excess is detected. However, the incidental detection of a pheochromocytoma can occur at any size. Pheochromocytomas tend to be dense and vascular. Therefore, they often have high attenuation on unenhanced CT imaging (>10 Hounsfield units) or high contrast avidity (often with heterogeneous enhancement) on CT imaging done with intravenous contrast, as in this patient's case, or they have poor delayed contrast washout when CT imaging is performed with an adrenal washout protocol. On MRI, pheochromocytomas tend to display hyperintensity on T2-weighted imaging and have features suggestive of low lipid content (no loss of signal on out-of-phase sequences).

Extra-adrenal metastases to the adrenal gland (Answer D) should be considered in this case. Metastatic lesions are usually dense with an attenuation of greater than 10 Hounsfield units on unenhanced CT imaging, and they often present with unusual and infiltration contours. However, they would not be associated with marked elevations in metanephrines.

The constellation of biochemical and radiographic findings in this vignette argues against a benign or malignant adrenocortical neoplasm (Answers A and C). There is no biochemical evidence of aldosterone or cortisol excess (Answer B).

This patient underwent a laparoscopic right adrenalectomy after preoperative α-adrenergic blockade, and pathologic examination revealed a 3.5-cm pheochromocytoma. Postoperatively, he did report a marked improvement in his overall anxiety level, which he had previously considered to be normal.

Educational Objective
Diagnose pheochromocytoma on the basis of radiographic and biochemical characteristics, even if a patient does not have classic adrenergic symptoms or spells.

UpToDate Topic Review(s)
Clinical presentation and diagnosis of pheochromocytoma

Reference(s)

Lenders JW, Duh QY, Eisenhofer G, et al; Endocrine Society. Pheochromocytoma and paraganglioma: an Endocrine Society clinical practice guideline. *J Clin Endocrinol Metab*. 2014;99(6):1915-1942. PMID: 24893135

Fassnacht M, Arlt W, Bancos I, et al. Management of adrenal incidentalomas: European Society of Endocrinology clinical practice guideline in collaboration with the European Network for the Study of Adrenal Tumors. *Eur J Endocrinol*. 2016;175(2):G1-G34. PMID: 27390021

7 **ANSWER: D) Measure sodium again in 2 weeks**
Antiseizure medications can have profound effects on hormone replacement therapy used in hypopituitarism. This mandates an open line of communication between the endocrinologist prescribing hormonal therapies and the neurologist prescribing antiseizure drugs.

Carbamazepine and oxcarbazepine (a keto-derivate of carbamazepine) increase the sensitivity of the renal tubules to the effects of endogenous vasopressin and exogenous desmopressin. Indeed, these drugs are a known cause of syndrome of inappropriate antidiuretic hormone secretion in patients without pituitary disease. For this reason, the desmopressin requirements can be significantly reduced in patients with diabetes insipidus when one of these medications is started. Lamotrigine, perampanel, and felbamate can also enhance the effects of exogenous desmopressin and increase the subsequent potential risk of hyponatremia and water intoxication.

This patient's diabetes insipidus seems presently well controlled, and the fact that he experiences a daily polyuric phase is a good indicator that he is at low risk of developing hyponatremia. However, the addition of oxcarbazepine may enhance desmopressin's effect, placing him at higher risk of hyponatremia. Particular attention should be paid to elderly patients, especially those taking concomitant natriuretic drugs, because they are more likely to develop hyponatremia. A recent study documented that a significant percentage of patients with diabetes insipidus are overtreated and have frequent hyponatremia (27% with mild hyponatremia [sodium, 131-134 mEq/L (131-134 mmol/L)]; 14.6% with more significant hyponatremia [sodium $\leq$130 mEq/L ($\leq$130 mmol/L)]). In addition to the potential dangers of acute hyponatremia, chronic hyponatremia has been associated with subtle neurologic symptoms and increased risk of osteoporosis and fractures. Therefore, sodium measurement (Answer D) is the most important next step in this patient.

Oxcarbazepine does not affect the metabolism of hydrocortisone. Therefore, increasing the hydrocortisone dosage (Answer A) is not necessary. Oxcarbazepine and carbamazepine can increase the catabolism of levothyroxine, thereby reducing serum free T_4 and total T_4 (although to a much lesser degree than phenytoin), with variable effects on total T_3, free T_3, and thyroxine-binding globulin. Therefore, free T_4 should be measured about 1 month after starting the drug, but the risk of hyponatremia is a more urgent issue. Testosterone is only minimally influenced by oxcarbazepine (by an increase in sex hormone–binding globulin), but not by carbamazepine. Such effect is seen only at high oxcarbazepine dosages (>900 mg daily). Thus, decreasing the testosterone dosage (Answer B) is not necessary. While it may be indicated to repeat the testosterone measurement at some point, the desmopressin dosage is a more important issue. Measuring free T_4 and testosterone again in 2 weeks (Answer E) is an incorrect next step. Modification of the levothyroxine dosage (Answer C) should be guided by the free T_4 level and, if anything, the dosage will need to be increased, not decreased.

Educational Objective
Explain how some antiseizure medications can cause hyponatremia and water intoxication in patients on desmopressin by increasing the responsiveness of the renal collecting duct system to antidiuretic hormone.

UpToDate Topic Review(s)
Antiseizure drugs: mechanism of action, pharmacology, and adverse effects

Reference(s)

Paragliola RM, Prete A, Kaplan PW, Corsello SM, Salvatori R. Treatment of hypopituitarism in patients receiving antiepileptic drugs. *Lancet Diabetes Endocrinol.* 2015;3(2):132-140. PMID: 24898833

Behan LA, Sherlock M, Moyles P, et al. Abnormal plasma sodium concentrations in patients treated with desmopressin for cranial diabetes insipidus: results of a long-term retrospective study. *Eur J Endocrinol.* 2015;172(3):243-250. PMID: 25430399

Usala RL, Fernandez SJ, Mete M, et al. Hyponatremia is associated with increased osteoporosis and bone fractures in a large US health system population. *J Clin Endocrinol Metab.* 2015;100(8):3021-3031. PMID: 26083821

8 **ANSWER: B) Start a statin**
This patient is seeking advice on cardiovascular risk management. Her lipid panel is fairly unremarkable, but advanced lipoprotein testing obtained in view of her family history of atherosclerotic cardiovascular disease revealed elevated levels of lipoprotein (a).

The 2013 American College of Cardiology/American Heart Association guidelines for cholesterol lowering, which have been adopted widely in the United States, focus on global cardiovascular risk assessment. For primary prevention of atherosclerotic cardiovascular disease in adults, as in this patient, the cardiovascular risk calculator uses age, sex, race, systolic blood pressure, diabetes status, total cholesterol level, and HDL-cholesterol level as variables to calculate 10-year cardiovascular disease risk. Moderate- to high-intensity statin therapy is recommended for

10-year cardiovascular risk greater than 7.5%. This patient's calculated risk is less than 5% and she does not necessarily need to be treated. However, family history and other advanced lipid measurements are not considered in the risk calculator. This patient indeed has a strong family history of cardiovascular disease.

Lipoprotein (a) is characterized as an LDL-like particle in which apolipoprotein B is covalently bound by a single disulfide bond to apolipoprotein (a). It has high homology to plasminogen. Plasma concentrations of lipoprotein (a) are genetically determined and vary markedly among individuals. Lipoprotein (a) has a longer plasma residence time than LDL, and mechanisms by which lipoprotein (a) is cleared from the circulation are unclear. On average, persons of African descent have 2- to 3-fold higher lipoprotein (a) plasma concentrations than most persons of European and Asian descent. The exact physiologic function of lipoprotein (a) is still elusive, but it has been associated with wound healing and interaction with vascular wall matrix. Several lines of evidence, both epidemiologic and genetic, now conclusively suggest that lipoprotein (a) is independently associated with cardiovascular disease risk. This increased risk is irrespective of LDL concentration and increases linearly with increasing lipoprotein (a) concentration. Elevated lipoprotein (a) increases lifetime risk for myocardial infarction, stroke, and peripheral arterial disease. Genetic variation in the *LPA* gene is also strongly associated with aortic valve calcification and stenosis. For routine clinical care, currently available assays are considered fairly accurate for separating low-risk patients from high-risk patients. Because circulating lipoprotein (a) levels are genetically determined, there is little influence from diet and environment and plasma levels do not fluctuate significantly from a preset baseline over a lifetime.

Currently, there is no consensus on when to measure lipoprotein (a). Lipoprotein (a) measurement is not commonly included in routine testing. There is no clinical trial evidence supporting a decrease in cardiovascular risk with lipoprotein (a) reduction. No current therapies are approved to lower lipoprotein (a), and traditionally, clinicians treat to lower LDL cholesterol, not lipoprotein (a). Thus, whether lipoprotein (a) is a risk factor when LDL cholesterol is controlled or low as in the patient in this vignette is not known. Recent studies suggest that elevated lipoprotein (a) remains a risk factor even when LDL-cholesterol levels less than 70 mg/dL (<1.81 mmol/L) are achieved. Considering a patient-orientated approach, some authorities recommend lipoprotein (a) testing in certain clinical situations, such as in individuals with a personal or family history of premature coronary artery disease, in younger patients with recurrent cardiovascular events despite the use of high-intensity statins and good cardiovascular risk factor control, and in patients with familial hypercholesterolemia. In this patient, the history of cardiovascular disease in her father and uncle and valvular disease in her grandmother suggest the a predisposition for elevated lipoprotein (a), and treatment with an LDL-cholesterol–lowering agent, preferably statin therapy, is indicated (thus, Answer B is correct and Answer E is incorrect).

Aspirin (Answer A), an antiplatelet agent, has not been shown to be beneficial in individuals with elevated lipoprotein (a) levels. Among currently approved drugs, niacin (Answer C) and PCSK9 inhibitors (Answer D) can modestly lower lipoprotein (a) levels, but their use is limited.

Educational Objective
Manage increased cardiovascular risk in an individual with elevated lipoprotein (a) levels.

UpToDate Topic Review(s)
Lipoprotein (a) and cardiovascular disease

Reference(s)
Tsimikas S. A test in context: lipoprotein (a): diagnosis, prognosis, controversies, and emerging therapies. *J Am Coll Cardiol.* 2017;69(6):692-711. PMID: 28183512

Nordestgaard BG, Langsted A. Lipoprotein (a) as a cause of cardiovascular disease: insights from epidemiology, genetics, and biology. *J Lipid Res.* 2016;57(11): 1953-1975. PMID: 27677946

9 ANSWER: D) Start a third antihyperglycemic medication
The patient in this vignette has had type 2 diabetes for 8 years and is being treated with metformin and a thiazolidinedione. There is a discrepancy between his glycosylated hemoglobin and the glucose levels by fingerstick testing. The question is whether the hemoglobin A_{1c} or the fingerstick glucose results are more accurate.

Sickle cell trait is the most common hemoglobin variant in the United States and it affects between 8% and 10% of persons of African descent. Persons with sickle cell trait have 60% to 70% hemoglobin A and 30% to 40% hemoglobin S. It is theorized that patients with sickle cell trait have shortened red cell survival time, which results in less time for glycosylation of hemoglobin. This can lead to spuriously low hemoglobin A_{1c} levels in many African American patients who have sickle cell trait. A recent large retrospective trial reported that the hemoglobin A_{1c} level was lower at any concentration of fasting glucose or 2-hour glucose in patients with sickle cell trait compared with that in patients without sickle cell disease or sickle cell trait. Other conditions that shorten red cell survival, such as hemolytic anemia, recovery from acute blood loss, or stage IV or V chronic kidney disease, may also lead to spuriously low hemoglobin A_{1c} levels.

The hemoglobin A_{1c} value of 6.8% (51 mmol/mol), measured in this patient 2 weeks ago, is equivalent to an estimated average glucose level of 148.5 mg/dL (8.2 mmol/L), whereas the fingerstick glucose average of 187 mg/dL (10.4 mmol/L) is equivalent to a hemoglobin A_{1c} level of 8.1% (65 mmol/mol). In this case, the fingerstick glucose measurements are more accurate than the hemoglobin A_{1c}. The best next step in the management of this patient's diabetes is to refer him to a dietician for review of a diabetic meal plan and to start a third antihyperglycemic medication (Answer D). Referral for nutrition counseling alone (Answer E) is inadequate.

Ordering a complete blood cell count (Answer B) will most likely not provide any useful information given that the hemoglobin level was normal 9 months ago. Ordering hemoglobin electrophoresis (Answer C) is not necessary, as the patient has documented sickle cell trait and this testing will not help in diabetes management.

The patient started atorvastatin 3 months ago. Several large randomized controlled trials have shown that high-dosage treatment with statins such as atorvastatin (80 mg daily) or rosuvastatin (40 mg daily) can increase glucose levels more than moderate statin dosages. However, the cardiovascular risk reduction with these medications far outweighs any effect on elevated glucose levels. Therefore, stopping statin therapy in this case (Answer A) is not warranted.

In the future, management of this patient's diabetes should focus on fingerstick glucose values rather than hemoglobin A_{1c} measurement.

Educational Objective
Identify causes of spurious glycosylated hemoglobin readings.

UpToDate Topic Review(s)
Estimation of blood glucose control in diabetes mellitus

Reference(s)

International Expert Committee. International Expert Committee report on the role of the A1C assay in the diagnosis of diabetes. *Diabetes Care*. 2009;32(7): 1327-1334. PMID: 19502545

Lacy ME, Wellenius GA, Sumner AE, et al. Association of sickle cell trait with hemoglobin A1c in African Americans. *JAMA*. 2017;317(5):507-515. PMID: 28170479

Nathan DM, Kuenen J, Borg R, Zheng H, Schoenfeld D, Heine RJ; A1c-Derived Average Glucose Study Group. Translating the A1C assay into estimated average glucose values [published correction appears in *Diabetes Care*. 2009;32(1):207]. *Diabetes Care*. 2008;31(8):1473-1478. PMID: 18540046

Ridker PM, Pradhan A, MacFadyen JG, Libby P, Glynn RJ. Cardiovascular benefits and diabetes risks of statin therapy in primary prevention: an analysis from the JUPITER trial. *Lancet*. 2012;380(9841):565-571. PMID: 22883507

10 ANSWER: B) Measure free T_4

The clinical features of hyperthyroidism vary widely. Common symptoms include fatigue, anxiety, tremor, weight loss, palpitations, and heat sensitivity. Typical clinical signs include tachycardia, arrhythmia, and goiter. In patients with Graves disease, eye features such as soreness and grittiness, conjunctival and periorbital edema, proptosis, vision disturbance, and ophthalmoplegia may also be present. Studies have indicated a direct correlation between higher concentrations of circulating thyroid hormones and longer duration of Graves disease with more prominent clinical features. The influence of age on presentation of hyperthyroidism has also been evaluated in a number of studies. The largest study systematically evaluating the influence of a number of parameters on the clinical presentation of hyperthyroidism confirmed that patients older than 61 years presented with very few symptoms of hyperthyroidism. The prevalence of most typical symptoms was lower in this age group with the exception of weight loss and shortness of breath, which were more common in older persons. The risk of presenting with atrial fibrillation was increased in older patients, those with higher serum free T_4 concentrations, men, and patients with toxic nodular hyperthyroidism. Importantly, the relatively asymptomatic presentation of older patients with hyperthyroidism often results in delays in diagnosis and treatment, which leads to worse outcomes. Moreover, clinicians should be cautious not to automatically attribute symptoms to aging or other illnesses.

Life-threatening thyrotoxicosis or thyroid storm is a rare and potentially fatal complication of hyperthyroidism, and timely recognition and treatment is essential to reduce morbidity and mortality. This disorder is characterized by multisystem involvement, and mortality rates are as high as 8% to 25%, even in modern series. The Burch and Wartofsky Point Scale is a well-recognized diagnostic scoring system for thyroid storm. Criteria for diagnosis include hyperpyrexia, tachycardia, arrhythmias, congestive heart failure, agitation, delirium, psychosis, stupor, and coma, as well as nausea, vomiting, diarrhea, hepatic failure, and the presence of an identified precipitant. A total score of 45 points or higher is consistent with thyroid storm; 25 to 44 points is classified as impending thyroid storm, and fewer than 25 points makes thyroid storm unlikely. The American Thyroid Association guidelines provide a detailed overview of this point scale.

Apathetic hyperthyroidism is a rare presentation of thyroid storm that occurs most commonly in older persons, and apathy or coma is often the initial presentation. A diagnosis of thyroid storm could be easily missed in the patient in this vignette due to the apathetic presentation. However, her presentation scores more than 45 points on the Burch and Wartofsky Point Scale. The clinical features of tachycardia, weight loss, tremor, and goiter are consistent with a diagnosis of hyperthyroidism. While a suppressed serum TSH concentration may be a feature of nonthyroidal illness, it is pertinent to establish whether this patient has hyperthyroidism, so measurement of the serum free T_4 concentration (Answer B) is crucial. Thyroid ultrasonography (Answer E) can help identify the underlying etiology of hyperthyroidism, although this diagnosis must first be confirmed by free T_4 measurement. Measurement of serum cortisol (Answer A) can determine whether there is coexisting adrenal insufficiency, although her clinical presentation is not suggestive of this.

This patient is pyrexial and has a mildly elevated white blood cell count and C-reactive peptide level; therefore, a differential diagnosis of meningitis warranting a lumbar puncture (Answer D) should be considered. However, there is no neck stiffness, and the inflammatory indices would be expected to be higher if the patient had bacterial meningitis. The neurologic features in this patient are atypical and no clear pathology is identified on brain CT. Further evaluation with brain MRI (Answer C) may be informative if the neurologic features persist following restoration of euthyroidism.

Thyroid storm requires aggressive treatment including (1) therapy directed against thyroid hormone synthesis with antithyroid drugs and secretion with saturated solution of iodine; (2) measures directed against the peripheral action of thyroid hormone at the tissue level with β-adrenergic–blocking agents; (3) reversal of systemic decompensation; (4) treatment of the precipitating event or intercurrent illness; and (5) definitive therapy. Conversion of T_4 to T_3 is inhibited by the use of propylthiouracil, glucocorticoids, and β-adrenergic–blocking agents such as propranolol, with selective ability to inhibit type 1 deiodinase.

Educational Objective
Diagnose apathetic thyroid storm.

UpToDate Topic Review(s)
Thyroid storm

Reference(s)

Boelaert K, Torlinska B, Holder RL, Franklyn JA. Older subjects with hyperthyroidism present with a paucity of symptoms and signs: a large cross-sectional study. *J Clin Endocrinol Metab.* 2010;95(6):2715-2726. PMID: 20392869

Yang SP, Wu PH, Tey BH, Tan CK. A patient with thyroid storm presenting with apathetic thyrotoxicosis and features of meningoencephalitis. *Thyroid.* 2011;61 (6):675-678. PMID: 21449770

Ross DS, Burch HB, Cooper DS, et al. 2016 American Thyroid Association guidelines for diagnosis and management of hyperthyroidism and other causes of thyrotoxicosis. *Thyroid.* 2016;26(10):1343-1420. PMID: 27521067

11 ANSWER: B) Total testosterone by liquid chromatography–tandem mass spectrometry

How best to assess a patient's androgen status is an area of uncertainty in many respects. Free testosterone represents 1% to 4% of circulating testosterone with the remainder bound to SHBG, albumin, corticosteroid-binding globulin, and orosomucoid. SHBG is a homodimer that is produced in the liver, as well as locally in tissues such as the testes, uterus, and brain. SHBG contains 2 binding sites for sex hormones (testosterone and estrogen) and has a high binding affinity for testosterone. In contrast, albumin, corticosteroid-binding globulin, and orosomucoid have a low binding affinity for testosterone. The high concentration of albumin allows it to buffer fluctuations in testosterone levels. Orosomucoid is an acute-phase reactant, with its circulating concentrations increasing during infection. Bioavailable testosterone refers to the testosterone not bound to SHBG, namely albumin bound and free.

There is debate over what constitutes the biologically active fraction of circulating testosterone. One theory is that only free testosterone can diffuse into cells to exert a biologic effect. Another theory is that testosterone bound to albumin can dissociate in tissue capillaries to become biologically active. Yet a third theory is that testosterone bound to SHBG enters cells via endocytosis through a membrane protein called megalin.

The accuracy of various testosterone assays varies widely and is particularly important when measuring low levels of testosterone as seen in children, women, and severely hypogonadal men such as the patient in this vignette. For this reason, the Endocrine Society recommends measuring total testosterone by liquid chromatography–tandem mass spectrometry (LC-MS/MS) (Answer B). Automated immunoassays for total testosterone (Answer C) either overestimate or underestimate total testosterone when compared with (LC-MS/MS). Equilibrium dialysis (Answer A) is a technique used to measure free testosterone. In this technique, free testosterone equilibrates across a semipermeable membrane, whereas the bound testosterone cannot. Although free testosterone by equilibrium dialysis has been considered a gold standard for measurement, it is technically difficult, expensive, and not easily automated to run large numbers of samples. An analogue immunoassay for the measurement of free testosterone (Answer D) is incorrect, as commercially available kits for these assays are often inaccurate. In addition to using free testosterone assays, free testosterone can also be calculated with one of several formulas or calculations such as those by Vermeulen and Sodergard. These calculations should be based on an accurate measurement of total testosterone in addition to SHBG and albumin. Ammonium sulfate precipitation (Answer E) is a technique used to measure bioavailable testosterone as opposed to free testosterone.

The patient in this vignette turned out to have hypogonadotropic hypogonadism. He had a normal sense of smell and a normal 46,XY karyotype.

Educational Objective

Select the most accurate testosterone assay to assess androgen levels in patients with suspected low levels such as women, children, and severely hypogonadal men.

UpToDate Topic Review(s)

Clinical features and diagnosis of male hypogonadism

Reference(s)

Goldman AL, Bhasin S, Wu FCW, Krishna M, Matsumoto AM, Jasuja R. A reappraisal of testosterone's binding in circulation: physiological and clinical implications. *Endocr Rev.* 2017;38(4):302-324. PMID: 28673039

Matsumoto AM, Bremner WJ. Serum testosterone assays--accuracy matters. *J Clin Endocrinol Metab.* 2004;89(2):520-524. PMID: 14764756

12 ANSWER: E) Perform a transiliac bone biopsy

The woman described in this vignette has abnormally low bone mineral density for her age and gender, history of a wrist fracture, and end-stage renal disease. While this may be consistent with osteoporosis, one must consider renal osteodystrophy in such a scenario. Renal osteodystrophy refers to alterations in bone histology associated with chronic kidney disease and is one component of the entity chronic kidney disease–mineral and bone disorder (CKD-MBD), which also includes laboratory abnormalities of secondary hyperparathyroidism (increased PTH, increased fibroblast growth factor 23, decreased calcitriol, phosphate retention, and hypocalcemia), as well as extraskeletal calcification. The table lists the 4 main subtypes of renal osteodystrophy and provides an example of how the histologic classification differs among these forms based on the TMV (turnover/mineralization/volume) classification system.

Form of Renal Osteodystrophy	Turnover	Mineralization	Volume
Adynamic bone disease	Low	Normal	Low-normal
Osteitis fibrosa cystica	High	Normal	Variable
Osteomalacia	Low	Abnormal	Low-normal
Mixed uremic osteodystrophy	High	Abnormal	Normal

This patient's PTH level is only mildly elevated (<100 pg/mL), with a normal bone-specific alkaline phosphatase level, which should raise concern for underlying adynamic bone disease. Adynamic bone disease is the most common form of renal osteodystrophy observed in patients undergoing dialysis. Bone turnover is markedly reduced, with reduced osteoblast and osteoclast activity. This is typically due to an oversuppression of PTH release induced by the use of relatively high dosages of calcium-based phosphate binders and active vitamin D analogues, as well as possibly due to skeletal resistance to the effect of PTH. The initial treatment of adynamic bone disease is to allow the PTH level to rise by reducing the dosage of active vitamin D analogues and using non–calcium-containing phosphate binders rather than calcium-containing phosphate binders. Bone biopsy (Answer E), which is the gold standard for the diagnosis and classification of renal osteodystrophy, would be the best next step at this time to guide this patient's management. Other indications for bone biopsy include unexplained bone pain or fractures and progressive decreases in bone mineral density despite standard therapy. The most commonly used site for a bone biopsy is the anterior iliac crest because it is easily accessible and associated with the fewest complications. Before performing the transiliac bone biopsy, double-labeling of the bone with tetracycline should be completed to allow for calculation of kinetic indices of bone turnover.

Starting an antiresorptive agent (Answers A and B) to treat osteoporosis before excluding the other forms of renal osteodystrophy (such as adynamic bone disease) would not be appropriate now, as this would exacerbate low bone turnover. It is also important to keep in mind that there are no prospective data showing efficacy of any of the approved pharmacologic agents to treat osteoporosis in patients on hemodialysis, which renders this treatment off-label. In addition, one must remember that bisphosphonates (Answer A) are renally excreted and that denosumab (Answer B) may induce significant hypocalcemia in patients with renal impairment. The anabolic agent teriparatide (Answer C) may benefit patients with adynamic bone disease, but its use is still considered experimental for this indication. Furthermore, it is contraindicated in this patient with a history of radiation therapy to the skeleton. Finally, measurement of serum C-telopeptide (Answer D), which is a biochemical marker of bone resorption, is not recommended in patients with kidney disease. In addition to the analytic and biologic variability related to the measurement of this bone turnover marker, its clinical usefulness is significantly limited in the setting of CKD since it is cleared by the kidney.

Educational Objective
Explain the importance of bone biopsy in the evaluation of patients with low bone mineral density in the setting of end-stage renal disease before recommending therapeutic intervention.

UpToDate Topic Review(s)
Bone biopsy and the diagnosis of renal osteodystrophy
Overview of chronic kidney disease-mineral and bone disorder (CKD-MBD)

Reference(s)
Moe S, Drueke T, Cunningham J, et al; Improving Global Outcomes (KDIGO). Definition, evaluation, and classification of renal osteodystrophy: a position statement from Kidney Disease: Improving Global Outcomes (KDIGO). *Kidney Int.* 2006;69(11):1945-1953. PMID: 16641930

Miller PD. The role of bone biopsy in chronic renal failure. *Clin J Am Soc Nephrol.* 2008;3(Suppl 3):S140-S150. PMID: 18988699

Miller PD. Diagnosis and treatment of osteoporosis in chronic renal disease. *Semin Nephrol.* 2009;29(2):144-155. PMID: 19371805

Ketteler M, Block GA, Evenepoel P, et al. Executive summary of the 2017 KDIGO Chronic Kidney Disease-Mineral and Bone Disorder (CKD-MBD) Guideline Update: what's changed and why it matters. *Kidney Int.* 2017;92(1):26-36. PMID: 28646995

Isakova T, Nickolas TL, Denburg M, et al. KDOQI US Commentary on the 2017 KDIGO Clinical Practice Guideline Update for the Diagnosis, Evaluation, Prevention, and Treatment of Chronic Kidney Disease-Mineral and Bone Disorder (CKD-MBD). *Am J Kidney Dis.* 2017;70(6):737-751. PMID: 28941764

13 ANSWER: B) Discontinue all diabetes medications and order a nutrition consult

This patient has 2 current issues: an acute hypoglycemic event, most likely due to his sulfonylurea combined with poor food intake, and malnutrition. Discontinuing glyburide alone (Answer C) will not address the malnutrition. Malnutrition is surprisingly common in hospitalized patients with type 2 diabetes, especially in elderly patients. A number of tools are available to screen for malnutrition in the office or hospital. Most malnutrition screening tools evaluate whether the patient has:

- Recent weight loss: how much and over what period?
- Reduced appetite?

If both questions are answered affirmatively, the patient has a low BMI, and the physical examination shows muscle atrophy, the patient most likely has malnutrition. The current patient reports a 20-lb (9.1-kg) weight loss and no urge to eat. On physical examination, he is thin and cachectic and has poor muscle mass. His BMI is low. On the basis of these findings, he has severe malnutrition. His suspected depression most likely contributed to his weight loss, but his weight loss and poor appetite preceded the death of his spouse by 3 months. This finding should compel the clinician to search for another underlying cause.

Metformin reduces appetite in many patients. An unpleasant metallic taste in the mouth is described as a possible adverse effect. The mechanism appears to be mediated via the central nervous system, as rats injected with metformin into the lateral ventricle have reduced food consumption. Severe weight loss and anorexia are rare complications of metformin therapy, but it is noted to be a medication that can cause unintentional weight loss in older adults.

Wong et al describe 3 elderly patients with type 2 diabetes, all of whom presented with anorexia and unexplained weight loss. Extensive evaluations for malignancy and malabsorption were negative in all patients. The authors found that discontinuing metformin therapy resulted in return of appetite and weight regain in these 3 patients, suggesting that metformin was the cause of the unexplained weight loss.

Reducing the dosage of the metformin/glyburide combination (Answer A) or changing to metformin alone (Answer C) may not resolve the weight loss. Because the patient has some impairments in activities of daily living (eg, dressing and bathing), the target hemoglobin A_{1c} level should be less than 8.0% (<64 mmol/mol). On the basis of this target, it is premature to determine whether he requires any other diabetes medications such as an SGLT-2 inhibitor (Answer D) or a DPP-4 inhibitor (Answer E). The best choice is to discontinue all diabetes medications and request a nutritional assessment (Answer B). A plan for replenishing his protein and calorie deficit can then be initiated. Once his depression is addressed and he starts eating a healthful diet, the clinician can determine whether diabetes medication is needed.

Educational Objective
Manage malnutrition in an elderly patient with type 2 diabetes mellitus.

UpToDate Topic Review(s)
Treatment of type 2 diabetes mellitus in the older patient

Reference(s)

American Diabetes Association. 11. Older adults: standards of medical care in diabetes-2018. *Diabetes Care.* 2018;41(Suppl 1):S119-S125. PMID: 29222382

Lee CK, Choi YJ, Park SY, Kim JY, Won KC, Kim YW. Intracerebroventricular injection of metformin induces anorexia in rats. *Diabetes Metab J.* 2012;36(4): 293-299. PMID: 22950061

Stajkovic S, Aitken EM, Holroyd-Leduc J. Unintentional weight loss in older adults [published correction appears in *CMAJ.* 2011;183(8):935]. *CMAJ.* 2011; 183(4):443-449. PMID: 21324857

McMinn J, Steel C, Bowman A. Investigation and management of unintentional weight loss in older adults. *BMJ.* 2011;342:d1732. PMID: 21447571

Wong LL, Wong TC. Metformin induced anorexia and weight loss. *Hawaii Med J.* 2003;62(5):104-105. PMID: 12806790

14 **ANSWER: B) Sertraline**

The key to answering this question is to recognize that this patient has night eating syndrome (NES). NES is an eating disorder characterized by 2 or more episodes per week of eating after awakening from sleep or by excessive food consumption after the evening meal. Patients with NES have morning anorexia (usually skip breakfast), and they eat at least 25% of their daily calories after dinner. The prevalence of NES is 1.5% in the general population and up to 16% in obese individuals. Patients with NES have a delay in the circadian rhythm of food intake and usually have sleep disturbances such as insomnia or difficulty initiating or maintaining sleep. Such patients are aware of the eating episodes and this distinguishes them from patients with sleep-related eating disorder, as the latter group is unaware of nocturnal eating episodes. Patients with NES feel they have no control over their eating pattern and often experience shame about their condition. Tools used to screen for this eating disorder include self-report questionnaires such as the Night Eating Questionnaire.

Both nonpharmacologic (cognitive behavioral therapy) and pharmacologic therapies (selective serotonin reuptake inhibitors) are used to treat affected patients. Cognitive behavioral therapy for NES includes information on sleep hygiene, self-monitoring of eating habits, exercise, and relaxation strategies. Among selective serotonin reuptake inhibitors, sertraline (Answer B) has been the most studied drug in this setting. Small clinical trials have shown that patients treated with sertraline have a decrease in the number of awakenings, nocturnal food intake, and ingestion of food after the evening meal, as well as a 6.6- to 11-lb (3-to 5-kg) weight loss. Frequently, patients benefit from simultaneous nonpharmacologic and pharmacologic therapy. Other pharmacologic options currently being studied include topiramate and agomelatine. Weight-loss medications (Answers A, C, E) would not be beneficial now, as this patient needs treatment for NES. Tricyclic antidepressants (Answer D) have not been studied in this population. Sleep-related eating disorder is treated with benzodiazepines, mood stabilizers, or dopaminergic medications.

Educational Objective

Diagnose night eating syndrome and recommend appropriate treatment.

UpToDate Topic Review(s)

Eating disorders: Overview of epidemiology, clinical features, and diagnosis

Reference(s)

Cleator J, Abbott J, Judd P, Sutton C, Wilding JP. Night eating syndrome: implications for severe obesity. *Nutr Diabetes.* 2012;2:e44. PMID: 23446659

Kucukgoncu S, Midura M, Tek C. Optimal management of night eating syndrome: challenges and solutions. *Neuropsychiatr Dis Treat.* 2015;11:751-760. PMID: 25834450

Pinto TF, Silva FG, Bruin VM, Bruin PF. Night eating syndrome: how to treat it? *Rev Assoc Med Bras.* 1992;2016;62(7):701-707. PMID: 27925052

15 **ANSWER: E) No treatment required**

Central diabetes insipidus is a common complication of pituitary surgery or head trauma. Under these circumstances, the incidence of central diabetes insipidus ranges from 10% to 20% and can be as high as 60% to 80% after removal of very large tumors. The rate is lower with minimally invasive endoscopic pituitary surgery.

Typically, postoperative diabetes insipidus is transient and becomes a permanent phenomenon only in a minority of cases (0.5%-15%). It is characterized by the passing of large volumes (usually in excess of 3 L per day) of dilute urine (<200 mOsm/kg). The development of postoperative diabetes insipidus is usually early, occurring within the first 24 to 48 hours after surgery. It is important, however, to consider other causes of postoperative polyuria under these circumstances such as hyperglycemia (due to parenteral steroids) or excessive intraoperative or postoperative fluid administration.

The syndrome of inappropriate antidiuretic hormone secretion (SIADH) is another relatively common complication after neurosurgery. Sometimes this can be part of a classic triphasic response to surgery: an initial polyuric phase with inhibition of antidiuretic hormone release due to hypothalamic damage, followed by SIADH due to the slow release of antidiuretic hormone by the degenerating posterior pituitary, and then permanent diabetes insipidus after posterior pituitary antidiuretic hormone stores are depleted. However, more commonly, SIADH occurs independently from transient or permanent diabetes insipidus. In this situation, there is a significant risk of hyponatremia, which can be severe.

This vignette describes a typical case of central diabetes insipidus that has developed soon after pituitary surgery. However, the patient has a normal plasma sodium concentration, and the polyuria is not profound. Given that postoperative diabetes insipidus is very often transient, it is very important not to overtreat to minimize the risk of severe hyponatremia if the subsequent SIADH phase were to occur.

In this scenario, the patient is able to match fluid intake with losses and, as a result, has a normal serum sodium level and normal osmolality. In addition, the urine output remains less than 250 mL/h. Under these circumstances, it is reasonable to not administer synthetic vasopressin and to continue to monitor fluid balance, serum electrolytes, and serum and urine osmolality (Answer E). Administration of synthetic vasopressin (Answers A, B, and C) in this situation would lead to a significantly increased risk of more profound hyponatremia if SIADH were to subsequently develop.

However, if the patient had more significant polyuria (>250 mL/h), had an elevated serum sodium level, or could not match fluid intake with output, then administration of synthetic vasopressin would be indicated. However, this should be given only in single doses and not prescribed as a regular medication (Answer C), as diabetes insipidus is likely to be transient and there is a significant risk of hyponatremia. Thus, the optimal method of synthetic vasopressin administration under these circumstances is as a single subcutaneous injection (Answer A) with a further dose only if symptoms recur or persist. While intranasal desmopressin (Answer B) is a common method of managing permanent diabetes insipidus over the long term, it is not appropriate in this patient who has just undergone transsphenoidal surgery.

Reduced fluid intake or fluid restriction (Answer D) is a reasonable treatment strategy for the management of mild to moderate hyponatremia due to SIADH. However, the presented scenario is consistent with diabetes insipidus and not yet SIADH.

Educational Objective
Determine when and how to best treat diabetes insipidus occurring after pituitary surgery.

UpToDate Topic Review(s)
Clinical manifestations and causes of central diabetes insipidus

Reference(s)

Woodmansee WW, Carmichael J, Kelly D, Katznelson L; AACE Neuroendocrine and Pituitary Scientific Committee. American Association of Clinical Endocrinologists and American College of Endocrinology Disease State Clinical Review: postoperative management following pituitary surgery. *Endocr Pract.* 2015;21(7):832-838. PMID: 26172128

Seckl J, Dunger D. Postoperative diabetes insipidus. *BMJ.* 1989;298(6665):2-3. PMID: 2492841

16 **ANSWER: C) Cancellation of pituitary surgery until the results of serum TSH measurement are available**
Several aspects of this patient's case require attention before pituitary surgery is considered. First, if the patient is presumed to have a prolactinoma, dopamine agonist therapy rather than surgery would be the recommended therapy. Second, the magnitude of the prolactin elevation is in the range where other causes of the prolactin elevation (eg, medications or "stalk effect") should be considered. Third, although the patient has pituitary enlargement on MRI, no discrete adenoma is actually visualized. These are all reasons to cancel surgery and reevaluate the situation.

In addition, several clues in this patient's presentation should lead to consideration of a diagnosis of hypothyroidism. The patient has a goiter and several symptoms and physical examination findings suggestive of hypothyroidism. In fact, additional aspects of this case could also be explained by hypothyroidism. As a result of the high TSH levels being produced in response to primary hypothyroidism, hyperplasia of the pituitary thyrotropes can occur. This can lead to pituitary enlargement as shown in the image. In this situation, hyperprolactinemia may also occur. The causes of this are 2-fold. The pituitary hypertrophy can lead to pressure on the pituitary stalk and impaired delivery of dopamine to the anterior pituitary, with resultant prolactin elevation (the so-called "stalk effect"). Additionally, primary hypothyroidism may result in high levels of thyrotropin-releasing hormone, which then stimulate prolactin production.

Because this patient has findings suggestive of hypothyroidism, she should not undergo transsphenoidal surgery without excluding the possibility of primary hypothyroidism (thus, Answer A is incorrect and Answer C is correct). Initiation of levothyroxine is indicated if the patient is proven to have hypothyroidism, but as this would cause regression of pituitary hyperplasia, there would no longer be a need to consider pituitary surgery (thus, Answer D is incorrect). A dopamine agonist is the preferred therapy for a prolactin-secreting pituitary adenoma. However, if primary hypothyroidism is confirmed in this patient, dopamine agonist therapy is not indicated. Such therapy would normalize the prolactin without having an effect on the pituitary hypertrophy, which would only be reversed by thyroid hormone (thus, Answer E is incorrect). Rapid shrinkage of the pituitary can occur within as few as 6 days of initiating levothyroxine, with normalization of pituitary contours within 4 weeks to several months.

In a patient found to have elevated serum TSH in the setting of an enlarged pituitary, the diagnosis of a TSH-secreting pituitary adenoma may also be entertained. However, this diagnosis would be accompanied by symptoms and signs of hyperthyroidism, rather than hypothyroidism. In addition, the thyroid hormone levels would be low in the setting of primary hypothyroidism and high in the setting of a TSH-secreting pituitary adenoma. If a thyrotropin-releasing hormone stimulation test (Answer B) were performed, the response would be blunted in a patient with a TSH-secreting pituitary adenoma, but vigorous in primary hypothyroidism. However, this stimulation test is not required given that the thyroid hormone levels and constellation of symptoms should be sufficient for distinguishing these disorders.

The patient in this vignette did in fact have primary hypothyroidism, and her symptoms, signs, hyperprolactinemia, and pituitary hyperplasia all regressed with initiation of thyroid hormone therapy. The "before and after" images are from a case of pituitary hypertrophy associated with hypothyroidism reported in the literature. The image to the right demonstrates resolution of the pituitary enlargement following treatment of her hypothyroidism. Similar findings were seen in the patient reported in this vignette.

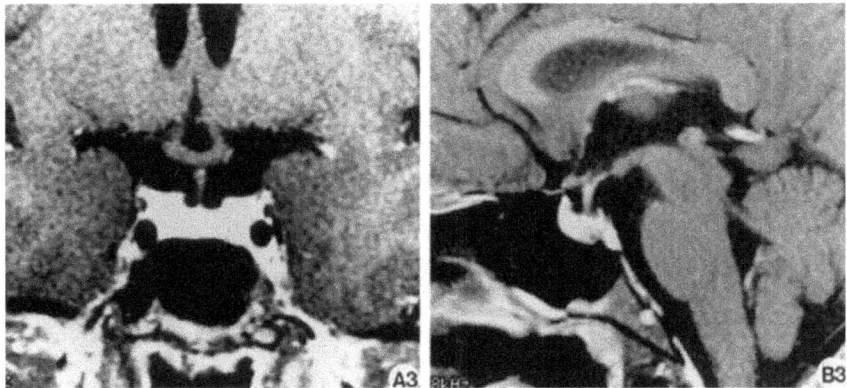

Reprinted from Sarlis NJ, Brucker-Davis F, Doppman JL, Skarulis MC. MRI-demonstrable regression of a pituitary mass in a case of primary hypothyroidism after a week of acute hormone therapy. *J Clin Endocrinol Metab.* 1997;82(3):808-811.

Educational Objective

Describe the potential presentation of untreated hypothyroidism with a goiter, hyperprolactinemia, and pituitary hyperplasia.

UpToDate topic review(s)
Clinical manifestations of hypothyroidism

Reference(s)

Joshi AS, Woolf PD. Pituitary hyperplasia secondary to primary hypothyroidism: a case report and review of the literature. *Pituitary.* 2005;8(2):99-103. PMID: 16195776

Passeri E, Tufano A, Locatelli M, Lania AG, Ambrosi B, Corbetta S. Large pituitary hyperplasia in severe primary hypothyroidism. *J Clin Endocrinol Metab.* 2011;96(1):22-23. PMID: 21209043

Sarlis NJ, Brucker-Davis F, Doppman JL, Skarulis MC. MRI-demonstrable regression of a pituitary mass in a case of primary hypothyroidism after a week of acute thyroid hormone therapy. *J Clin Endocrinol Metab.* 1997;82(3):808-811. PMID: 9062487

17 ANSWER: D) Review the DXA images to ensure valid assessment of the hip regions of interest

The proper acquisition and analysis of bone mineral density images is critical to the optimal management of patients with osteoporosis and other metabolic bone disease. Without the review of image data or access to the highest quality DXA interpretation, the clinician is basically "driving blind" in the care of such patients, especially given the high prevalence of errors in bone density testing and reporting. Specific attention to maintaining the regions of interest between baseline and follow-up DXA scans is essential to determining whether a significant change in bone mineral density has indeed occurred that would influence management decisions (Answer D).

In this patient, inconsistency in the region of interest of the right hip has yielded an apparent significant change in bone mineral density at the total hip. The region of interest numbers reflect the horizontal (first number) and vertical (second number) dimensions in millimeters of the scanned skeletal region. Specifically, the images shown (*see figures*) reveal changes in the regions of interest (108 x 136 vs 100 x 127) that disparately include a greater amount of femoral bone mineral density in the intertrochanteric region in the 2015 scan compared with the 2016 scan (*see difference in yellow shaded regions*). This makes it appear as though there was significant loss of bone mineral density at the right total hip. Importantly, the femoral neck bone mineral density is essentially unchanged between scans. It is important to note that there are intermanufacturer differences in the display of DXA regions of interest.

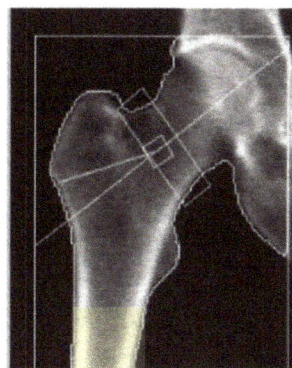 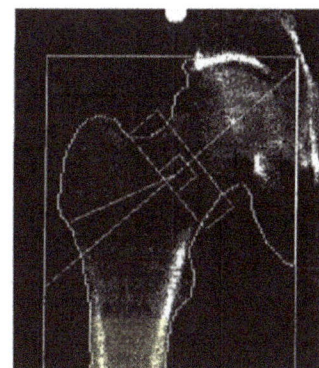

2015 scan   **2016 scan**

108 x 136   100 x 127
Neck: 49 x 15   Neck: 49 x 15

2015 scan

Region	Area, cm^2	BMD, g/cm^2	T-Score
Neck	5.80	0.582	−2.6
Troch	10.24	0.650	−1.0
Inter	30.91	1.064	−0.7
Total	46.96	0.914	−0.8

2016 scan

Region	Area, cm^2	BMD, g/cm^2	T-Score
Neck	5.76	0.595	−2.5
Troch	11.24	0.607	−1.3
Inter	26.69	0.999	−1.1
Total	43.70	0.845	−1.2

Given that the patient's hip and spine bone mineral density (not shown) are stable, and in light of his continued low absolute risk of fracture by FRAX calculation (National Osteoporosis Foundation treatment threshold recommendations for 10-year risk of hip and major osteoporotic fracture are 3% and 20%, respectively), pharmacologic antifracture therapy with an anabolic agent (Answer A) or an oral bisphosphonate (Answer B) is not indicated. Repeating the DXA scan (Answer C) to verify that a significant change in bone mineral density has occurred is reasonable, but it is indicated only if the baseline and follow-up scan have been properly performed and analyzed with comparable regions of interest, which is not the case in this vignette. Indeed, incorporation of another DXA scan of specific sites that exhibit greater than 10% decline between studies to confirm change is a reasonable practice for scans that are technically valid. Finally, repeating laboratory studies in the secondary evaluation of osteoporosis (Answer E) is not indicated or cost effective in this patient's clinical management.

Educational Objective

Explain the importance of region of interest change in DXA measurements of the proximal femur and the impact it can have on osteoporosis management.

UpToDate Topic Review(s)

Overview of dual-energy x-ray absorptiometry

Reference(s)

Messina C, Bandirali M, Sconfienza LM, et al. Prevalence and type of errors in dual-energy x-ray absorptiometry. *Eur Radiol.* 2015;25(5):1504-1511. PMID: 25428701

Lewiecki EM, Binkley N, Morgan SL, et al; International Society for Clinical Densitometry. Best practices for dual-energy x-ray absorptiometry measurement and reporting: International Society for Clinical Densitometry Guidance. *J Clin Densitom.* 2016;19(2):127-140. PMID: 27020004

18 ANSWER: A) Add liraglutide

Patients with type 2 diabetes are at increased risk for fractures. Direct effect of hyperglycemia on bone metabolism, effects of medications used for blood glucose management, and diabetes complications leading to increased risk of falls are all thought to contribute to this increased risk. As in the general population, there is an inverse correlation between bone mineral density and fracture risk in patients with diabetes. The FRAX score appears to underestimate the fracture risk in patients with type 2 diabetes. This has prompted some to suggest that type 2 diabetes should be included in the FRAX risk calculator.

A recent clinical practice guideline reviews medications and surgical intervention and effect on bone mineral density and fracture risk, although data in this area of study are limited. Observational studies suggest that metformin may have a beneficial effect on bone mineral density and fracture risk. In the Osteoporotic Fractures in Men study, older men with type 2 diabetes who were taking sulfonylureas had an increased fracture risk; however, other studies have shown beneficial or neutral effects on fracture risk and neutral effects on bone mineral density. The authors do note that sulfonylureas and insulin must be used with caution to avoid hypoglycemia, falls, and fractures.

Thiazolidinediones (Answer D) reduce bone mineral density and increase fracture risk in women and should be avoided in those at high fracture risk. Canagliflozin (Answer B) appears to decrease bone mineral density and increase fracture risk. Neither DPP-4 inhibitors (Answer C) nor GLP-1 receptor agonists (Answer A) have negative effects on bone mineral density or fracture, and both may be a reasonable choice from a bone health perspective. However, the hemoglobin A_{1c} reduction required in this patient exceeds the 0.5% expected from use of DPP-4 inhibitors. Liraglutide would be expected to reduce hemoglobin A_{1c} by 1% to 1.5% and is therefore the better choice.

This patient's hemoglobin A_{1c} level is significantly above normal, she has no complications from diabetes, renal function is normal, and she has no history of hypoglycemia, Thus, tighter hemoglobin A_{1c} control is reasonable despite her history of osteoporosis. Simply continuing her current regimen (Answer E) is incorrect.

Educational Objective
Recommend the best treatment approach for type 2 diabetes mellitus in a patient with osteoporosis.

UpToDate Topic Review(s)
Bone disease in diabetes mellitus

Reference(s)

Paschou SA, Dede AD, Anagnostis PG, Vryonidou A, Morganstein D, Goulis DG. Type 2 diabetes and osteoporosis: a guide to optimal management. *J Clin Endocrinol Metab.* 2017;102(10):3621-3634. PMID: 28938433

Giangregorio LM, Leslie WD, Lix LM, et al. FRAX underestimates fracture risk in patients with diabetes. *J Bone Miner Res.* 2012;27(2):301-308. PMID: 22052532

19 ANSWER: E) Increase the testosterone dosage

In this case, masculinizing hormone therapy induced cessation of menstrual bleeding within the expected time frame of the first 6 months on testosterone. Persistent or recurrent uterine bleeding should be evaluated for structural and nonstructural causes similar to the evaluation in a cisgender woman. For transgender patients, consideration of patient comfort and dysphoria might lead to selection of different exam and imaging techniques—for example, choosing transabdominal instead of transvaginal ultrasonography.

Management strategies for persistent or recurrent uterine bleeding in transgender men should also take into account patient preference and tolerance for different hormonal options. In cisgender women, use of oral estrogen (Answer A) can more rapidly stop abnormal uterine bleeding. However, this option would most likely worsen this patient's dysphoria.

Progesterone (Answer B)—orally, injected, implanted, or by intrauterine system—would be another option to stop bleeding, and the injected or intrauterine device forms would also provide contraceptive benefit, as ovulation can still occur despite male physiologic testosterone levels. A levonorgestrel-releasing intrauterine device would be a good option to decrease bleeding and induce amenorrhea, but it was not provided as a choice. The copper intrauterine device (Answer D) would not induce amenorrhea and could be associated with abnormal or heavy uterine bleeding.

Testosterone injections administered subcutaneously are just as effective as intramuscular dosing in achieving therapeutic concentrations in cisgender men with hypogonadism and in transgender men. Advantages to subcutaneous dosing include decreased anxiety and less pain during and after the injection. Subcutaneous doses are initiated at 50% of doses used intramuscularly (50 mg instead of 100 mg weekly and 100 mg instead of 200 mg every 2 weeks). Switching to the intramuscular route (Answer C) might not necessarily increase testosterone concentrations in this patient unless the dosage were increased as well.

Higher testosterone dosages and shorter intervals between doses are correlated with faster time to amenorrhea when initiating masculinizing therapy. Interestingly, physiologic male testosterone concentrations and low estradiol levels are not requirements for the development of amenorrhea. Increasing this patient's testosterone dosage (Answer E) has the added benefit of improving gender dysphoria (compared with progesterone [Answer B]). With the midpeak testosterone concentrations on the low end of the male reference range, the best choice in this case would be to increase the testosterone dosage.

Educational Objective

Counsel transgender men taking masculinizing hormone therapy regarding management options for persistent or recurrent uterine bleeding.

UpToDate Topic Review(s)

Transgender men: Evaluation and management

Reference(s)

Deutsch MB. *Guidelines for the Primary and Gender-Affirming Care of Transgender and Gender Nonbinary People.* 2nd ed. Center of Excellence for Transgender Health, Department of Family and Community Medicine, University of California San Fransisco. June 2016. Available at www.transhealth.ucsf.edu/guidelines.

Hembree WC, Cohen-Kettenis PT, Gooren L, et al. Endocrine treatment of gender-dysphoric/gender-incongruent persons: an Endocrine Society Clinical Practice Guideline. *J Clin Endocrinol Metab.* 2017;102(11):3869-3903. PMID: 28945902

20 ANSWER: A) Referral for adrenalectomy

The radiographic characteristics of an adrenal mass are critical in evaluating whether the mass is benign or potentially malignant. Reassuring features that are suggestive of a benign adrenal mass include small size (generally <4 cm), round and uniform shape, homogenous appearance, and high lipid content (such as low attenuation on unenhanced CT [<10 Hounsfield units] or loss of signal on out-of-phase sequencing on MRI), and high contrast washout on delayed contrast CT imaging. Features that raise concern for a malignant process include larger size (generally >4 or 6 cm), irregular shape or contours, heterogeneous content, calcifications, low lipid content on CT or MRI, and poor washout on delayed contrast CT imaging. A benign pheochromocytoma may have poor lipid content and poor washout on delayed contrast CT imaging, but it generally presents with a round contour and shape and with substantial elevations in metanephrines.

The initial characteristics of this patient's mass on enhanced CT were concerning because the mass was medium-to-large (just under 4 cm) and had an irregular shape. The subsequent imaging confirmed reasons for concern since the unenhanced CT attenuation was 23 Hounsfield units, suggesting a lipid-poor mass, and there was high avidity for contrast on a washout protocol. Benign adrenal neoplasms generally display greater than 60% absolute and greater than 40% relative washout of contrast on 15-minute delayed CT imaging. The most concerning potential diagnosis in this case is a primary adrenal malignancy, such as an adrenocortical carcinoma.

The role of adrenal biopsy is limited to 2 scenarios: (1) confirmation of an extra-adrenal metastasis to determine staging and consequent management and (2) confirmation of an invasive infectious infiltration of the adrenal glands. Both scenarios can be either unilateral or bilateral processes. The absence of a known history of, or risk for, extra-adrenal malignancy makes an adrenal metastasis unlikely in this patient. There is no reason to suspect an infiltrating fungal or tuberculous infection based on the current history. Therefore, biopsy was not indicated for this patient. The use of a biopsy to confirm an adrenocortical carcinoma is not recommended, in part because of the theoretical risk for seeding the malignant tumor in the needle track, but also because of the risk of false-negative results. Adrenocortical carcinomas can be large and heterogeneous, and sampling of a small segment can show normal-appearing tissue that provides false reassurance. Thus, repeated biopsy in 1 year (Answer D) is incorrect.

In this vignette, the best management would be to proceed with a radical adrenalectomy (Answer A) to conduct a cancer-focused surgery with planned lymphadenectomy for a presumptive adrenocortical carcinoma. Given the concern for a primary adrenal malignancy, delayed imaging surveillance (Answer C) or proceeding with no surveillance (Answer E) is not reasonable. The results of the dexamethasone suppression test already suggest that this is a nonfunctional tumor, and further assessment of cortisol (Answer B) is not likely to change this interpretation or influence the ultimate management decision.

This patient's biopsy result inappropriately provided reassurance to her providers that the tumor was benign, even though the radiographic characteristics were concerning for a malignancy. One year later, the patient's imaging showed that the tumor had grown by 1 cm and a surgical resection was performed, which revealed a high-grade stage II adrenocortical carcinoma.

Educational Objective
Determine the malignant potential of an adrenal mass on the basis of radiographic characteristics and explain the role of adrenal biopsy.

UpToDate Topic Review(s)
Clinical presentation and evaluation of adrenocortical tumors

Reference(s)
Fassnacht M, Arlt W, Bancos I, et al. Management of adrenal incidentalomas: European Society of Endocrinology clinical practice guideline in collaboration with the European Network for the Study of Adrenal Tumors. *Eur J Endocrinol*. 2016;175(2):G1-G34. PMID: 27390021

21   ANSWER: B) Mammography
This patient is wondering whether he may have a pituitary tumor given a low testosterone level and a family history of a pituitary tumor. An appropriate way to address his concern is to explain why a pituitary tumor is unlikely given a lack of relevant symptoms (headache, galactorrhea, visual field deficits) and the normal values of free T_4 and gonadotropins. Ordering additional laboratory tests to assess for hypopituitarism (Answer A) or a subset of pituitary tumors (Answer E) would be low yield. Although some clinicians might be inclined to order a pituitary MRI (Answer C) to placate the patient or to rule out a pituitary tumor, it would not be clinically indicated and is not a cost-effective use of health care resources. Appropriate settings in which to order pituitary imaging include persistent hyperprolactinemia, symptoms of a pituitary tumor due to mass effect, or confirmed secondary hypogonadism with total testosterone concentrations less than 150 ng/dL (<5.2 nmol/L).

The patient is self-conscious about the appearance of his chest. Distinguishing between gynecomastia and pseudogynecomastia on physical examination can be difficult. Pseudogynecomastia refers to subareolar fat without actual glandular breast tissue. It is commonly seen in overweight and obese men. Gynecomastia is typically located under the nipple-areola complex in a concentric pattern and may be unilateral or bilateral. Given the patient's concern and uncertain findings on physical examination, ordering mammography (Answer B) is the best next step in his management. Whether he has gynecomastia or pseudogynecomastia, cessation of marijuana should be discussed, as it has been associated with gynecomastia.

His borderline serum total testosterone concentration is most likely attributable to his overweight status or normal variability. Normal testicular volumes and gonadotropins rule out primary hypogonadism. Ordering testicular ultrasonography (Answer D) is not clinically indicated given normal testicular volumes, normal gonadotropins, and no abnormalities noted on physical examination.

Educational Objective
Determine when it is appropriate to order pituitary MRI in the evaluation of hypogonadism and distinguish between gynecomastia and pseudogynecomastia.

UpToDate Topic Review(s)
Clinical features and diagnosis of male hypogonadism
Clinical features, diagnosis, and evaluation of gynecomastia in adults

Reference(s)

Bhasin S, Brito JP, Cunningham GR, et al. Testosterone therapy in men with hypogonadism: an Endocrine Society clinical practice guideline. *J Clin Endocrinol Metab.* 2018;103(5):1715-1744. PMID: 29562364

Braunstein GD. Clinical practice. Gynecomastia. *N Engl J Med.* 2007;357(12):1229-1237. PMID: 17881754

22 ANSWER: B) Antiinsulin receptor antibodies

This patient exhibits extreme insulin resistance, often described functionally as a requirement of greater than 200 units or 3 units/kg of insulin per day. Common causes of insulin resistance are obesity, pregnancy, exposure to excess glucocorticoids, acromegaly, and underlying metabolic stressors such as infection. In most circumstances, the etiology is unknown. This patient has several unusual features, namely substantially increased insulin requirements, extensive acanthosis, and low levels of serum triglycerides. A rare cause of severe insulin resistance is an autoimmune condition in which antibodies to the insulin receptor develop (Answer B), known as type B insulin resistance. Affected persons are typically middle-aged, nonobese black women with acanthosis nigricans, and they often have other rheumatologic conditions. In typical cases of severe insulin resistance, one might expect to see elevated triglyceride levels. But in cases of type B insulin resistance, interestingly, serum triglyceride levels are low, as in the described patient. Similarly, circulating levels of the adipokine adiponectin, which often varies inversely with insulin sensitivity, are lower than anticipated for the degree of insulin resistance.

While there are reports of antiinsulin antibodies (Answer A) being associated with severe insulin resistance, this is more rare than the classic type B insulin resistance, especially when use of animal insulins is excluded. It appears that antiinsulin antibodies as a cause of severe insulin resistance may occur equally in patients with type 1 or type 2 diabetes. Aside from a male predominance, few distinguishing features exist. Interestingly, patients with antiinsulin antibodies may have worse outcomes than those with classic type B insulin resistance and still require insulin after treatment with immunosuppressive regimens, presumably due to the underlying diagnosis of diabetes.

Regarding partial lipodystrophy (Answer D), one would expect triglycerides to be elevated. Also, loss of fat in a specific distribution was not described on physical examination, making this diagnosis unlikely. While infection (Answer C) can exacerbate hyperglycemia in patients with diabetes, it would not explain the underlying cause of diabetes in this patient. Occult malignancy (Answer E) would not explain this clinical presentation.

Type B insulin resistance is important to recognize, as it is associated with high mortality—as high as 54% in one series. The National Institutes of Health has reported a protocol involving rituximab, cyclophosphamide, and dexamethasone followed by maintenance azathioprine that is associated with long-term remission of diabetes and freedom from insulin requirement.

Educational Objective

Identify severe insulin resistance and the clinical and laboratory findings that suggest type B insulin resistance as a cause.

UpToDate Topic Review(s)
Insulin resistance: Definition and clinical spectrum

Reference(s)

Semple RK, Cochran EK, Soos MA, et al. Plasma adiponectin as a marker of insulin receptor dysfunction: clinical utility in severe insulin resistance. *Diabetes Care.* 2008;31(5):977-979. PMID: 18299442

Flier JS, Kahn CR, Roth J, Bar RS. Antibodies that impair insulin receptor binding in an unusual diabetic syndrome with severe insulin resistance. *Science.* 1975; 190(4209):63-65. PMID: 170678

Arioglu E, Andewelt A, Diabo C, Bell M, Taylor SI, Gorden P. Clinical course of the syndrome of autoantibodies to the insulin receptor (type B insulin resistance): a 28-year perspective. *Medicine (Baltimore).* 2002;81(2):87-100. PMID: 11889410

Malek R, Chong AY, Lupsa BC, et al. Treatment of type B insulin resistance: a novel approach to reduce insulin receptor autoantibodies. *J Clin Endocrinol Metab.* 2010;95(8):3641-3647. PMID: 20484479

23 ANSWER: B) Perform fasting lipid testing after a 10- to 12-hour fast at the end of shift

Historically, a fasting lipid panel has been used for assessment of atherosclerotic cardiovascular disease risk. The Friedewald formula developed in the 1970s allows for estimation of LDL-cholesterol levels by correcting for nonfasting changes in plasma triglycerides. This equation estimates LDL cholesterol after measuring total cholesterol, HDL cholesterol, and triglycerides, and then subtracting from the total cholesterol concentration the HDL cholesterol plus VLDL cholesterol, which is estimated by triglycerides divided by 5. The formula is not used when plasma triglycerides are greater than 400 mg/dL (>4.52 mmol/L) because in this setting VLDL particles contain relatively less cholesterol and the calculated LDL-cholesterol value is falsely low.

The significance of fasting vs nonfasting is that food consumption results in variable increases in plasma triglycerides, with contributions from both dietary fat and carbohydrate. Carbohydrate intake increases VLDL triglyceride secretion within 30 to 90 minutes after ingestion, whereas fat ingestion increases plasma triglycerides via chylomicron assembly and secretion from the small intestine over an interval up to 8 hours. Even in the fasting state, triglycerides are subject to substantial biologic variability (~30%). Since LDL cholesterol is a calculated number, the value can be inaccurate after food intake.

Large epidemiologic studies have established the power to predict cardiovascular disease by the use of nonfasting triglycerides. The Copenhagen City Heart Study has demonstrated that elevated nonfasting triglycerides are associated with an increased risk of myocardial infarction, ischemic heart disease, and death in men and women. A meta-analysis of 29 prospective studies has shown that fasting and nonfasting triglycerides are similarly predictive of fatal and nonfatal coronary events. Results from the Women's Health Study suggest that triglycerides measured 2 to 4 hours postprandially might be a better predictor of cardiovascular disease than fasting triglycerides.

In certain countries, especially in Europe, nonfasting lipid profiles have become the norm. The argument for a nonfasting lipid measurement is that it allows patients to eat normally before blood sampling and allows physicians to determine the lipid profile at any random moment. This may prevent long waiting times for venipunctures in the early morning.

Nevertheless, it is important to focus on the question to be answered with the lipid panel results. For assessment of initial cardiovascular risk for primary prevention in an untreated individual, fasting or nonfasting states are acceptable. If there is a family history of a genetic hyperlipidemia or premature atherosclerotic cardiovascular disease, a fasting lipid panel is recommended to distinguish the nature of the underlying lipid disorder. To assess patients at risk for or who have pancreatitis, fasting lipids can help evaluate whether hypertriglyceridemia is the cause. In this vignette, limited family history is available before the visit. The patient already had a nonfasting panel in the past 6 months, which revealed moderate hypertriglyceridemia. Another lipid panel with a sample drawn in the nonfasting state (Answer A) is unnecessary. For further risk stratification, a fasting lipid panel is needed (Answer B). While this patient will eventually need therapy for moderate hyperlipidemia, there are insufficient clinical data to initiate therapy at this time (thus, Answers C, D, and E are incorrect).

Educational Objective
Explain the utility of assessing lipid values from samples drawn in a fasting vs nonfasting state.

UpToDate Topic Review(s)
Measurement of blood lipids and lipoproteins

Reference(s)

Driver SL. Fasting or nonfasting lipid measurement: it depends on the question. *J Am Coll Cardiol.* 2016;67(10):1227-1234. PMID: 26965545

Nordestgaard BG. A test in context: lipid profile, fasting versus Nonfasting. *J Am Coll Cardiol.* 2017;70(13):1637-1646. PMID: 28935041

24 ANSWER: B) Liraglutide

This middle-aged man has a longstanding history of diabetes and has suboptimal glycemic control. Given his comorbidities, an appropriate hemoglobin A_{1c} goal is in the 7.5% range (58 mmol/mol). He should be referred to a nutritionist to review a diabetic meal plan, and a third antiglycemic medication should be started to improve glucose control. Options include basal insulin (not listed as a choice in this vignette), a thiazolidinedione, a DPP-4 inhibitor, a GLP-1 receptor agonist, an SGLT-2 inhibitor, or an α-glucosidase inhibitor.

Liraglutide (Answer B) is the best treatment option listed in this vignette. Liraglutide has been shown to reduce cardiovascular events in a large randomized controlled trial of patients with type 2 diabetes who had at least 1 additional cardiovascular risk factor or coexisting coronary artery disease (LEADER Trial). After a mean follow-up of 3.8 years, the primary endpoint of a composite of death from cardiovascular causes, nonfatal myocardial infarction, or nonfatal stroke occurred in significantly fewer patients in the liraglutide-treated group (hazard ratio, 0.87; 95% confidence interval, 0.78-0.97) than in the placebo group. GLP-1 receptor agonists can be safely used in patients with stage 3 chronic kidney disease, as long as renal function is monitored. Liraglutide should be potent enough to achieve the hemoglobin A_{1c} goal set for this patient.

When used as add-on therapy for patients with type 2 diabetes, DPP-4 inhibitors such as saxagliptin (Answer C) lower hemoglobin A_{1c} by 0.5% to 0.7% and would not be potent enough to adequately lower this patient's glucose levels.

Pioglitazone (Answer A) is a treatment option. However, the patient has significant pedal edema and a history of diastolic dysfunction. Thiazolidinediones are relatively contraindicated under these circumstances.

In a large randomized controlled trial, patients with type 2 diabetes mellitus and increased cardiovascular risk or a history of coronary heart disease (CANVAS trial) were randomly assigned to canagliflozin (Answer D) or placebo. The primary outcome was a composite of death from cardiovascular cause, nonfatal myocardial infarction, or nonfatal stroke. After a mean of 3.6 years, the hazard ratio was 0.86 (95% confidence interval, 0.75-0.97; $P < .001$ for noninferiority; $P = .02$ for superiority) in the patients assigned treatment with canagliflozin vs the placebo-treated group. Secondary analysis revealed a lower rate of hospitalization for treatment of heart failure in the patients treated with canagliflozin (hazard ratio, 0.67; 95% confidence interval, 0.52-0.97). A second trial with canagliflozin (CANVAS-Renal or CANVAS-R) demonstrated a decrease in the composite outcome of a 40% reduction in the estimated glomerular filtration rate, the need for renal replacement treatment, or death from renal causes (hazard ratio, 0.60; 95% confidence interval, 0.47-0.77) compared with the placebo-treated group.

An unexpected outcome of the combined analysis of the CANVAS and CANVAS-R trials was that canagliflozin doubled the risk of lower-limb amputation in patients with type 2 diabetes. This risk has not been demonstrated in large randomized controlled trials with other SGLT-2 inhibitors. An analysis of the US FDA Adverse Event Reporting System (FAERS) reported on 66 cases of amputations in patients treated with SGLT-2 inhibitors through March 31, 2017. Use of canagliflozin was reported in 86% of the cases. On average, the patients who required amputation were 60 years or older and most cases were reported in men. Toe amputations were the most common type, but above ankle or lower-limb amputations were also reported. In a significant number of cases in this series, altered foot anatomy, lower-limb ischemia, or diabetic foot wounds were also documented. The patient in this vignette has a Charcot joint involving the left foot, peripheral neuropathy, and peripheral arterial disease. Canagliflozin is relatively contraindicated given the increased risk for amputation.

Acarbose (Answer E), an α-glucosidase inhibitor, is another treatment option, but it would not be the best choice in this case. Use of acarbose is limited by gastrointestinal adverse effects such as excess gas, diarrhea, and abdominal pain. These symptoms usually prevent titration of the drug, and glucose-lowering effects are therefore limited.

Although this patient has stage 3 chronic kidney disease, continuing metformin should be safe as long as kidney function is monitored.

Educational Objective
Describe the glycemic benefit and the adverse effects and potential complications of each class of antihyperglycemic medication.

UpToDate Topic Review(s)
Management of persistent hyperglycemia in type 2 diabetes mellitus

Reference(s)

Neal B, Perkovic V, Mahaffey KW, et al; CANVAS Program Collaborative Group. Canagliflozin and cardiovascular and renal events in type 2 diabetes. *N Engl J Med*. 2017;377(7):644-657. PMID 28605608

Fadini GP, Avogaro A. SGLT2 inhibitors and amputations in the US FDA Adverse Event Reporting System. *Lancet Diabetes Endocrinol*. 2017;5(9):680-681. PMID: 28733172

Marso SP, Daniels GH, Brown-Frandsen K, et al; LEADER Steering Committee; LEADER Trial Investigators. Liraglutide and cardiovascular outcomes in type 2 diabetes. *N Engl J Med*. 2016;375(4):311-322. PMID: 27295427

25 ANSWER: C) Measure GH after an oral glucose load

Surgery is the first-line therapy for acromegaly unless there are obvious contraindications or the adenoma is not surgically resectable. Surgery can provide permanent cure and avoid the need for lifetime medical treatment. Most studies have shown that the cure rate in acromegaly depends on the size and location of the adenoma. For microadenomas and intrasellar macroadenomas without cavernous sinus invasion, such as the one described here, the cure rate in the hands of an experienced pituitary neurosurgeon is greater than 70%. Several studies have shown that the surgeon's experience in pituitary surgery increases the cure rate and reduces the complication rate. Therefore, it is the job of the endocrinologist to know the neurosurgeon's experience and outcomes and to refer a patient with surgically curable disease to a neurosurgeon who is experienced in pituitary surgery.

While the decline of GH in patients with surgically cured acromegaly is very rapid (and patients often notice reduced hand swelling within 1 to 2 days), it may take several months for serum IGF-1 to normalize. The reason for this observation is not completely clear. This patient has noted symptomatic improvement, and his IGF-1 level 12 weeks after surgery has declined significantly compared with his presurgical level, albeit not yet reaching the normal range. His random GH level is nondiagnostic. At this point, it is important to determine whether he is fully cured. Therefore, measuring a nadir GH following an oral glucose load (Answer C) is the best next step. If his GH suppression is normal (<0.4 ng/mL with modern assays), he can be reassured and told that his IGF-1 level will very likely normalize in the next few months. Some studies have shown that the degree of suppression may also help predict the risk of recurrence, with the lowest risk if GH suppresses to less than 0.14 ng/mL.

If the GH value after an oral glucose load suppresses to less than 0.4 ng/mL, there is no need to perform pituitary MRI or to refer him back to neurosurgery (Answer A). Similarly, cabergoline or somatostatin analogues (Answers B and D) are possible therapies for active acromegaly (with response rates of about 20% and 50%, respectively), but they would be considered only if the patient has not been cured by surgery. IGFBP-3 (Answer E) is a GH-dependent protein that binds to IGF-1 in a ternary complex with acid-labile subunit. Although its levels are higher in acromegaly, at this point, there is no evidence that it is useful in determining whether a patient with acromegaly is cured by surgery.

Educational Objective

Recommend GH measurement following an oral glucose load as the gold standard to determine whether a patient with acromegaly has been cured by surgery.

UpToDate Topic Review(s)
Treatment of acromegaly

Reference(s)

Nomikos P, Buchfelder M, Fahlbusch R. The outcome of surgery in 668 patients with acromegaly using current criteria of biochemical 'cure'. *Eur J Endocrinol.* 2005;152(3):379-387. PMID: 15757854

Ahmed S, Elsheikh M, Stratton IM, Page RC, Adams CB, Wass JA. Outcome of transphenoidal surgery for acromegaly and its relationship to surgical experience. *Clin Endocrinol (Oxf).* 1999;50(5):561-567. PMID: 10468920

Giustina A, Chanson P, Bronstein MD, et al; Acromegaly Consensus Group. A consensus on criteria for cure of acromegaly. *J Clin Endocrinol Metab.* 2010;95(7): 3141-3148. PMID: 20410227

Shin MS, Yu JH, Choi JH, et al. Long-term changes in serum IGF-1 levels after successful surgical treatment of growth hormone-secreting pituitary adenoma. *Neurosurgery.* 2013;73(3):473-479. PMID: 23728452

Kinoshita Y, Tominaga A, Usui S, et al. Clinical features and natural course of acromegaly in patients with discordance in the nadir GH level on the oral glucose test and the IGF-1 value at 3 months after adenomectomy. *Neurosurg Rev.* 2016;39(2):313-318. PMID: 26785642

26 ANSWER: C) Measure urinary metanephrine in 6 months

The patient in this vignette has had a good surgical outcome so far. He has no clinical, biochemical, or radiologic evidence of recurrent pheochromocytoma. The major learning point from this case is that unlike most other solid-organ tumors, the histopathology of pheochromocytoma does not reliably predict malignant potential, meaning that patients require long-term (usually lifelong) follow-up by regular assessment of metanephrine production (Answer C). If a genetic cause for pheochromocytoma had been found (as is now the case in at least 20%

of pheochromocytomas and up to 40% of paragangliomas), then regular MRI imaging (every 2 to 3 years) would also be indicated, as well as biochemical follow-up.

In 2002, the Pheochromocytoma of the Adrenal Gland Scaled Score (PASS) was introduced as part of histopathologic assessment. PASS examines histopathologic parameters such as vascular, capsular, or periadrenal adipose tissue invasion; necrosis; high cellularity; cellular monotony; >3 mitoses/10 per high-power field; atypical mitotic figures; nuclear pleomorphism; and hyperchromasia. Using this tool, it was proposed that a score of 4 or more was predictive of the likelihood of malignancy. The tumor described in this vignette would score at least 4 according to this scale (although there is insufficient information in the histopathology report to give a final PASS score), which suggests an increased malignant potential. However, this scoring system lacks reliability and sensitivity. According to the 2004 World Health Organization assessment criteria, metastatic spread is the only reliable indicator of malignancy in pheochromocytoma/paraganglioma. There is currently no evidence of this in the vignette. Moreover, the Ki67 index is relatively low at 2.5% (>3% is more suggestive of higher-grade activity).

^{131}I-MIBG radionuclide therapy (Answer A) and platinum-based adjuvant chemotherapy (Answer D) are therapeutic options for malignant pheochromocytoma but they are not appropriate in this case where there is no evidence of malignant disease.

Chromogranins (designated as A, B, and C) are proteins that are stored and released with peptides and amines in a variety of neuroendocrine tissues, including the adrenal medulla. Pheochromocytoma can be associated with elevated blood concentrations of chromogranin A (Answer B), which increases with larger tumor burden. However, this is not a diagnostic or screening test for pheochromocytoma, as it lacks sufficient sensitivity in comparison with urinary metanephrines and would not be appropriate as a means of follow-up in this case.

While ^{123}I-MIBG scintigraphy (Answer E) is a legitimate imaging modality for pheochromocytoma (particularly if metastatic disease is suspected), the optimal follow-up for this patient is regular biochemical screening by measurement of either urine or plasma metanephrines. Only if this screening is abnormal would further imaging be indicated. It should also be noted that 50% of anatomically normal adrenal glands demonstrate significant MIBG avidity, leading to misinterpretation.

Educational Objective
Explain the pitfalls in histopathology reporting of pheochromocytoma and recognize that the presence of distant metastases is the only reliable method of identifying malignant disease.

UpToDate Topic Review(s)
Treatment of pheochromocytoma in adults

Reference(s)

Thompson LD. Pheochromocytoma of the Adrenal Gland Scaled Score (PASS) to separate benign from malignant neoplasms. *Am J Surg Path*. 2002;26(5):551-566. PMID: 11979086

Lenders JW, Duh QY, Eisenhofer G, et al; Endocrine Society. Pheochromocytoma and paraganglioma: an Endocrine Society Clinical Practice Guideline. *J Clin Endocrinol Metab*. 2014;99(6):1915-1942. PMID: 24893135

27 ANSWER: D) Thymoma
The thymus is a specialized organ in the immune system whose primary function is to educate T cells. Thymomas are uncommon neoplasias derived from the epithelial cells of the thymus. They are the most common mediastinal mass in adults, representing up to 50% of anterior mediastinal masses. The most common autoimmune condition associated with thymoma is myasthenia gravis, which may improve or remit following thymectomy. Thymoma has also been associated with other autoimmune diseases, including autoimmune thyroid diseases, pure red-cell aplasia, systemic lupus erythematosus, pemphigus, rheumatoid arthritis, and autoimmune hepatitis. In a series of 85 cases of thymoma, autoimmune thyroid disease was the second most commonly associated autoimmune condition following myasthenia gravis. Links with both Hashimoto thyroiditis and Graves disease have been described, which occur in 2% to 4% and 5% to 8% of patients with myasthenia gravis, respectively. Importantly, the association with thymic hyperplasia and thymoma is particularly strong in patients with coexisting thyroid autoimmunity and myasthenia gravis. The thymic hyperplasia seen in patients with Graves disease has both a

thyroid hormone–dependent and immunologic pathogenesis caused in part by activation of TSH receptors in thymic cells. Rarely, malignant thymic tumors have been found in patients with Graves disease.

The patient in this vignette presents with typical features of thyrotoxicosis. The clinical and biochemical findings are consistent with a diagnosis of Graves thyrotoxicosis, and the technetium scan provides further confirmation. The chest CT shows a large, homogeneous, noncystic, anterior mediastinal mass without calcification and not invading adjacent structures, which is most likely caused by a thymoma (Answer D).

The differential diagnosis includes lymphoma (Answer A), and the patient's symptoms could be consistent with this. However, the absence of lymphadenopathy elsewhere, either clinically or on CT, and the normal lactate dehydrogenase concentration indicate that this diagnosis is less likely. The differential diagnosis of a well-demarcated mediastinal mass should include the possibility of a germinoma (Answer B), although typically there would be variable attenuation on the CT scan consistent with different tissues: fat, water-density cystic spaces, fat-fluid levels, homogeneous soft-tissue density, and calcification. Moreover, the normal β-hCG concentration would argue against this diagnosis. The presence of ectopic thyroid tissue (Answer E) in the mediastinum is a possible cause, but this would be identified on the technetium scan, which shows diffuse thyroid uptake only. Ectopic parathyroid tissue (Answer C) may occur in the mediastinum, although the size of the mass and the normal serum calcium concentration are not consistent with this diagnosis.

In many cases, the discovery of an anterior mediastinal mass prompts surgical resection via median sternotomy. If such a mass is found in association with Graves disease, then further evaluation with CT scanning is warranted. If suspicious radiologic features such as inhomogeneity, calcification, or invasion into surrounding structures are present, further evaluation with MRI or thymic biopsy may be indicated. If suspicion for malignancy is low and findings are consistent with thymic hyperplasia in the context of Graves disease, then it is reasonable to treat the thyrotoxicosis for 6 months before repeating the imaging. In most cases, there will 50% or more regression in area or volume of the thymic hyperplasia if euthyroidism is achieved and often surgical resection is not needed. If significant regression is not seen after 6 months of euthyroidism, thymic biopsy could be considered, even when the index of suspicion for malignancy is low.

Educational Objective
Explain the association between Graves disease and thymoma.

UpToDate Topic Review(s)
Clinical presentation and management of thymoma and thymic carcinoma

Reference(s)

Bernard C, Frih H, Pasquet F, et al. Thymoma associated with autoimmune diseases: 85 cases and literature review. *Autoimmun Rev.* 2016;15(1):82-92. PMID: 26408958

Haider U, Richards P, Gianoukakis AG. Thymic hyperplasia associated with Graves' disease: pathophysiology and proposed management algorithm. *Thyroid.* 2017;27(8):994-1000. PMID: 28578595

28   ANSWER: B) Polycystic ovary syndrome

This patient presents with secondary amenorrhea. Premature ovarian insufficiency (Answer A) is diagnosed by the presence of elevated FSH and low estradiol. Instead, this patient has a profile of FSH and estradiol concentrations that could be considered normal. However, she failed to have withdrawal bleeding with progesterone therapy, and pelvic ultrasonography demonstrates a uterine lining less than 4 mm. Both of these findings are more suggestive of secondary hypogonadism. In some cases, there can be overlap in the presentations of functional hypothalamic amenorrhea (Answer C) and polycystic ovary syndrome (Answer B). An initial suggestion of functional hypothalamic amenorrhea might evolve into a presentation of androgen excess and anovulatory cycles with recovery of the hypothalamic-pituitary-gonadal axis. Because both conditions are diagnosed based on excluding other potential causes, further evaluation was indicated before initiating therapy.

An elevated LH-to-FSH ratio is not diagnostic of polycystic ovary syndrome, but it can be suggestive of or consistent with LH-driven excess androgen production. Androstenedione and antimullerian hormone concentrations were both elevated in this patient. Androstenedione is a precursor for estrogens and androgens that can originate from either the ovary or adrenal gland and be converted to DHEA or testosterone in the periphery and target tissues (*see figure*).

Antimullerian hormone is secreted by antral follicles in the ovary and is a measure of ovarian reserve in ovulatory women. It tends to be elevated or on the higher end of normal in women with polycystic ovary syndrome. Taken together, the evidence in this case is suggestive of polycystic ovary syndrome rather than secondary hypogonadism. Metformin was prescribed for this patient, which can increase ovulatory frequency, even in lean women with polycystic ovary syndrome. Within

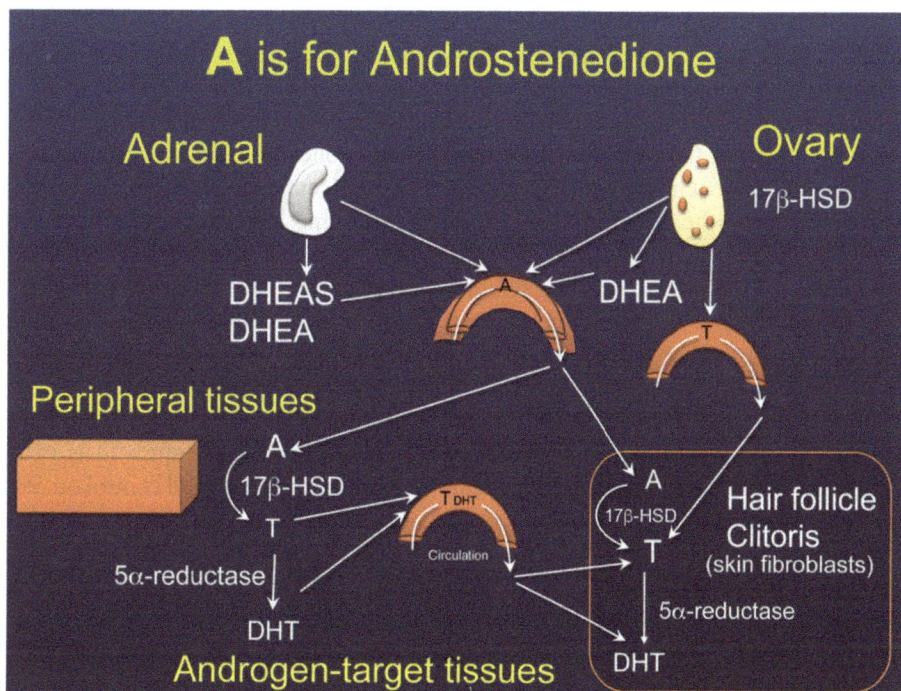

A is for Androstenedione

3 months, she reported a withdrawal bleed and resumed monthly menses. With this diagnosis, she preferred to restart oral contraceptives for birth control, and metformin was discontinued.

Asherman syndrome (Answer E) describes amenorrhea resulting from intrauterine adhesions or fibrosis of the endometrium associated with a uterine procedure, such as dilation and curettage, uterine infection, or severe postpartum hemorrhage. This patient has no history of pelvic procedures, infection, or pregnancy.

Empty sella syndrome describes the appearance of a flattened pituitary gland on the floor of the sella, and in some cases the pituitary might not be visible. In partial empty sella syndrome (Answer D), the pituitary gland is more visible within the sella. The patient's MRI shows a normal-sized and normally enhancing pituitary gland within the sella.

Educational Objective
Distinguish between polycystic ovary syndrome and hypothalamic amenorrhea in a woman with secondary amenorrhea.

UpToDate Topic Review(s)
Diagnosis of polycystic ovary syndrome in adults
Functional hypothalamic amenorrhea: Evaluation and management

Reference(s)

Gordon CM, Ackerman KE, Berga SL, et al. Functional hypothalamic amenorrhea: an Endocrine Society Clinical Practice Guideline. *J Clin Endocrinol Metab*. 2017;102(5):1413-1439. PMID: 28368518

Legro RS, Arslanian SA, Ehrmann DA, et al; Endocrine Society. Diagnosis and treatment of polycystic ovary syndrome: an Endocrine Society Clinical Practice Guideline. *J Clin Endocrinol Metab*. 2013;98(12):4565-4592. PMID: 24151290

Wang JG, Lobo RA. The complex relationship between hypothalamic amenorrhea and polycystic ovary syndrome. *J Clin Endocrinol Metab*. 2008;93(4):1394-1397. PMID: 18230664

29   ANSWER: D) Start rhPTH (1-84) injections once daily
The patient described in this vignette has permanent postsurgical hypoparathyroidism currently treated with calcium and active vitamin D supplementation. In patients with chronic hypoparathyroidism, the goals of therapy are to relieve symptoms and maintain the serum calcium concentration in the mildly low to low-normal

range, while avoiding hyperphosphatemia and hypercalciuria (defined as a 24-hour urinary calcium excretion >300 mg or more than 4 mg/kg). Patients with chronic hypoparathyroidism excrete more calcium than normal persons at the same serum calcium concentration due to the lack of the effect of PTH at the kidney level. The reason to avoid complete correction of hypocalcemia in such patients is that this would typically lead to worsening hypercalciuria with the potential of causing kidney stones or other kidney disease.

Since this patient has chronic symptomatic hypocalcemia, not changing her current medications to address this (Answer E) would be incorrect. She is already exhibiting hypercalciuria on her current replacement regimen; therefore, increasing the calcitriol dosage (Answer A) or elemental calcium intake (Answer B) would not be appropriate, as this would only worsen the hypercalciuria. Increasing the calcitriol dosage (Answer A) can also be associated with worsening hyperphosphatemia, because active vitamin D therapy also increases intestinal phosphate absorption. Starting a phosphate-binding agent (Answer C) would be helpful to treat hyperphosphatemia, but it would not correct her symptomatic hypocalcemia or hypercalciuria.

In 2015, the US FDA approved recombinant human PTH (1-84) for the management of chronic hypoparathyroidism not well controlled with conventional therapy. Approved as an adjunct to calcium and vitamin D, rhPTH (1-84) is recommended for patients who cannot achieve good control on conventional therapy alone. Use of rhPTH (1-84) injections once daily (Answer D) is effective in reducing the dosages of oral calcium and active vitamin D supplementation in patients with hypoparathyroidism while maintaining stable serum calcium levels within the normal range. Similar to teriparatide or PTH (1-34), rhPTH (1-84) has a black box warning for osteosarcoma, as this has also been observed in rat studies with rhPTH (1-84). This medication is only available through a restricted program under a Risk Evaluation and Mitigation Strategy (REMS). Prescribers are required to complete an online or paper-based training process (available at http://www.natpararems.com), after which they will become certified and enrolled in the REMS Program. Prescribers must also counsel patients on the benefits and risks of rhPTH (1-84) before initiating treatment.

Educational Objective
Recommend PTH replacement therapy as an adjunct to calcium and vitamin D to control hypocalcemia in a patient with postsurgical hypoparathyroidism.

UpToDate Topic Review(s)
Hypoparathyroidism

Reference(s)

Shoback D. Clinical practice. Hypoparathyroidism. *N Engl J Med*. 2008;359(4):391-403. PMID: 18650515

Mannstadt M, Clarke BL, Vokes T, et al. Efficacy and safety of recombinant human parathyroid hormone (1-84) in hypoparathyroidism (REPLACE): a double-blind, placebo-controlled, randomised, phase 3 study [published correction appears in *Lancet Diabetes Endocrinol*. 2014;2(1):e3]. *Lancet Diabetes Endocrinol*. 2013;1(4):275-283. PMID: 24622413

Bilezikian JP, Brandi ML, Cusano NE, et al. Management of hypoparathyroidism: present and future. *J Clin Endocrinol Metab*. 2016;101(6):2313-2324. PMID: 26938200

Marcucci G, Della Pepa G, Brandi ML. Drug safety evaluation of parathyroid hormone for hypocalcemia in patients with hypoparathyroidism. *Expert Opin Drug Saf*. 2017;16(5):617-625. PMID: 28332412

30 ANSWER: A) Hepatic embolization of liver metastases

This patient has metastatic insulinoma. Although it is not curable, a number of new interventions are available that can reduce tumor burden and reverse hypoglycemia. Somatostatin receptor analogues such as octreotide are not FDA approved for insulinoma, but these drugs are commonly used to reduce insulin secretion. Octreotide and other long-acting analogues (eg, lantreotide) and new analogues (eg, pasireotide) are used to provide short-term reduction of insulin production. Diazoxide (Answer C) is approved for treatment of insulinoma, but it may not be effective for patients with large tumor burden and it is associated with edema. Continuous glucose monitoring (Answer D) will aid in monitoring for hypoglycemia, but it will do nothing to reduce the frequency or severity of the hypoglycemia. Chemotherapy with various agents such as everolimus (Answer E) is effective, but the resolution of hypoglycemia may be delayed. Performing pancreatectomy (Answer B) will do little to reduce the tumor burden or reduce hypoglycemia risk because most of the tumor is in the liver.

In contrast, hepatic embolization via the hepatic arteries (Answer A) can rapidly reduce tumor burden. Metastases from neuroendocrine tumors derive a large amount of their blood supply from the hepatic artery. Three techniques for hepatic embolization are currently used: transarterial bland embolization, transarterial chemoembolization, and embolization using drug-eluting beads. For embolization using drug-eluting beads, 500 to 700 small beads are loaded with chemotherapeutic drug (usually doxorubicin), which elutes into the liver parenchyma over a period of 7 to 14 days. There are no head-to-head studies comparing these techniques.

Educational Objective
Manage hypoglycemia caused by metastatic insulinoma.

UpToDate Topic Review(s)
Insulinoma

Reference(s)

Hendren NS, Panach K, Brown TJ, et al. *Clin Endocrinol (Oxf)*. 2018;88(2):341-345. PMID: 29055143

Lee E, Leon Pachter H, Sarpel U. Hepatic arterial embolization for the treatment of metastatic neuroendocrine tumors. *Int J Hepatol*. 2012;2012:471203. PMID: 22319651

31 ANSWER: D) Combined effect of nonthyroidal illness and steroid therapy

This vignette illustrates the superimposed effects of illness and sex steroid therapy on thyroid function tests. The effect of the patient's estrogen therapy has been to obscure one of the characteristic features of nonthyroid illness, namely a fall in the total T_4.

Thyroxine-binding globulin is the main transport protein for thyroid hormones and it carries about 75% of circulating T_4. The free fraction of hormone is responsible, however, for its physiologic function. Several drugs, including gonadal steroids, can affect the secretion or metabolism of thyroxine-binding globulin. Estrogen administration is associated with a rise in thyroxine-binding globulin. It is thought that this is due to increased sialylation of thyroxine-binding globulin, which results in slowed clearance by the liver and an increased half-life. The stimulatory effect of estrogen on thyroxine-binding globulin is particularly notable with oral conjugated equine estrogens, which result in higher levels of thyroxine-binding globulin and total T_4 than does transdermal estradiol. This patient, who has no history of thyroid dysfunction and is taking oral conjugated estrogen, would therefore be expected to have had a rise in her total T_4 after starting hormone replacement therapy. However, she would be anticipated to have normal free T_4 and TSH levels because following pituitary adjustment to a transient drop in free T_4, a new steady state is achieved with normal free T_4 and TSH concentrations. Consistent with this, the patient did have a normal TSH level documented before her hospitalization.

The effect of illness on thyroid function tests is complex and influenced by illness severity, the stage of the illness (whether the patient's illness is progressing or the patient is recovering), drug treatment regimens, and whether the patient is receiving parenteral nutrition. For these reasons, it is unwise to order thyroid function tests in a hospitalized patient unless there is a high index of suspicion for thyroid disease or preexisting thyroid disease. Without parenteral nutrition, as critical illness progresses there is a decline in total T_3, TSH, and total T_4. These changes may be adaptive (as the lowered T_3 limits catabolism) and may be mediated by changes in the activity of the type 1 and type 3 deiodinases and suppression of pituitary TSH production. Generally, the more severe the illness and the longer its duration, the more pronounced these changes are. Increased mortality in such patients is predicted by the magnitude of the drop in T_3 and TSH. These changes are often of lesser magnitude if macronutrient supplementation is initiated early in the course of the illness. Iodine administration, for example, if given for imaging studies, can also have various effects on thyroid function, including inducing either hypothyroidism or hyperthyroidism. A TSH-lowering effect may also be seen if drugs such as high-dosage glucocorticoids, dopamine, or dobutamine are administered. On the basis of this patient's hospital course, lack of parenteral nutrition, and glucocorticoid treatment, she would be expected to have a low TSH, low T_3, high reverse T_3 (if that were measured), and low T_4 level. However, superimposed on this pattern of thyroid function tests is the effect of the patient's estrogen therapy. Oral conjugated estrogen can occasionally raise total T_4 levels to as high as 15 µg/dL (193 nmol/L). In this vignette, the patient's estrogen therapy has increased her total T_4 levels to the upper end of the normal range. Thus, Answer

D is correct in fully explaining the pattern of this patient's thyroid function parameters, with the combination of illness, glucocorticoids, and sex steroids in play.

When a patient is transitioned out of the intensive care unit setting and/or is being discharged following recovery from nonthyroidal illness (Answer C), there can be a transient increase in the TSH level as the pituitary gland resumes its function. TSH values as high as 20 mIU/L may be seen. This patient is most likely not yet recovering sufficiently for this phenomenon to be observed.

Glucocorticoid therapy (Answer E) can explain the lowering of the patient's serum TSH, but it does not explain the high-normal total T_4 value. Central hypothyroidism (Answer B) is typically characterized by low or low-normal TSH and low or low-normal T_4 and may be considered in the differential diagnosis, along with the effects of nonthyroidal illness, in patients with these 2 laboratory observations. However, this patient's T_4 is actually at the upper end of the normal range. The pattern of her TSH and T_4 (low TSH and high-normal T_4) is certainly consistent with subclinical hyperthyroidism (Answer A). However, it would be unwise to make this diagnosis based on a single TSH value obtained in the intensive care unit setting, particularly when the patient had a normal TSH value before hospitalization. A low TSH value obtained in the outpatient setting when the patient has fully recovered would suggest subclinical hyperthyroidism.

Educational Objective
Explain the effect of nonthyroidal illness on thyroid function tests and how the characteristic changes may be obscured by estrogen as a result of thyroxine-binding globulin stimulation.

UpToDate Topic Review(s)
Thyroid function in nonthyroidal illness

Reference(s)
Mebis L, Van den Berghe G. Thyroid axis function and dysfunction in critical illness. *Best Pract Res Clin Endocrinol Metab*. 2011;25(5): 745-757. PMID: 21925075

Shifren JL, Desindes S, McIlwain M, Doros G, Mazer NA. A randomized, open-label, crossover study comparing the effects of oral versus transdermal estrogen therapy on serum androgens, thyroid hormones, and adrenal hormones in naturally menopausal women. *Menopause*. 2007;14(6):985-994. PMID: 17507833

Tahboub R, Arafah BM. Sex steroids and the thyroid. *Best Pract Res Clin Endocrinol Metab*. 2009;23(6):769-780. PMID: 19942152

Van den Berghe G. Non-thyroidal illness in the ICU: a syndrome with different faces. *Thyroid*. 2014;24(10):1456-1465. PMID: 24845024

32 ANSWER: C) A switch in the mode of estradiol delivery from oral to sublingual

Estrogen therapy for transgender women is the mainstay to promote feminization. Transgender women should be counseled to expect physical changes including breast tissue growth, change in body composition, as well as a decrease in facial and body hair, oiliness of skin, sexual desire, and spontaneous erections. Estrogen therapy also induces psychological changes and usually improves gender dysphoria and depression and/or anxiety, if present.

The most well-studied estrogen regimens for transgender women include oral estradiol, transdermal estradiol, and intramuscular estradiol valerate or cypionate. The dosages used for transgender women are considerably higher than those used for postmenopausal women. Typical dosages are 2 to 6 mg daily for oral estradiol, 0.025 to 0.2 mg daily for transdermal estradiol, and 5 to 30 mg every 2 weeks for intramuscular estradiol valerate or cypionate. Transgender women are often part of a community where information is shared, including doses and regimens of estrogen. Many transgender women have learned that they can increase their serum estrogen levels by taking estradiol sublingually. In a randomized clinical trial of 6 postmenopausal women who were given 1 mg estradiol, the maximum serum concentration was 34.0 ± 20.4 pg/mL with the oral route and 451 ± 162 pg/mL with the sublingual route. The area under the curve for 24 hours was 2.6 times higher for the sublingual dosing vs the oral dosing. The half-lives for the 1-mg dose were 18.0 ± 2.5 hours vs 20.1 ± 14.2 hours for the sublingual and oral routes, respectively.

In this case, switching estradiol from oral to sublingual (Answer C) is the most likely explanation for the nearly 10-fold increase in serum estradiol concentration that would not be expected from simply doubling the oral dose or taking 6 mg orally (Answer B). The serum estradiol concentration of 56 pg/mL is consistent with taking the 2 mg daily oral dose of estradiol, so a missed dose of estrogen at the time of the blood draw 3 months ago (Answer A) is unlikely. There is no evidence to suggest a pharmacy or laboratory error (Answers D and E), and a more likely explanation exists.

Physicians should ask transgender women how they take their estrogen pills. Compared with the oral route, the sublingual route has the advantage of bypassing the first-pass metabolism in the liver, which presumably carries a lower risk of venous thromboembolism. The disadvantage of sublingual dosing is that monitoring can be more difficult given the rapid peak within the first 6 hours of administration.

Educational Objective
Explain how different routes of estradiol administration affect serum estradiol levels in transgender women.

UpToDate Topic Review(s)
Transgender women: Evaluation and management

Reference(s)
Hembree WC, Cohen-Kettenis PT, Gooren L, et al. Endocrine Treatment of Gender-Dysphoric/Gender-Incongruent Persons: an Endocrine Society Clinical Practice Guideline. *J Clin Endocrinol Metab*. 2017;102(11):3869-3903. PMID: 28945902

Price TM, Blauer KL, Hansen M, Stanczyk F, Lobo R, Bates GW. Single-dose pharmacokinetics of sublingual versus oral administration of micronized 17 beta-estradiol. *Obstet Gynecol*. 1997;89(3):340-345. PMID: 9052581

33 ANSWER: E) Discontinue denosumab and start zoledronic acid once yearly

Denosumab is a human monoclonal antibody to RANK ligand that was approved by the US FDA in 2010 for the treatment of postmenopausal osteoporosis. It has also received US FDA approval for the prevention of bone loss in women and men who take gonadal deprivation therapies. Randomized controlled trials have confirmed a vertebral and nonvertebral antifracture benefit of the drug when given as a 60-mg dose twice yearly for postmenopausal osteoporosis. It is generally well tolerated, and it may be given to patients with impaired renal function (due to nonrenal clearance of the drug). However, in clinical trials, it has been associated with a higher rate of serious infections. In addition, studies have shown that the drug is entirely reversible, in that there is rapid bone mineral density decline within the first year of drug discontinuation that has been associated with multiple vertebral fractures in some patients.

Given these observations, discontinuation of denosumab without initiation of pharmacologic therapy (Answer C) is not recommended. This patient cannot tolerate risedronate, which, based on its chemical structure (pyridinyl bisphosphonate vs amino bisphosphonate [ie, alendronate and ibandronate]), is typically the most well-tolerated oral bisphosphonate from an upper gastrointestinal standpoint. Therefore, an appropriate option for her would be intravenous zoledronic acid, 5 mg annually (Answer E). She has no active dental concerns (ie, risk for osteonecrosis of the jaw) or renal concerns that would preclude its use. Indeed, zoledronic acid would have been a reasonable initial alternative therapy in this woman who had upper gastrointestinal intolerance to an oral bisphosphonate. This patient has experienced a repeated cutaneous reaction to denosumab, which was observed more frequently in the pivotal randomized clinical trial compared with the occurrence in the placebo group. Therefore, the drug should not be continued (Answer A) due to safety concerns. Denosumab must be given every 6 months for therapeutic effect based on the biologic and pharmacokinetic profile of the drug, so decreasing administration to once yearly (Answer B) would also be incorrect.

While raloxifene (Answer D)—the alternative but known to be weaker antiresorptive agent—could be considered, the patient's age and underlying atrial fibrillation substantially increase her risk of stroke. Pertinent to this concern, the RUTH trial (Raloxifene Use in The Heart) demonstrated a higher risk for fatal stroke in women at higher baseline risk (ie, those with hypertension, diabetes mellitus, atrial fibrillation). Thus, risk-benefit assessment would not favor the use of raloxifene for this patient. It is important to note that neither oral nor intravenous bisphosphonates have been associated with an increased risk of atrial fibrillation.

Educational Objective
In a postmenopausal woman with osteoporosis, determine the need to start zoledronic acid based on the risk-benefit assessment upon discontinuation of denosumab.

UpToDate Topic Review(s)
Overview of the management of osteoporosis in postmenopausal women

Reference(s)

Tsourdi E, Langdahl B, Cohen-Solal M, et al. Discontinuation of denosumab therapy for osteoporosis: a systematic review and position statement by ECTS. *Bone*. 2017;105:11-17. PMID: 28789921

Bone HG, Bolognese MA, Yuen CK, et al. Effects of denosumab treatment and discontinuation on bone mineral density and bone turnover markers in postmenopausal women with low bone mass. *J Clin Endocrinol Metab*. 2011;96(4):972-980. PMID: 21289258

34 ANSWER: E) Lorcaserin

Pharmacotherapy for obesity should be considered for patients with a BMI of 27 kg/m^2 or greater who have comorbidities or for patients with a BMI greater than 30 kg/m^2. These medications should be used in addition to diet, exercise, and behavioral modification. Factors to be considered when deciding which medication is the best for a given patient include adverse effects, comorbidities, contraindications, patient preference, and cost.

Lorcaserin (Answer E) is a serotonin (5HT2c) receptor agonist. It decreases appetite by stimulating pro-opimelanocortin neurons in the arcuate nucleus. The recommended dosage is 20 mg daily. There are no contraindications to use of lorcaserin, but physicians should be cautious when patients are also taking serotonergic medications due to the risk of serotonin syndrome or neuroleptic malignant syndrome. Adverse effects of this medication include headache, back pain, and upper respiratory tract infection. Lorcaserin seems to be the safest option for this patient now.

Phentermine (Answer A) is a norepinephrine-releasing agent approved for short-term use (3 months). The increase in norepinephrine in the hypothalamus leads to appetite suppression. In clinical practice, it is prescribed off label for a longer duration. The recommended dosage is 15 to 37.5 mg daily. The most common adverse effects include dry mouth, tachycardia, anxiety, insomnia, and hypertension. This patient has uncontrolled hypertension, so starting phentermine alone would not be the best option.

The combination of phentermine and topiramate extended release (Answer C) was approved by the US FDA in 2012. Topiramate reduces appetite through its action on GABA receptors. The starting dosage of this medication is 3.75 mg/23 mg daily for 14 days, after which patients are transitioned to the recommended dosage of 7.5 mg/46 mg daily. If after 12 weeks patients have not lost 3% of their baseline weight, the medication can be discontinued or the dosage can be increased to its maximum of 15 mg/92 mg daily. Patients take an escalation dose of 11.25 mg/69 mg daily for 14 days before starting the maximum dosage. Contraindications to phentermine/topiramate are glaucoma, hyperthyroidism, use during or within 14 days following monoamine oxidase inhibitor therapy, or pregnancy. Adverse effects related to topiramate include paresthesias, somnolence, and increased risk of developing kidney stones. This patient's history of kidney stones makes phentermine/topiramate not the best first choice for weight-loss management.

Naltrexone/bupropion extended release (Answer D) is a combination pill with an opioid antagonist and a reuptake inhibitor of dopamine and norepinephrine. Bupropion stimulates pro-opiomelanocortin neurons that release α-melanocyte–stimulating hormone, which binds to melanocortin 4 receptors, thus inducing satiety. Naltrexone blocks μ-opioid receptors, which blocks the binding of β-endorphins. β-Endorphins are responsible of providing inhibitory feedback and limiting the release of α-melanocyte–stimulating hormone. The pill has 8 mg of naltrexone and 90 mg of bupropion. Patients take 1 tablet daily for the first week and then add a tablet weekly until they achieve the approved dosage of 2 tablets twice daily. Uncontrolled hypertension is one of this medication's contraindications. Thus, it would be a poor choice for this patient. The most common reported adverse effects include headache, sleep disorders, nausea, constipation, and vomiting.

Liraglutide (Answer B) is a long-acting GLP-1 receptor agonist approved for long-term weight loss. This medication decreases food intake by slowing gastric emptying and by activating hypothalamic and extrahypothalamic nuclei in the brain. The starting dosage is 0.6 mg daily. Patients increase the dosage by 0.6 mg on a weekly basis until they achieve the recommended dosage of 3 mg daily. It is contraindicated when patients have a personal or family history of medullary thyroid carcinoma or multiple endocrine neoplasia type 2. The most common adverse effects include nausea, diarrhea, and increased heart rate (>10 beats per min from baseline). Cases of acute and chronic pancreatitis have been reported. A personal history of pancreatitis is not an absolute contraindication to the use of liraglutide, as it is not known whether this medication increases risk of pancreatitis in this setting. Given this patient's history of pancreatitis, liraglutide is not his best option, but it could be considered if it were his only option.

Educational Objective

Prescribe an appropriate weight-loss medication, bearing in mind various contraindications.

UpToDate Topic Review(s)

Obesity in adults: Drug therapy

Reference(s)

Apovian CM, Aronne LJ, Bessesen DH, et al; Endocrine Society. Pharmacological management of obesity: an Endocrine Society clinical practice guideline. *J Clin Endocrinol Metab.* 2015;100(2):342-362. PMID: 25590212

Bray GA, Fruhbeck G, Ryan DH, Wilding JP. Management of obesity. *Lancet.* 2016;387(10031):1947-1956. PMID: 26868660

Garvey WT, Mechanick JI, Brett EM, et al; Reviewers of the AACE/ACE Obesity Clinical Practice Guidelines. American Association of Clinical Endocrinologists and American College of Endocrinology comprehensive clinical practice guidelines for medical care of patients with obesity. *Endocr Pract.* 2016;22(Suppl 3):1-203. PMID: 27219496

35 ANSWER: C) Repaglinide

Pharmacologic management of diabetes must be adjusted if the patient has evidence of renal compromise. Patients with chronic kidney disease who are not on dialysis can be managed with insulin or certain oral agents with appropriate dosage adjustments. Most patients undergoing hemodialysis will be switched to insulin.

In this vignette, an oral agent is considered because of patient preference. The National Kidney Disease Outcomes Quality Initiative (KDOQI) guideline from 2012 gives guidance on choice of agent. Sulfonylureas act on the β cells of the pancreas to release insulin. Most sulfonylurea agents are metabolized in the liver, but some of them have active metabolites that are excreted in the urine. These active metabolites can accumulate in patients with chronic kidney disease. Sulfonylureas should therefore be used with caution, especially since the sulfonylurea class of agents cannot be dialyzed. Short-acting sulfonylureas such as glipizide can be considered. Dosage-adjusted glimepiride (1 mg daily) would also be a reasonable choice. However, glyburide (Answer A) is not recommended because of risk of hypoglycemia with its active metabolites, and it would not be the safest choice.

Meglitinides are sulfonylurea-like and they release insulin from the β cells of the pancreas. Repaglinide (Answer C) is hepatically metabolized and less than 10% is renally excreted. A conservative repaglinide dosage of 0.5 mg with meals is therefore the preferred meglitinide in the setting of chronic kidney disease. Nateglinide is more likely than repaglinide to lead to accumulation of active metabolites in patients with chronic kidney disease. With its shorter half-life, hepatic metabolism, and lower risk of active metabolites in chronic kidney disease, repaglinide would be a safer choice than glyburide.

Thiazolidinediones are synthetic ligands for peroxisome proliferator–activated receptors. These agents reduce blood glucose by improving peripheral and hepatic insulin resistance. Although thiazolidinediones do not cause hypoglycemia, there is concern for fluid retention with their use. Pioglitazone (Answer B) could be prescribed, but repaglinide would be a safer choice.

GLP-1 receptor agonists exert an influence on blood glucose levels in a number of ways, including decreased weight, decreased appetite, slowing gastric motility, improved insulin resistance, etc. Clearance of exenatide (Answer D) is reduced by about 60% if the glomerular filtration rate is less than 30 mL/min per 1.73 m². The use of GLP-1 receptor agonists in patients with end-stage renal disease is not well studied and is not currently recommended.

SGLT-2 inhibitors (Answer E) lower plasma glucose levels by changing the renal threshold for glucose excretion. Renal effects of these agents are complex. There is a reduction in the estimated glomerular filtration rate after SGLT-2 inhibitors are initiated; however, there may be a renal protective effect as well. These agents may reduce proteinuria and the need for renal replacement therapy. SGLT-2 inhibitors may have an increasing role in the management chronic kidney disease; however, more data are needed regarding the choice of patient, appropriate agent, and optimal dosage. At this time, there are few data on SGLT-2 use in patients undergoing dialysis. The 2012 KDOQI guideline does not comment on SGLT-2 inhibitors.

Of all the choices offered, repaglinide (Answer C) would be the safest choice based on currently available data.

Educational Objective

Recommend appropriate pharmacotherapy for diabetes management in patients with end-stage renal disease.

UpToDate Topic Review(s)
Management of hyperglycemia in patients with type 2 diabetes and pre-dialysis chronic kidney disease or end-stage renal disease

Reference(s)

National Kidney Foundation. KDOQI Clinical Practice Guideline for Diabetes and CKD: 2012 Update [published correction appears in *Am J Kidney Dis*. 2013;61 (6):1049]. *Am J Kidney Dis*. 2012;60(5):850-886. PMID: 23067652

Rhee CM, Leung AM, Kovesdy CP, Lynch KE, Brent GA, Kalantar-Zadeh K. Updates on the management of diabetes in dialysis patients. *Semin Dial*. 2014;27(2): 135-145. PMID: 24588802

36 ANSWER: B) Switch from cabergoline to temozolomide

Most patients with prolactinomas (>90%) respond well to dopaminergic therapy and, if the prolactin level is well controlled by a low dosage, patients can sometimes be weaned from medication after 2 years of therapy. However, there is a subset of patients who fail to respond or with time become unresponsive to dopaminergic therapy. In these patients, mass effect on surrounding structures may threaten their vision and eventually their life. Dopamine agonist resistance is defined as the failure to achieve normal prolactin levels and failure to achieve tumor size reduction of at least 50% with maximal conventional medication dosages (7.5 mg daily of bromocriptine or 2.0 mg weekly of cabergoline). Despite being on a high dosage of cabergoline, this patient's prolactin level is increasing and the mass is enlarging and threatening his vision. Therefore, his prolactinoma is cabergoline resistant. A further increase in the cabergoline dosage is unlikely to be successful and would have the potential risk of causing heart valve damage (by activation of serotonin receptor 2B, a mechanism similar to that of fenfluramine).

In some patients with resistance to dopamine agonists, a clinically significant response to the oral chemotherapy agent temozolomide (Answer B) has been reported. Temozolomide is an alkylating agent commonly used in the treatment of gliomas. The DNA repair enzyme methylguanine methyltransferase (MGMT) counteracts the effect of temozolomide. Therefore, tumors low in MGMT generally respond better to such treatment. Whitelaw et al documented that 15 of 20 resistant prolactin-secreting macroadenomas responded to temozolomide. This drug is administered orally during 5-day monthly cycles, and it is best if one can consult with a neuro-oncologist who has expertise with its use. Unfortunately, many of these very aggressive tumors escape from the suppressive effects of temozolomide after 6 months to 2 and a half years. A second treatment cycle has been reported to be successful in 1 patient after relapse.

Bromocriptine (Answer A) is generally less effective and less well tolerated than cabergoline; it would be extremely unlikely to work in a patient who is not responding to such a high cabergoline dosage. This patient has already received fractionated radiation relatively recently, so more radiation therapy now, within such a short time interval (Answer E), would potentially risk his vision. Somatostatin analogues (Answers C and D) are effective in treating GH- and TSH-secreting pituitary tumors, but they have not been documented to be useful for prolactinomas. The somatostatin receptor subtype 5 (SSTR5) is the most important receptor in the regulation of prolactin secretion, and of the 3 approved somatostatin analogues, only pasireotide binds significantly to this receptor. However, no published data are available regarding the effect of pasireotide on aggressive prolactinomas.

Educational Objective

Recommend chemotherapy with temozolomide for patients with aggressive macroprolactinomas that are resistant to dopaminergic therapy after surgical and radiotherapy options have been exhausted.

UpToDate Topic Review(s)
Management of hyperprolactinemia

Reference(s)

Whitelaw BC, Dworakowska D, Thomas NW, et al. Temozolomide in the management of dopamine agonist-resistant prolactinomas. *Clin Endocrinol (Oxf)*. 2012; 76(6):877-886. PMID: 22372583

Molitch ME. Management of medically refractory prolactinoma. *J Neurooncol*. 2014;117(3):421-426. PMID: 24146188

Strowd RE, Salvatori R, Laterra JJ. Temozolomide retreatment in a recurrent prolactin-secreting pituitary adenoma: hormonal and radiographic response. *J Oncol Pharm Pract.* 2016;22(3):517–522. PMID: 25616657

37 ANSWER: A) Anteroposterior and lateral radiographs of the thoracic and lumbar spine

This patient has established hypercalcemia and biochemical evidence of hyperparathyroidism. What is unclear is whether she is best served by medical management or by referral for parathyroidectomy. On the basis of clinical history, she is asymptomatic without evident renal or skeletal complications. Since 1990, the National Institutes of Health has periodically convened an expert panel to review the existing evidence base and provide guidelines on indications for surgical referral of patients with asymptomatic primary hyperparathyroidism. The most recent guidelines were issued in 2014 and addressed emerging data on the importance of identifying "subclinical" end-organ disease. Specifically, the revised guidelines recommend screening for the presence of nephrolithiasis and vertebral compression fractures. This patient has physical examination findings suggestive of existing vertebral fractures (historical height loss of greater than 4 cm and thoracic kyphosis). Given this aggregate clinical information, plain radiography of the thoracic and lumbar spine (Answer A) is indicated to establish her potential candidacy for surgical referral. Recommended screening for asymptomatic nephrolithiasis includes plain radiography, ultrasonography, or CT.

This patient does not meet bone mineral density criteria for surgical referral based on DXA images, which demonstrate osteopenia at all diagnostic sites, including the lumbar spine. Although localizing studies such as neck ultrasonography (Answer E), CT, and parathyroid scintigraphy (Answer D) are commonly used and have been shown to reduce operative time and cost, they may yield false-negative findings (~80% sensitivity for technetium ^{99m}Tc parathyroid scanning) that would not preclude surgical intervention in a patient with clinical indications for parathyroidectomy.

Measurement of plasma ionized calcium (Answer B) is more sensitive in detecting hypercalcemia than albumin-adjusted serum calcium, but this patient has unequivocal evidence for serum calcium elevation.

The 24-hour urine calcium and calculated fractional excretion of calcium are not low (<0.01 for the latter). Thus, sequencing the *CASR* gene (Answer C) to confirm the presence of familial hypocalciuric hypercalcemia is not indicated for this patient.

Educational Objective

Explain the importance of vertebral fracture identification in patient assessment for the surgical management of primary hyperparathyroidism.

UpToDate Topic Review(s)
Primary hyperparathyroidism: Management

Reference(s)

Bilezikian JP, Brandi ML, Eastell R, et al. Guidelines for the management of asymptomatic primary hyperparathyroidism: summary statement from the Fourth International Workshop. *J Clin Endocrinol Metab.* 2014;99(10):3561-3569. PMID: 25162665

Green AD, Colón-Emeric CS, Bastian L, Drake MT, Lyles KW. Does this woman have osteoporosis? *JAMA.* 2004;292(23):2890-2900. PMID: 15598921

38 ANSWER: B) Start glyburide

Neonatal diabetes is a rare cause of diabetes (1 in 90,000 to 160,000 live births) and is diagnosed in the first few months of life. To meet the diagnostic criteria, patients must have persistent hyperglycemia for at least 2 weeks and be treated with insulin. Most patients diagnosed with neonatal diabetes before 6 months of age have a monogenic form of diabetes rather than autoimmune type 1 diabetes.

Pathogenic variants in the genes encoding the subunits of the adenosine triphosphate (ATP)-sensitive potassium channel are commonly found in persons with neonatal diabetes. Activating pathogenic variants in the *KCNJ11* gene lead to formation of abnormal Kir6.2 subunits of the ATP-sensitive channel, an increased number of open KATP channels, hyperpolarization of the plasma membrane, and impaired insulin release in response to hyperglycemia. This most commonly results in permanent diabetes mellitus and less often in transient neonatal diabetes. Affected infants are usually small for gestational age and about 20% have neurologic deficits. Pathogenic variants in the *ABCC8* gene more typically lead to transient neonatal diabetes rather than permanent diabetes.

More than 20 distinct pathogenic variants resulting in neonatal diabetes have been described, including pathogenic variants in the following genes: *GATA6*, *PDX1* (formerly *IPF1*), *GCK*, *FOXP3*, and *INS*. Patients with transient diabetes have remission of diabetes after treatment with insulin for a mean of about 12 weeks, but they usually redevelop diabetes later in life.

The patient in this vignette has been treated with insulin since the time diabetes was diagnosed in infancy. Glutamic acid decarboxylase antibodies and other autoimmune markers are negative in patients with a history of permanent neonatal diabetes. In about 90% of cases, patients who have activating pathogenic variants in the gene encoding the ATP-sensitive potassium channel can be switched from insulin to treatment with a relatively high dosage of a sulfonylurea. Most of the clinical research in permanent neonatal diabetes has been with use of glyburide (Answer B), as it blocks the KATP channels containing both SUR1 and SUR2 types. The starting glyburide dosage is 0.1 mg/kg per day, and the dosage is increased by 0.1 mg/kg per day on a weekly basis. Initiation of glyburide and tapering of insulin should be conducted in a supervised setting in the clinic or hospital due to the increased risk of developing marked hyperglycemia. Patients who have been successfully transitioned to glyburide generally have improved and quite stable glycemic control over time. The risk of hypoglycemia in these patients is markedly lower than it is with insulin therapy. Compared with insulin treatment, sulfonylurea treatment is associated with cost savings, a better quality of life, and lower rates of complications in patients with a history of permanent neonatal diabetes.

The patient in this case could be started on insulin pump therapy (Answer A). However, this is a more complicated and expensive treatment, and there is no guarantee of improved glucose control over that of basal-bolus insulin. Similarly, switching the patient to alternative insulin therapy with insulin degludec and insulin lispro (Answer E) is not the best next step.

Metformin's primary mechanism of action is to reduce glucose output from the liver and, secondarily, to reduce insulin resistance. Metformin (Answer C) is not the treatment of choice in a patient with an insulin secretion defect.

There is no literature available on using sodium-glucose cotransporter 2 inhibitors such as empagliflozin (Answer D) in patients with monogenic forms of diabetes.

Educational Objective
Distinguish monogenic forms of diabetes from other types of diabetes and recommend appropriate treatment.

UpToDate Topic Review(s)
Classification of diabetes mellitus and genetic diabetic syndromes

Reference(s)
Von Muhlendahl KE, Herkenhoff H. Long-term course of neonatal diabetes. *N Engl J Med*. 1995;333(11):704-708. PMID: 7637748

Pearson ER, Flechtner I, Njolstad PR, et al; Neonatal Diabetes International Collaborative Group. Switching from insulin to oral sulfonylureas in patients with diabetes due to Kir6.2 mutations. *N Engl J Med*. 2006;355(5):467-477. PMID: 16885550

Carmody D, Bell CD, Hwang JL, et al. Sulfonylurea treatment before genetic testing in neonatal diabetes: pros and cons. *J Clin Endocrinol Metab*. 2014;99(12): E2709-E2714. PMID: 25238204

39 **ANSWER: D) Increase the estradiol dosage**

Estrogen therapy in a female with delayed puberty should be initiated slowly and with dosages lower than those used in adults to optimize breast and uterine development. In older adolescents and young adults, estrogen therapy might start as low as 25 to 50 mcg daily transdermally or 0.5 mg to 1 mg daily with oral estradiol and would be gradually increased every 6 months over the course of 2 years. The best next step in this patient's management is to increase the estradiol dosage (Answer D).

Progesterone is initiated only after significant breast development is achieved, as progesterone might interfere with optimal breast growth. Cyclic progesterone therapy is generally initiated after about 2 years of estrogen therapy or when breakthrough bleeding occurs. Therefore, since she has only advanced to Tanner stage 2, it would be too early to move to oral contraceptives (Answer A) or to add micronized progesterone (Answer B). Progesterone would also be added only for days 1 through 12 of a 28-day cycle, not daily as listed in Answer B.

Girls with delayed puberty due to Turner syndrome often present with short stature, so delaying bone maturation might be important to improve growth potential. In contrast, the steady linear growth rate in idiopathic hypogonadotropic hypogonadism is associated with taller than normal achieved height. In this case, although she has not achieved midparental height, she is only showing signs of early pubertal development with a bone age younger than chronologic age. Even in cases of constitutional delay of puberty, serum GH and IGF-1 concentrations might be low but will increase in response to estrogen (or testosterone therapy in males). Patients with idiopathic hypogonadotropic hypogonadism, as in this patient with a normal IGF-1 level, are not typically GH deficient and will continue to grow when treated with sex steroids alone. While GH (Answer C) is less likely to lead to epiphyseal closure than estrogen replacement, there is no evidence that patients with idiopathic hypogonadotropic hypogonadism benefit from GH therapy as opposed to women with Turner syndrome and primary hypogonadism.

Before age 18 years, estrogen therapy might be discontinued periodically after optimal breast development has occurred to determine whether spontaneous ovulatory cycles occur as in constitutional delay. Persistent hypogonadotropic hypogonadism is highly likely if spontaneous pubertal progression does not occur by age 18. Because this patient is older than 18 and her breast development has not progressed beyond Tanner stage 2, discontinuing estradiol (Answer E) is not recommended.

Educational Objective

Select the appropriate hormone therapy when a woman with delayed puberty and idiopathic hypogonadotropic hypogonadism presents as an adult.

UpToDate Topic Review(s)

Isolated gonadotropin-releasing hormone deficiency (idiopathic hypogonadotropic hypogonadism)
Management of Turner syndrome in adults

Reference(s)

Boehm U, Bouloux PM, Dattani MT, et al. Expert consensus document: European Consensus Statement on congenital hypogonadotropic hypogonadism--pathogenesis, diagnosis and treatment. *Nat Rev Endocrinol.* 2015;11(9):547-564. PMID: 26194704

Davenport ML. Approach to the patient with Turner syndrome. *J Clin Endocrinol Metab.* 2010;95(4):1487-1495. PMID: 20375216

40 ANSWER: A) Annual evaluation of full pituitary function indefinitely

As a result of the significant improvement in survival outcomes after childhood cancer, it is increasingly recognized that treatment of malignancy in childhood can lead to lifelong consequences. In particular, survivors of childhood cancer are at risk of developing a spectrum of neuroendocrine abnormalities, primarily because of the effect of radiation therapy on the hypothalamus. Indeed, hypothalamic and pituitary endocrinopathies occur in up to 80% of adults following radiotherapy to these areas; even doses as low as 20 Gy can cause pituitary dysfunction.

All pituitary hormones can be affected, but GH production is most commonly impaired as is the case in this vignette. For example, in one study of 748 childhood cancer survivors treated with cranial irradiation and observed for a mean of 27.3 years, 46.5% developed GH deficiency, 10.8% developed LH/FSH deficiency, 7.5% developed TSH deficiency, and 4% developed ACTH deficiency. In this study and others, cumulative incidence of pituitary dysfunction increased throughout the follow-up period. Therefore, it is recommended that individuals who have undergone pituitary radiation at a dose greater than 30 Gy undergo lifelong annual surveillance of all pituitary axes, even if they are symptom-free (thus, Answer A is correct and Answers B and C are incorrect).

The patient feels well and has thyroid function testing within normal limits (albeit with a TSH and free T_4 at the low end of the normal range). Therefore, this does require re-evaluation in the next round of pituitary function testing. A thyrotropin-releasing hormone stimulation test (Answer D) is not (and is unlikely to ever be) required. In this vignette, the patient has an early-morning cortisol level of 15 µg/dL (413.8 nmol/L), which probably indicates sufficient ACTH secretion, although a level greater than 18 µg/dL (>496.6 nmol/L) would be required to be entirely reassuring. In contrast, a serum cortisol value less than 3 µg/dL (<82.8 nmol/L) is highly suggestive of cortisol deficiency. Therefore, it is reasonable for this patient to undergo further evaluation of ACTH reserve, although there is no definitive recommendation as to the gold standard stimulation test to use. The ACTH stimulation test is done by many; however, it can miss cases of partial or early ACTH deficiency that may respond normally to cosyntropin. Other options include the metyrapone stimulation test or the insulin-induced hypoglycemia test (insulin tolerance test) (Answer E). The latter test is performed by administering insulin (0.1 units/kg) and measuring serum glucose and cortisol at regular intervals for 120 minutes after the injection. A normal response is characterized by a serum glucose value less than 50 mg/dL (<2.8 mmol/L) and a cortisol value greater than 18 μg/dL (>496.6 mmol/L). While the insulin tolerance test is considered to be the gold standard test of pituitary reserve and could also reassess GH status, it is unpleasant, and hypoglycemia can be dangerous in elderly patients and in those with an underlying seizure disorder as this patient has. Therefore, it would be contraindicated in this scenario.

This patient developed GH deficiency after pituitary irradiation, which is the most common endocrine abnormality in this setting. GH replacement therapy was started after completion of cancer treatment in order to optimize skeletal growth during puberty and was discontinued some time after growth had ceased. There is good evidence that continuation of GH therapy into adulthood in such individuals can provide further benefits for bone density and could be considered in this case (especially if age-adjusted bone mineral density is low). If this were to be considered, further evaluation of the GH axis may well be required given that pituitary function is otherwise intact and there is no structural pituitary lesion. The glucagon stimulation test would be the test of first choice in this circumstance as the GHRH-arginine test may be falsely reassuring within the first 10 years after radiation therapy.

Educational Objective
Counsel patients who have undergone cranial irradiation regarding the need for long-term (usually lifelong) screening of pituitary function.

UpToDate Topic Review(s)
Delayed complications of cranial irradiation

Reference(s)

Darzy KH. Radiation-induced hypopituitarism after cancer therapy: who, how and when to test. *Nat Clin Pract Endocrinol Metab*. 2009;5(2):88-99. PMID: 19165221

Children's Oncology Group. Children's Oncology Group long-term follow-up guidelines for survivors of childhood, adolescent, and young adult cancer. Version 4.0, October 2013. Available at: www.survivorshipguidelines.org.

Molitch ME, Clemmons DR, Malozowski S, Merriam GR, Vance ML; Endocrine Society. Evaluation and Treatment of Adult Growth Hormone Deficiency: an Endocrine Society Clinical Practice Guideline. *J Clin Endocrinol Metab*. 2011;96(6):1587-1609. PMID: 21602453

41 ANSWER: B) Serum PSA measurement

The patient described in this vignette has bony pain associated with a markedly elevated bone-specific alkaline phosphatase level; diffuse sclerosis involving the pelvis and visualized portions of the proximal femurs on his pelvis x-ray; and diffusely scattered foci of radionuclide uptake involving the skull, sternum, bilateral ribs, humerus, pelvic bones, and femora on his bone scan. Although the scintigraphic pattern in this patient's pelvic bones may be partially explained by Paget disease, it is important to consider other conditions that may also be present or have overlapping features with Paget disease, given that he has had significant weight loss and appears ill. Specifically, metastatic prostate cancer should be considered. This patient had a serum PSA level measured (Answer B), which turned out to be 1743 ng/mL (≤5.3 ng/mL). A subsequent CT of his abdomen and pelvis revealed diffuse osteoblastic sclerotic osseous metastases with iliac and retroperitoneal lymphadenopathy, consistent with metastatic prostate cancer.

The radiographic appearance of Paget disease on x-ray may be difficult to distinguish from metastatic malignancy in some patients, and in such cases, CT or MRI may be helpful. A bone biopsy (Answer E) may sometimes be required if imaging studies are unable to distinguish these conditions with sufficient confidence, but it would be premature to recommend a bone biopsy at this time.

Serum protein electrophoresis (Answer A) to test for possible multiple myeloma is unlikely to be diagnostic in this scenario. This patient has sclerotic as opposed to "punched out" lytic lesions on his x-ray, which would not be consistent with multiple myeloma. Furthermore, the absence of hypercalcemia and renal impairment on his biochemistry argue against this diagnosis. Standard bone scans tend to underestimate the extent and severity of disease in multiple myeloma and may even be normal. Therefore, these are not performed routinely in the workup of patients with suspected or established multiple myeloma.

There are several different etiologies of elevated bone-specific alkaline phosphatase isoenzyme, which is a result of increased osteoblastic activity. Causes other than Paget disease and metastatic cancer to bone include hyperparathyroidism and osteomalacia. This patient has normal calcium, phosphate, 25-hydroxyvitamin D, and kidney function; therefore, measuring PTH (Answer C) would not be indicated. Similarly, there is no reason to suspect that he has tumor-induced osteomalacia in the absence of hypophosphatemia, so measuring FGF-23 (Answer D) would also not be appropriate.

Educational Objective
Explain how the clinical presentation of metastatic prostate cancer (to bone) may mimic Paget disease of bone.

UpToDate Topic Review(s)
Clinical manifestations and diagnosis of Paget disease of bone

Reference(s)

Singer FR, Bone HG 3rd, Hosking DJ, et al; Endocrine Society. Paget's disease of bone: an Endocrine Society clinical practice guideline. *J Clin Endocrinol Metab.* 2014;99(12):4408-4422. PMID: 25406796

Sonoda LI, Balan KK. Co-existent Paget's disease of the bone, prostate carcinoma skeletal metastases and fracture on skeletal scintigraphy-lessons to be learned. *Mol Imaging Radionucl Ther.* 2013;22(2):63-65. PMID: 24003400

42 ANSWER: D) No further testing needed; initiate statin therapy now

This patient is seeking appropriate management of cardiovascular risk after undergoing an extensive evaluation for atypical chest pain. The coronary artery calcium (CAC) score is determined by performing a noncontrast, limited chest CT acquired with a 3- to 5-second breath hold, and it measures calcium in the epicardial coronary system. Radiation exposure is now comparable to that of a mammogram. By comparing a patient's calcium score with that of others of the same age, sex, and ethnicity through the use of large databases of asymptomatic patients, a calcium percentile is generated; higher than the 75th percentile is considered high risk irrespective of the score, and this indicates premature atherosclerosis. Variations according to sex and ethnicity have also been described. There are no randomized controlled trials demonstrating clinical benefit of this assessment.

CAC is a good tool for elucidating decision-making when the decision to treat with statins or combination therapy remains uncertain for the provider or the patient. CAC scoring has been proposed as a method to identify individuals who may not always require lifelong statin treatment. CAC scores increase with age and are higher in men. Coronary mortality risk is low among individuals with CAC scores of 0 even when multiple risk factors are present, and several retrospective and prospective studies and meta-analyses have shown that asymptomatic individuals with a CAC score of 0 are very unlikely to have clinically important coronary heart disease events despite the presence of clinical risk factors.

Conversely, patients with higher CAC scores have event rates more similar to those in secondary prevention. CAC scores higher than 100 or higher than the 75th percentile are associated with a high risk (>2% annual risk) of a coronary heart disease event and provide a rationale for intensifying LDL-cholesterol–lowering therapy. Therefore, this man should be offered statin therapy for cardiovascular risk reduction (thus, Answer D is correct and Answer E is incorrect). Whether assessment of CAC score progression improves cardiovascular risk prediction is currently unclear. No randomized controlled trial data to date suggest that statin therapy slows the progression of CAC. Cumulative radiation exposure from repeated CT studies can occur. Therefore, routine serial CAC quantification (Answer A) is not recommended in clinical practice.

Chronic inflammation is a recognized contributor to the initiation and progression of the atherosclerotic disease process and it increases plaque vulnerability and rupture. C-reactive protein (CRP) is the best-studied marker of chronic inflammation. It is an acute-phase reactant protein synthesized by the liver in response to cytokines such as TNF-α and interleukin-6 and is a nonspecific marker of inflammation. Evidence from epidemiologic studies suggests an association between elevated CRP levels and the presence of atherosclerosis. A highly sensitive assay that can accurately detect very low CRP levels is used to determine cardiovascular risk. CRP levels are influenced by genetics, sex, ethnicity, and lifestyle factors. Currently, there is no conclusive evidence to recommend the routine measurement of CRP in the process of cardiovascular risk prediction or to use it to determine whether to initiate statin therapy. Statins benefit individuals with or without elevated CRP levels (thus, Answer B is incorrect).

Measuring LDL particle number is an alternative way to quantify LDL burden. There is significant interindividual and intraindividual variability in the amount of cholesterol carried by LDL particles. Usually, LDL cholesterol and LDL particle number are correlated; however, there is occasional discordance between the two, especially when plasma triglyceride levels are elevated. In patients with elevated triglycerides and/or low HDL-cholesterol levels, LDL-cholesterol levels are often lower compared with LDL particle number. Currently, LDL particle number can be quantified directly by nuclear magnetic resonance spectroscopy. Measurement is not widely available, is not standardized, and is costly. Several studies have shown that LDL particle number is more strongly associated with atherosclerotic cardiovascular disease than LDL cholesterol. However, in most studies, the predictive strength of LDL particle number is very similar to that of non-HDL cholesterol (part of the standard lipid panel). Also, LDL particle number correlates with apolipoprotein B measurement, which is more widely available. Thus, at this time, there is no evidence that measuring LDL particle number (Answer C) provides a substantial amount of information beyond what is provided by non-HDL cholesterol and standard risk factor assessment.

Educational Objective
Appropriately use coronary artery calcium scores in cardiovascular risk assessment.

UpToDate Topic Review(s)
Diagnostic and prognostic implications of coronary artery calcification

Reference(s)

Hecht HS. Coronary artery calcium scanning: past, present, and future. *JACC Cardiovasc Imaging*. 2015;8(5):579-596. PMID:25937196

Benzaquen LR, Yu H, Rifai N. High sensitivity C-reactive protein: an emerging role in cardiovascular risk assessment. *Crit Rev Clin Lab Sci*. 2002;39(4-5): 459-497. PMID: 23727085

Allaire J, Vors C, Couture P, Lamarche B. LDL particle number and size and cardiovascular risk: anything new under the sun? *Curr Opin Lipidol*. 2017;28(3): 261-266. PMID: 28460374

43 ANSWER: C) Glutamic acid decarboxylase antibody assessment

This patient was diagnosed with type 2 diabetes, but her course has not been typical. She has had a poor response to sulfonylureas and metformin and it would be reasonable to start insulin on the basis of this presentation. However, the time course raises the possibility that she has an atypical form of diabetes.

Reasonable diagnostic considerations are Cushing syndrome and acromegaly, which may worsen insulin resistance, but the information provided suggests no specific findings for these conditions. Hemochromatosis may cause a so-called bronze diabetes, but there are no other clinical indications for this condition. Maturity-onset diabetes of the young (MODY), a group of monogenetic disorders, is often considered in younger adults who are lean and diagnosed with mild diabetes. Most patients with MODY can be treated with oral agents. Some forms of MODY do progress to the point that insulin is required, but the time course described for this patient would be very unusual. Thus, genetic testing for MODY (Answer E) is not indicated.

An autoimmune basis for diabetes would be reasonable to consider, especially given her diagnoses of Crohn disease and hypothyroidism. Patients who have diabetes diagnosed in adulthood, for whom there is evidence of an autoimmune basis for their disease, represent a heterogeneous population. While some have classic type 1 diabetes requiring insulin from the time of diagnosis, others have a slower progression to insulin requirement. In the 1990s, the term latent autoimmune diabetes in adults (LADA) was used to describe patients diagnosed with type 2 diabetes but for whom antibodies typically found in patients with type 1 diabetes were present. Other terms include type 1.5 diabetes and non–insulin-requiring autoimmune diabetes. The American Diabetes Association and World Health Organization do not recognize LADA as a distinct clinical entity. The Immunology of Diabetes Society has provided criteria for the diagnosis of LADA: age at diagnosis older than 30 years, presence of any islet autoantibody, and at least 6 months of no insulin treatment after diagnosis.

Prevalence of glutamic acid decarboxylase (GAD) antibodies in adult-onset autoimmune diabetes is not affected by the age at presentation. In contrast, there is a decreasing prevalence of insulin, ZnT8, and IA-2 antibodies with older age at diagnosis. Therefore, GAD antibody testing (Answer C) assesses the most sensitive antibody marker for autoimmune diabetes in adulthood. Additionally, some groups have suggested that higher GAD antibody titers are associated with other organ-specific antibodies. Therefore, the GAD titer may help tune the clinical suspicion for other autoimmune conditions.

The degree of β-cell dysfunction at the time of diagnosis is more severe with younger age of onset. Fasting C-peptide levels are positively correlated with age at diagnosis. Therefore, fasting C-peptide measurement (Answer

A) would not be a sensitive way to detect whether there is an autoimmune basis for this patient's diabetes. Additionally, because her hemoglobin A_{1c} level is greater than 10%, there is the likelihood of glucose toxicity, which may falsely lower the C-peptide level. Lastly, in patients diagnosed with LADA, decline in C-peptide occurs more slowly. Fasting insulin levels (Answer B) may be used in a clinical research setting to calculate indices of insulin sensitivity, but insulin measurement is not an appropriate choice to confirm the diagnosis.

While hemochromatosis can cause diabetes, there is nothing to indicate hemochromatosis clinically in this vignette and ferritin measurement (Answer D) is unnecessary. Further, the presence of an autoimmune condition (ie, Crohn disease) makes LADA more likely.

Educational Objective
Differentiate among atypical presentations of diabetes mellitus presenting in adulthood.

UpToDate Topic Review(s)
Classification of diabetes mellitus and genetic diabetic syndromes

Reference(s)
Buzzetti R, Zampetti S, Maddaloni E. Adult-onset autoimmune diabetes: current knowledge and implications for management. *Nat Rev Endocrinol*. 2017;13(11): 674-686. PMID: 28885622

44 ANSWER: D) Development of hypothyroidism

Patients with Graves disease may have orbitopathy that can run a varying course, with worsening, stabilization, or resolution. As the use of radioactive iodine can be associated with the onset of orbitopathy or worsening orbitopathy, other treatment options such as antithyroidal agents or thyroidectomy are often desirable in those with risk factors for orbitopathy or who already have this condition. Radioactive iodine therapy without concurrent steroids is considered a reasonable therapeutic option in patients without apparent orbitopathy. However, radioactive iodine therapy is not recommended in those patients with moderate to severe orbitopathy. If radioactive iodine is selected as a treatment option for patients with mild orbitopathy who have risk factors such as high TRAb levels, high T_3 levels, or cigarette smoking, concurrent glucocorticoid administration is recommended. In addition, glucocorticoids should be considered in patients with mild orbitopathy, even if there are no underlying risk factors for deterioration of Graves orbitopathy. An example of a glucocorticoid regimen is starting with 30 mg prednisone daily and tapering off within 6 to 8 weeks. The patient described in this vignette has at least one risk factor for orbitopathy: high pretreatment T_3 levels. His pretreatment TRAb value is elevated at 5.0 IU/L, with greater than 8.8 IU/L generally being considered high risk for progression of orbitopathy. As he also has mild orbitopathy, use of glucocorticoids while administering radioactive iodine would have been a reasonable option.

In addition to cigarette smoking, high pretreatment TRAb levels, and high pretreatment T_3 levels, other risk factors for worsening orbitopathy are untreated hyperthyroidism and delay in treating hypothyroidism that develops after radioiodine administration. This patient was rendered euthyroid with methimazole before radioactive iodine therapy, so untreated hyperthyroidism was not a contributing factor in his case. Pretreatment with methimazole (Answer B) does not trigger worsening orbitopathy, although in some studies it may predict failure to respond to radioactive iodine therapy. However, the main culprit with respect to such treatment failure is propylthiouracil. Several studies have shown that delay in treating hypothyroidism when this develops as a result of radioactive iodine therapy is linked with worsening orbitopathy. This patient unfortunately developed profound hypothyroidism (Answer D) that was probably uncorrected for several months and this has likely contributed to his worsening orbitopathy. Use of sunglasses (Answer A) and raising the head of the bed (Answer C) are considered to be useful local measures that may improve symptoms of Graves orbitopathy and would not be expected to cause progression.

Male sex, older age (Answer E), and white ancestry are all risk factors for Graves orbitopathy. However, given the degree of this patient's hypothyroidism, this is probably the most relevant risk factor in this vignette.

Educational Objective
Identify factors that can contribute to worsening orbitopathy after radioactive iodine treatment.

UpToDate topic review(s)
Clinical features and diagnosis of Graves' orbitopathy (ophthalmopathy)

Reference(s)

Stan MN, Durski JM, Brito JP, Bhagra S, Thapa P, Bahn RS. Cohort study on radioactive iodine-induced hypothyroidism: implications for Graves' ophthalmopathy and optimal timing for thyroid hormone assessment. *Thyroid.* 2013;23(5):620-625. PMID: 23205939

Perros P, Kendall-Taylor P, Neoh C, Frewin S, Dickinson J. A prospective study of the effects of radioiodine therapy for hyperthyroidism in patients with minimally active graves' ophthalmopathy. *J Clin Endocrinol Metab.* 2005;90(9):5321-5323. PMID: 15985483

Ross DS, Burch HB, Cooper DS, et al. 2016 American Thyroid Association Guidelines for Diagnosis and Management of Hyperthyroidism and Other Causes of Thyrotoxicosis. *Thyroid.* 2016;26(10):1343-1421. PMID: 27521067

Tallstedt L, Lundell G, Blomgren H, Bring J. Does early administration of thyroxine reduce the development of Graves' ophthalmopathy after radioiodine treatment? *Eur J Endocrinol.* 1994;130(5):494-497. PMID: 8180678

45 ANSWER: A) Start testosterone replacement therapy

Exogenous testosterone can have numerous physiologic effects, including a decrease in proinflammatory cytokines and HDL cholesterol and an increase in hemoglobin/hematocrit, salt retention, water retention, interleukin 10, and platelet thromboxane A2 receptor density. The effects of exogenous testosterone may also be mediated by its conversion to estradiol and dihydrotestosterone.

Studies have shown conflicting results regarding the potential cardiovascular risks of testosterone replacement therapy (TRT). A sufficiently powered, long-term, randomized controlled trial of TRT has not been conducted to determine whether it increases or decreases the rates of outcomes such as myocardial infarction, stroke, or venous thromboembolism. Nonetheless, an overview of 7 systematic reviews can help inform clinical practice regarding the risk of myocardial infarction with TRT. Seven systematic reviews of 6 to 75 randomized controlled trials estimated the odds ratios or relative risks of cardiovascular events with TRT as follows (95% confidence intervals in parentheses): 1.14 (0.59-2.20), 1.82 (0.78-4.23), 0.91 (0.29-2.82), 1.54 (1.09-2.18), 1.28 (0.76-2.13), 1.07 (0.69-1.65), and 1.10 (0.86-1.41). Six of the 7 systematic reviews concluded that TRT was not statistically associated with cardiovascular events (thus, Answer E is incorrect). In subgroup analyses, 2 of the systematic reviews reported increased risk with oral testosterone only and within the first 12 months of TRT.

A trial of testosterone therapy (Answer A) is the correct recommendation for this patient, as it is a reasonable option in the setting of multiple sexual symptoms, confirmed low levels of serum testosterone, and the patient's inclination to try TRT. TRT may or may not improve his symptoms, which may not be related to his androgen levels. If there is no improvement in his symptoms after 3 to 6 months, the TRT can be discontinued.

There is no solid evidence that TRT should be avoided in men older than a certain age or should not be offered to men with a positive family history of heart disease. Regardless of whether he is prescribed TRT, the cardiovascular risk of this 69-year-old man should be assessed given his age, hypertension, and positive family history. There is no evidence that adding an aromatase inhibitor (Answer B) to lower estradiol levels would be safer than TRT alone. In fact, the Framingham Heart Study demonstrated that men with endogenous estradiol levels in the highest quartile had a lower 10-year incidence of cardiovascular disease. Prescribing a phosphodiesterase 5 inhibitor alone would also be reasonable as there are no contraindications. Adding a phosphodiesterase 5 inhibitor, such as tadalafil, after he has been on TRT would be reasonable, but prescribing both at the same time (Answer C) would make it difficult to assess which medication could be improving his erectile dysfunction. Yohimbine (Answer D) is a plant alkaloid with α2-adrenergic–blocking activity and is considered a second-line treatment for erectile dysfunction.

Educational Objective
Counsel a man on the potential cardiovascular effects of testosterone replacement therapy.

UpToDate Topic Review(s)
Testosterone treatment of male hypogonadism

Reference(s)

Arnlöv J, Pencina MJ, Amin S, et al. Endogenous sex hormones and cardiovascular disease incidence in men. *Ann Intern Med.* 2006;145(3):176-184. PMID: 16880459

Bhasin S, Brito JP, Cunningham GR, et al. Testosterone therapy in men with hypogonadism: an Endocrine Society clinical practice guideline. *J Clin Endocrinol Metab*. 2018;103(5):1715-1744. PMID: 29562364

Onasanya O, Iyer G, Lucas E, Lin D, Singh S, Alexander GC. Association between exogenous testosterone and cardiovascular events: an overview of systematic reviews. *Lancet Diabetes Endocrinol*. 2016;4(11):943-956. PMID: 27669646

46 ANSWER: C) Biopsy of the adrenal mass

This patient presented with widespread lymphadenopathy due to lymphoma, which resolved on surveillance imaging with appropriate lymphoma-directed therapy. However, the focus of decision-making now involves a new large left adrenal mass that is heterogeneous with lipid-poor content (as evidenced by high attenuation [>10 Hounsfield units] on unenhanced CT). The radiographic characteristics of an adrenal mass are critical in evaluating whether the mass is benign or potentially malignant. Reassuring features that are suggestive of a benign adrenal mass include small size (generally <4 cm), round and uniform shape, homogenous appearance, and high lipid content (such as low attenuation on unenhanced CT [<10 Hounsfield units] or loss of signal on out-of-phase sequencing on MRI), and high contrast washout on delayed contrast CT imaging. Features that raise concern for a malignant process include larger size (generally >4 or 6 cm), irregular shape or contours, heterogeneous content, calcifications, low lipid content on CT or MRI, and poor washout on delayed contrast CT imaging. A benign pheochromocytoma may have poor lipid content and poor washout on delayed contrast CT imaging, but it generally presents with a round contour and shape and with substantial elevations in metanephrines. Thus, this patient's new adrenal mass is concerning for a potentially malignant process and the main issue at hand is whether this process represents a metastatic lymphoma or a primary adrenal malignancy (such as adrenocortical carcinoma). A more distant consideration, particularly since the patient was treated with medications that can suppress the immune system, is whether this mass may represent a fungal or tuberculous infection. However, the round shape and contour of the mass is atypical for infiltrative adrenal infections.

The role of adrenal biopsy is limited to 2 scenarios: (1) confirmation of an extra-adrenal metastasis to determine staging and consequent management and (2) confirmation of an invasive infectious infiltration of the adrenal glands. Both scenarios can be either unilateral or bilateral processes. If this adrenal mass represents a metastatic lymphoma, a decision to surgically debulk the disease or give systemic medical therapy could be made. However, if this mass represents an adrenocortical carcinoma, the treatment of choice would be a radical adrenalectomy. Thus, an adrenal biopsy (Answer C) to confirm or exclude a lymphoma would provide critical data to inform the subsequent staging and treatment decisions.

Further imaging with MRI (Answer A) or PET-CT (Answer B) is unlikely to distinguish a lymphoma from an adrenocortical carcinoma. Proceeding to surgery without confirming the diagnosis (Answers D and E) could be problematic since this could result in the inappropriate approach to a cancer-focused surgical adrenalectomy or the unnecessary removal of a lymphoma that could be medically treated.

In this case, the mass was ultimately confirmed to be a high-grade stage III adrenocortical carcinoma and the patient underwent appropriate surgical resection. Although this vignette represents the rare confluence of 2 uncommon diagnoses, it highlights the value in approaching the evaluation of an adrenal mass in a systematic manner.

Educational Objective

Determine when an adrenal biopsy is indicated to assess for a potential invasive infection or an extra-adrenal malignancy.

UpToDate Topic Review(s)

Clinical presentation and evaluation of adrenocortical tumors

Reference(s)

Fassnacht M, Arlt W, Bancos I, et al. Management of adrenal incidentalomas: European Society of Endocrinology clinical practice guideline in collaboration with the European Network for the Study of Adrenal Tumors. *Eur J Endocrinol*. 2016;175(2):G1-G34. PMID: 27390021

47 ANSWER: E) Referral to gynecology for bilateral oophorectomy

New or significantly worsening hirsutism with a rapid pace in a premenopausal or postmenopausal woman can be a symptom of a tumor producing excess androgens. In a postmenopausal woman, the normal range for total testosterone is not clearly defined and should be on the lower end of the reference range given the known decline in ovarian androgens produced during menopause. Therefore, the mild elevation in total testosterone in this case is more notable than in a premenopausal woman. In addition, what is considered a normal-sized ovary in a premenopausal woman might be considered larger than normal in a postmenopausal woman.

Menopause can be associated with symptoms of mild hirsutism because of an excess of ovarian androgen production from high postmenopausal gonadotropin levels compared to the more abrupt menopausal fall in estrogens. In this case, the patient's terminal hair distribution across the upper back, buttocks, and chest with a Ferriman-Gallwey score above 15 and rapid pace of symptom development demonstrate a more severe presentation that requires further evaluation. The presence of virilization signs—voice deepening, male-pattern alopecia, and clitoromegaly—would be additional indications of a severe presentation requiring assessment for an androgen-producing tumor. Simply reassuring this patient that her symptoms are due to menopause (Answer C) would be inappropriate.

Even though a tumor is not specifically identified on ovarian ultrasonography, ovarian pathology could still be the source of androgen excess. Leydig-cell tumors can present with symptoms of androgen excess even when not visible by imaging. Ovarian hyperthecosis is a nonneoplastic condition of androgen excess classically described by the presentation of significant and progressive hirsutism or virilization due to differentiation of ovarian interstitial cells into active luteinized theca cells capable of producing androstenedione and testosterone. It is more common in postmenopausal women with more severe, progressive hirsutism or even virilization. Premenopausal women with ovarian hyperthecosis tend to also have more severe hirsutism or virilization with even higher total testosterone concentrations. In some cases, the ultrasound might demonstrate homogeneous, hyperechogenic ovarian stroma. Especially in a postmenopausal woman, this might be more difficult to appreciate, and the diagnosis is often made on the basis of pathology. Although the gold standard is a histologic diagnosis with nests of steroidogenically active luteinized stromal cells throughout the ovarian stroma, cases have also been described with normal ovarian histology. Other clinical features suggestive of ovarian hyperthecosis include postmenopausal status with symptoms of hyperandrogenism, ovarian volume of 6 cc or greater, or total testosterone concentration of 150 ng/dL or greater ($\geq$5.2 nmol/L). Yet, as many as 50% of androgen-secreting tumors are associated with total testosterone levels less than 150 ng/dL and can be associated with normal ovarian volume.

Ovarian and adrenal venous sampling (Answer D) can be particularly helpful to distinguish between an ovarian or adrenal source when an adrenal nodule/adenoma is present, especially in a premenopausal woman. This is a technically difficult test that should only be performed in a tertiary care center by an experienced interventional radiologist. However, adrenal tumors are a very rare cause of hirsutism in women. The diagnosis of ovarian hyperthecosis is more likely in this patient with more rapidly progressive hirsutism, ovarian volume of 6 cc or greater, and total testosterone level above the normal range generally defined in premenopausal women.

Although medical treatment with spironolactone (Answer B), GnRH agonists, or oral contraceptives (Answer A) might be considered in suspected ovarian hyperthecosis, this patient is very symptomatic and distressed. The best recommendation would be referral for bilateral oophorectomy (Answer E), which will be both diagnostic and therapeutic.

Educational Objective
Diagnose and treat ovarian hyperthecosis in a postmenopausal woman with hirsutism.

UpToDate Topic Review(s)
Ovarian hyperthecosis

Reference(s)

Alpañés M, González-Casbas JM, Sánchez J, Pián H, Escobar-Morreale HF. Management of Postmenopausal Virilization. *J Clin Endocrinol Metab*. 2012;97(8): 2584-2588. PMID: 22669303

Markopoulos MC, Kassi E, Alexandraki KI, Mastorakos G, Kaltsas G. Hyperandrogenism after menopause. *Eur J Endocrinol*. 2015;172(2):R79-R91. PMID: 25225480

Giacobbe M, Mendes Pinto-Neto A, Simoes Costa-Paiva LH, Martinez EZ. The usefulness of ovarian volume, antral follicle count and age as predictors of menopausal status. *Climacteric*. 2004;7(3):255-260. PMID: 15669549

48 ANSWER: E) Liraglutide

Inadequate weight loss after bariatric surgery can be due to insufficient initial weight loss after surgery (defined as losing <50% of excess weight at 12 months) or due to progressive weight regain (defined as gaining ≥15% of maximal initial weight lost). The patient described achieved an initial successful weight loss; however, she has now regained most of her weight. Weight regain after bariatric surgery is multifactorial and is associated with recurrence of presurgical comorbid conditions. Up to 35% of patients experience weight regain 2 to 5 years after their initial bariatric surgery. Therapeutic interventions for weight regain after bariatric surgery include lifestyle modification, endoscopic therapies, and revisional surgery. Successful management of weight regain with lifestyle modification alone is difficult, as weight regain usually results from nonadherence to dietary and physical activity recommendations. Endoscopic procedures such as stoma reductions, pouch plications, and sclerotherapy are not effective over the long term. Revisional surgery is an effective approach; however, it has substantially higher morbidity.

In clinical practice, patients who experience weight regain after bariatric surgery are often prescribed weight-loss medications to aid with their weight-loss efforts. On average, an additional 7.6% weight loss occurs when a weight-loss medication is added after bariatric surgery. Small clinical studies with short follow-up periods have been published regarding phentermine, phentermine/topiramate, and liraglutide. Patients who experienced weight regain or weight loss plateau after bariatric surgery and took phentermine or phentermine/topiramate for 90 days lost 12.8% and 12.9% of their excess weight, respectively. A study of liraglutide, 1.8 mg daily for 12.5 weeks, documented weight loss of 7.3%. The recommended liraglutide dosage for chronic weight management is 3.0 mg daily. Although data are limited, these medications are the preferred weight-loss agents for patients who experience weight regain after bariatric surgery. The patient described in this vignette is a candidate for liraglutide (Answer E) for management of her weight regain. Phentermine (Answer B) could be an option if her blood pressure were controlled.

Data are insufficient, regarding both efficacy and safety, to recommend lorcaserin (Answer A) or naltrexone/bupropion (Answer D) as first-line treatment in this patient population. Also, this patient takes opioids regularly, so naltrexone/bupropion would be contraindicated. Her use of fluoxetine is not a contraindication for lorcaserin; however, concomitant use of both medications may increase her risk of developing serotonin syndrome. Metformin (Answer C) is a drug approved for treatment of type 2 diabetes and is associated with mild weight loss (<5%). This patient does not have diabetes, so metformin would not be a drug of choice.

Educational Objective
Recommend treatment options for patients who regain weight after bariatric surgery.

UpToDate Topic Review(s)
Late complications of bariatric surgical operations

Reference(s)

Schwartz J, Chaudhry UI, Suzo A, et al. Pharmacotherapy in conjunction with a diet and exercise program for the treatment of weight recidivism or weight loss plateau post-bariatric surgery: a retrospective review. *Obes Surg*. 2016;26(2):452-458. PMID: 26615406

Pajecki D, Halpern A, Cercato C, Mancini M, de Cleva R, Santo MA. Short-term use of liraglutide in the management of patients with weight regain after bariatric surgery. *Rev Col Bras Cir*. 2013;40(3):191-195. PMID: 23912365

Garvey WT, Mechanick JI, Brett EM, et al; Reviewers of the AACE/ACE Obesity Clinical Practice Guidelines. American Association of Clinical Endocrinologists and American College of Endocrinology comprehensive clinical practice guidelines for medical care of patients with obesity. *Endocr Pract*. 2016;22(Suppl 3):1-203. PMID: 27219496

49 ANSWER: A) Use of exogenous insulin

Hypoglycemia is an uncommon condition in patients without diabetes mellitus. The correct diagnosis can be determined by ordering appropriate laboratory tests at the time of hypoglycemia. Only those patients who fulfill the Whipple triad should undergo further evaluation. The Whipple triad consists of having symptoms suggestive of hypoglycemia, documentation of a low plasma glucose level, and resolution of hypoglycemic symptoms after treatment of the hypoglycemia.

The patient in this vignette has developed recurrent severe hypoglycemia and has no history of diabetes. Fortunately, he has undergone evaluation in the emergency department and, for the most part, the laboratory workup has been completed. In a patient with hypoglycemia due to a neuroendocrine insulin-secreting tumor, the insulin level should be elevated (≥3.0 μIU/mL [≥20.8 pmol/L]) at the time of hypoglycemia (plasma glucose ≤55 mg/dL [≤3.1 mmol/L]). The C-peptide and proinsulin levels should also be elevated. The β-hydroxybutyrate level should be in the normal range due to the effects of endogenous insulin on suppression of ketone body production by the liver. Surreptitious use of an insulin secretogue (sulfonylurea or glinide) leads to identical results. Therefore, assessment for insulin secretagogues must be part of the complete evaluation of hypoglycemia.

In this case, the patient's plasma insulin value is elevated at the time of frank hypoglycemia. Therefore, this represents insulin-mediated hypoglycemia (thus, Answer E is incorrect). However, the C-peptide level is in the low-normal range and the proinsulin level is frankly low. This excludes endogenous hyperinsulinism from an insulin-secreting neuroendocrine tumor (Answer D) as the cause of the hypoglycemia. Even though an insulin secretagogue screen was not completed in this case, the low or low-normal proinsulin and C-peptide values rule out surreptitious use of a sulfonylurea or meglitinide (Answer B).

Non-insulinoma pancreatogenous hypoglycemia syndrome (Answer C) has been described in a small subset of patients who have undergone Roux-en-Y gastric bypass surgery. Affected patients present with postprandial hypoglycemia rather than fasting hypoglycemia. The laboratory findings are identical to that of a neuroendocrine insulin-secreting tumor. This type of hypoglycemia is thought to be due to islet-cell hyperplasia or nesidioblastosis, which does not lead to tumor formation, so anatomic imaging studies are therefore negative. In this setting, the C-peptide and proinsulin levels are not elevated, thus ruling out non-insulinoma pancreatogenous hypoglycemia syndrome as the cause of this patient's hypoglycemia.

The results of the biochemical evaluation are consistent with factitious hypoglycemia (Answer A). The patient has been given exogenous insulin, either intentionally or by accident. The insulin level is elevated at the time of hypoglycemia; however, the C-peptide and proinsulin values are low or undetectable. Given the scenario, the patient was most likely given a long-acting insulin such as insulin glargine, detemir, or degludec. An immunoassay for insulin can be ordered to detect exogenously administered insulin. However, not all of the newer recombinant insulin analogues can be detected by a given commercially available assay.

Educational Objective
Explain the differential diagnosis of hypoglycemia in a patient without diabetes mellitus and correctly interpret the laboratory results in the setting of hypoglycemia.

UpToDate Topic Review(s)
Factitious hypoglycemia

Reference(s)

Cryer PE, Axelrod L, Grossman AB, et al; Endocrine Society. Evaluation and management of adult hypoglycemic disorders: an Endocrine Society Clinical Practice Guideline. *J Clin Endocrinol Metab*. 2009;94(3):709-728. PMID: 19088155

Grunberger G, Weiner JL, Silverman R, Taylor S, Gorden P. Factitious hypoglycemia due to surreptitious administration of insulin. Diagnosis, treatment, and long-term follow-up. *Ann Intern Med*. 1988;108(2):252-257. PMID: 3277509

Neal JM, Han W. Insulin immunoassays in the detection of insulin analogues in factitious hypoglycemia. *Endocr Pract*. 2008;14(8):1006-1010. PMID: 19095600

50 ANSWER: C) Cumulative ^{131}I dose of 458 mCi

The primary goal of radioiodine (RAI) administration following total thyroidectomy for differentiated thyroid cancer includes (1) *RAI thyroid remnant ablation* to facilitate detection of recurrence and to improve initial staging with serum thyroglobulin measurements or whole-body RAI scans, (2) *RAI adjuvant therapy* to improve disease-free survival by destroying suspected, but unproven, residual disease, especially in patients at increased risk of disease recurrence, or (3) *RAI therapy* to improve disease-specific and disease-free survival by treating persistent disease in patients at higher risk. Other factors influencing decision-making processes regarding RAI in thyroid cancer include comorbidities, preferred disease surveillance procedures, and patient preferences. Following total thyroidectomy, RAI ablation is routinely recommended for patients deemed to be at high risk by the American Thyroid Association guidelines and it should be considered for patients at medium risk. For regional nodal metastases discovered on diagnostic whole-body scan, RAI may be used in patients with low-volume disease or in combination with surgery, although surgery is typically preferred in the presence of bulky disease or when disease is amenable to surgery.

Current guidelines recommend RAI therapy for pulmonary micrometastases (<2 mm), and this therapy should be repeated every 6 to 12 months as long as the disease continues to concentrate RAI and respond clinically. Radioiodine-avid macronodular metastases can be treated with RAI, and treatment may be repeated when objective benefit, including decrease in lesion size and/or decrease in thyroglobulin, is demonstrated. However, complete remission is rare and survival remains poor. While RAI appears to be a reasonably safe therapy, it is associated with a cumulative dose-related low risk of early- and late-onset complications such as salivary gland damage, dental caries, nasolacrimal duct obstruction, secondary malignancies and effects on fertility. A risk to benefit ratio should be established on an individual basis.

The patient in this vignette has thyroid cancer that was classified as stage IVa according to the American Joint Committee on Cancer 7th Edition TNM classification. Using the revised 8th Edition, this would be classified as stage II disease. An ablative dose of RAI was administered immediately after thyroidectomy because of the finding of a moderate-risk tumor according to the American Thyroid Association risk stratification (aggressive histologic characteristics: tall-cell variant papillary carcinoma). In view of pulmonary metastases, 2 therapeutic doses of RAI were also administered.

While patients should be counseled regarding the risks of developing secondary primary malignancies, the absolute risk in patients who have undergone RAI treatment is small and generally does not warrant screening to any extent greater than age-appropriate general population health screening. Large retrospective studies have estimated the relative risk of second malignancies in patients with thyroid cancer treated with RAI to be 1.19 (95% confidence interval, 1.04-1.36; $P<.010$) and that of leukemia to be 2.5 (95% confidence interval, 1.13-5.53; $P<.024$) compared with risk in patients with thyroid cancer not treated with RAI. The risk of secondary malignancies is dose related, with an excess absolute risk of 14.4 for solid cancers and 0.8 for leukemias per gigabecquerel (1 GBq = 27 mCi) of RAI at 10,000 person-years of follow-up. The risk is clearly increased in patients who have been treated with large cumulative activity that is higher than 500 to 600 mCi, which suggests a dose–effect relationship. The cumulative dose of 458 mCi of RAI administered (Answer C) is most likely to have contributed to this patient's risk of developing leukemia.

An excess risk of second hematologic malignancies is observed more commonly in patients younger than 45 years when treated with RAI compared with those older than 45 (thus, Answer D is incorrect). There is no evidence that sex (Answer A), family history of malignancy (Answer B), and the histologic subtype of thyroid cancer (Answer E) are associated with varied risks of developing secondary malignancies following RAI treatment of thyroid cancer. Epidemiologic studies have shown an increased risk of breast cancer in women with thyroid cancer. It is unclear whether this is due to screening bias, RAI therapy, or other factors.

Educational Objective
Assess the risk of secondary malignancy in patients treated with radioiodine for thyroid cancer.

UpToDate Topic Review(s)
Differentiated thyroid cancer: Radioiodine treatment

Reference(s)

Rubino C, de Vathaire F, Dottorini ME, et al. Second primary malignancies in thyroid cancer patients. *Br J Cancer.* 2003;89(9):1638-1644. PMID: 14583762

Sawka AM, Thabane L, Parlea L, et al. Second primary malignancy risk after radioactive iodine treatment for thyroid cancer: a systematic review and meta-analysis. *Thyroid.* 2009;19(5):451-457. PMID: 19281429

Haugen BR, Alexander EK, Bible KC, et al. 2015 American Thyroid Association Management Guidelines for Adult Patients with Thyroid Nodules and Differentiated Thyroid Cancer: the American Thyroid Association Guidelines Task Force on Thyroid Nodules and Differentiated Thyroid Cancer. *Thyroid.* 2016;26(1):1-133. PMID: 26462967

51 ANSWER: B) Perform DXA scanning to include measurement of the nondominant, proximal one-third radius

Bone and mineral disturbances are common following bariatric surgical procedures, and they appear to correlate with the degree of malabsorption induced by the specific surgical approach (ie, greater effects with duodenal switch and Roux-en-Y than with gastric restrictive procedures). The most pronounced effects of such procedures appear to be on PTH secretion and, most likely related, increases in markers of bone formation and resorption. As a result of these changes, and expectedly paralleling the skeletal effects of patients with primary hyperparathyroidism, significantly greater declines occur in cortical-rich skeletal sites (femoral neck and proximal one-third radius) than in cancellous-rich sites (lumbar spine). These biochemical and skeletal changes are very likely related to the increase in nonvertebral fracture risk that has been observed following bariatric surgery, particularly in patients who undergo Roux-en-Y vs gastric restriction such as sleeve gastrectomy. Given this evidence, it is critical to measure bone mineral density in patients who have undergone bariatric surgery, and this assessment should include the proximal one-third radius as a DXA skeletal site (Answer B).

This patient has a mid-range normal albumin-adjusted calcium level, thus markedly reducing the clinical suspicion for primary hyperparathyroidism. As such, neither nuclear parathyroid imaging (Answer C) as an attempt to localize a candidate parathyroid adenoma nor referral to endocrine surgery for consideration of neck exploration (Answer D) is indicated for this patient. Although he does have a sibling with a history of primary hyperparathyroidism, the high prevalence of the condition in the general population makes this a most likely unrelated finding.

Although calcitriol (Answer E) and other vitamin D analogues may lower PTH levels, there is no evidence that they reduce the risk of nonvertebral fractures in patients with osteoporosis.

Finally, this patient is already sufficient in 25-hydroxyvitamin D, and further increases in serum 25-hydroxyvitamin D by increasing his cholecalciferol dosage (Answer A) would not be expected to reduce his PTH level nor enhance intestinal calcium absorption. The low urinary calcium should prompt the clinician to confirm that the patient is adherent to supplemental calcium. Of note, this patient is already on calcium citrate, which has been proven to be more bioavailable than calcium carbonate in patients who have undergone Roux-en-Y gastric bypass.

Educational Objective
Manage secondary hyperparathyroidism following bariatric surgery.

UpToDate Topic Review(s)
Bariatric surgery: Postoperative nutritional management

Reference(s)

Liu C, Wu D, Zhang JF, et al. Changes in bone metabolism in morbidly obese patients after bariatric surgery: a meta-analysis. *Obes Surg*. 2016;26(1):91-97. PMID: 25982806

Yu EW, Lee MP, Landon JE, Lindeman KG, Kim SC. Fracture risk after bariatric surgery: Roux-en-Y gastric bypass versus adjustable gastric banding. *J Bone Miner Res*. 2017;32(6):1229-1236. PMID: 28251687

Tondapu P, Provost D, Adams-Huet B, Sims T, Chang C, Sakhaee K. Comparison of the absorption of calcium carbonate and calcium citrate after Roux-en-Y gastric bypass. *Obes Surg*. 2009;19(9):1256-1261. PMID: 19437082

52 ANSWER: E) Cortisol, low; ACTH, normal; DHEA-S, low

Surgical cure of an ACTH-secreting adenoma is invariably followed by the development of central adrenal insufficiency. This is due to the chronic suppression of the function of the normal corticotroph cells. For this reason, patients must be promptly placed on glucocorticoid replacement therapy. It may take many months or years for the hypothalamic-pituitary-adrenal (HPA) axis to recover. A similar hormonal pattern during HPA axis recovery is seen after unilateral adrenalectomy for cortisol-secreting adenomas and after successful surgery that removes the source of ACTH in the ectopic ACTH secretion syndrome. However, the length of time until the HPA axis recovers seems shorter in Cushing disease (mean, 1.4 years [interquartile range, 0.9-3.4 years]) than in adrenal Cushing syndrome (mean, 2.5 years [interquartile range, 1.6-5.4 years]). During this period, patients should be educated about adrenal insufficiency management and sick day rules and should wear a medical alert tag.

While the time necessary for HPA axis recovery is highly variable, its pattern is quite typical. After an initial phase during which both ACTH and cortisol are low, ACTH starts rising and often goes through a period of supraphysiologic levels. Cortisol lags behind the ACTH increase, as it takes a period of ACTH stimulation for the atrophied adrenal gland(s) to start working again. Eventually, both ACTH and cortisol normalize. Typically, during this period, one should check early-morning serum cortisol and plasma ACTH (before the hydrocortisone dose) every 8 to 12 weeks. If the previous day's afternoon hydrocortisone dose was taken before 3 PM, it does not interfere with the morning cortisol measurement. When cortisol starts rising, one can start reducing the replacement dose, as well as add DHEA-S serum measurement to periodic blood draws. When the cortisol concentration is above 15 µg/dL (>413.8 nmol/L), hydrocortisone can be stopped. For cortisol levels between 10 and 15 µg/dL (275.9-413.8 nmol/L), one should consider ordering an ACTH stimulation test to verify recovery of the axis before completely stopping replacement.

DHEA-S is the last hormone level to normalize, often remaining low for years. Unless the patient's Cushing disease recurs, DHEA-S never becomes elevated. Therefore, any of the listed answers with a pattern of elevated DHEA-S (Answers A, B, D) is incorrect.

The patient in this vignette is doing well, and it is impossible to predict with certainty whether her HPA axis has now recovered or is still recovering, or whether she still has adrenal insufficiency. The patterns in both Answer C and Answer E are possible. However, the most likely scenario is Answer E, as it would be very unlikely that ACTH would still be suppressed 11 months after surgery and with a nonsuppressive dose of hydrocortisone (particularly because her normal menstrual pattern indicates that the pituitary gland was not damaged during surgery).

Educational Objective
Explain the pattern of recovery of the hypothalamic-pituitary-adrenal axis after successful surgery for Cushing disease.

UpToDate Topic Review(s)
Primary therapy of Cushing's disease: transsphenoidal surgery and pituitary irradiation

Reference(s)

Fitzgerald PA, Aron DC, Findling JW, et al. Cushing's disease: transient secondary adrenal insufficiency after selective removal of pituitary microadenomas; evidence for a pituitary origin. *J Clin Endocrinol Metab*. 1982;54(2):413-422. PMID: 6274904

Prete A, Paragliola RM, Bottiglieri F, et al. Factors predicting the duration of adrenal insufficiency in patients successfully treated for Cushing disease and nonmalignant primary adrenal Cushing syndrome. *Endocrine*. 2017;55(3):969-980. PMID: 27395418

Berr CM, Di Dalmazi G, Osswald A, et al. Time to recovery of adrenal function after curative surgery for Cushing's syndrome depends on etiology. *J Clin Endocrinol Metab*. 2015;100(4):1300-1308. PMID: 25546155

53 ANSWER: D) Duloxetine

Approximately 1% of patients with diabetes mellitus experience diabetic amyotrophy and present with subacute or acute, progressive, asymmetric pain and then weakness of the proximal lower extremities. Pain is the initial symptom followed by weakness, and the symptoms can become more symmetric over time. Weight loss is also associated with this process. It is most often observed in older patients with fairly well-controlled type 2 diabetes. Affected patients do not usually have evidence of retinopathy or nephropathy.

This entity has a number of names, including diabetic amyotrophy, Bruns-Garland syndrome, diabetic myelopathy, diabetic polyradiculopathy, diabetic radiculoplexus neuropathy, diabetic lumbosacral plexopathy, and diabetic lumbosacral radiculoplexus neuropathy. The various names assigned to it reflect the debate about its neuroanatomic location and physiologic underpinnings. The etiology is thought to be ischemia due to microscopic polyangiitis. Thus, there has been interest in immunotherapy for the management of diabetic amyotrophy.

Some retrospective studies have reported clinical improvement with immune suppression. Therapies such as oral prednisone, intravenous methylprednisolone (Answer A), intravenous immunoglobulin (Answer B), and cyclophosphamide (Answer C) have all been considered as possible useful treatment options. A Cochrane database systematic review in 2017 identified 73 relevant articles on initial search. Only 1 randomized controlled trial in abstract form showed no benefit from the use of methylprednisolone for diabetic amyotrophy. Immunotherapy has not clearly been shown to be effective in this patient population. There are also no data showing that tighter blood glucose control (Answer E) changes the course of the disorder.

Typically, patients with diabetic amyotrophy show clinical improvement over time without specific disease-altering therapy. It is therefore difficult to determine whether any of the agents tested impacts outcomes or whether improvement is simply due to the natural history of the disorder. Patients are often left with some residual symptoms such as foot drop. Currently, symptomatic management is recommended with agents such as tricyclic antidepressants, pregabalin, duloxetine (Answer D), and gabapentin. Thus, duloxetine is the best option for this patient.

Educational Objective
Recommend appropriate management of diabetic amyotrophy.

UpToDate Topic Review(s)
Diabetic amyotrophy and idiopathic lumbosacral radiculoplexus neuropathy

Reference(s)
Chan YC, Lo YL, Chan ES. Immunotherapy for diabetic amyotrophy. *Cochrane Database Syst Rev.* 2017;7:CD006521. PMID: 28746752

Dyck JB, O'Brien P, Bosch EP, et al. The multi-center double-blind controlled trial of IV methylprednisolone in diabetic lumbosacral radiculoplexus neuropathy. *Neurology.* 2006;66(5):A191.

54 ANSWER: A) Decrease his dietary oxalate intake
The patient in this vignette has recurrent kidney stones composed primarily of calcium oxalate, which is the most common type of kidney stones. His biochemical workup reveals hypercalciuria along with an elevated urinary calcium oxalate saturation ratio. Because the risk of stone formation increases with increasing urinary oxalate, a lower intake of dietary oxalate and vitamin C is prudent (vitamin C is metabolized into oxalate); thus, Answer A is correct and Answer C is incorrect. Examples of oxalate-rich foods and beverages to avoid include beets, nuts (eg, peanuts, almonds, walnuts, cashews, pecans), peanut butter, rhubarb, spinach, sweet potatoes, wheat bran, strawberries, kiwi, soy products, chocolate/cocoa, chocolate milk, tea, and draft beer.

Other dietary risk factors for recurrent nephrolithiasis include lower fluid intake and higher sodium intake (thus, Answer D is incorrect). The effect of dietary calcium intake is paradoxical, as increased dietary calcium intake is associated with a decreased risk of kidney stones (thus, Answer B is incorrect). Examples of calcium-rich foods and beverages include dairy products (eg, cheese, yogurt, ice cream, milk).

Drug therapy such as hydrochlorothiazide (Answer E) is indicated if the stone disease remains active or if there is insufficient improvement in the urine chemistries despite dietary modification over a 3- to 6-month period. It would be premature to initiate this drug now before first attempting dietary changes.

Educational Objective
Identify risk factors for calcium oxalate stone formation in a patient with recurrent nephrolithiasis and provide appropriate counseling.

UpToDate Topic Review(s)
Prevention of recurrent calcium stones in adults

Reference(s)
Massey LK, Liebman M, Kynast-Gales SA. Ascorbate increases human oxaluria and kidney stone risk. *J Nutr.* 2005;135(7):1673-1677. PMID: 15987848

Heilberg IP, Goldfarb DS. Optimum nutrition for kidney stone disease. *Adv Chronic Kidney Dis.* 2013;20(2):165-174. PMID: 23439376

National Institute of Diabetes and Digestive and Kidney Diseases. Eating, diet, and nutrition for kidney stones. Available at: https://www.niddk.nih.gov/health-information/urologic-diseases/kidney-stones/eating-diet-nutrition. Accessed for verification April 3, 2018.

55 ANSWER: E) Pursue no further evaluation or treatment
Identification of adrenal insufficiency in acute illness is controversial. Patients with significant intercurrent illness should, in theory, undergo activation of the hypothalamic-pituitary-adrenal axis, resulting in significant elevation of free plasma cortisol levels and enhanced responsiveness to ACTH stimulation. Insufficient cortisol production during septic shock has been termed functional or relative adrenal insufficiency. However, there is no consensus about the diagnostic criteria or indications for treatment of this entity. In addition,

there exists considerable disagreement over what cortisol level is normal or appropriate in the setting of septic shock, what constitutes an adequate response to ACTH, and what dose of synthetic ACTH should be used for stimulation testing. Two very recent placebo-controlled trials have further examined this concept and continue to show conflicting results. In one trial, hydrocortisone did not reduce mortality at 28 or 90 days, while in the other trial, in more unwell patients, hydrocortisone plus fludrocortisone reduced mortality at 90 and 180 days, but not at 28 days. In both trials, hydrocortisone resulted in faster resolution of shock and was not harmful, but it did cause hyperglycemia.

In this vignette, there is very little clinical evidence to support adrenal insufficiency. The patient is recovering well, she is hemodynamically stable with satisfactory urine output, and she does not require inotropic support. In addition, she has no major risk factors for adrenal insufficiency: no recent use of glucocorticoids and no family history of autoimmune disease. While the anesthetic agent etomidate can cause temporary adrenal insufficiency due to its inhibition of the enzyme 11β-hydroxylase, this only lasts for a maximum of 24 hours. Therefore, the best advice in this situation is not to look for adrenal insufficiency in the first place (Answer E).

Both the high-dose (250 mcg) and low-dose (1 mcg) ACTH-stimulation tests (Answers A and B) have been studied in the context of septic shock, which is not analogous to the situation outlined above. Overall, the results have been inconsistent, particularly when a postcosyntropin increment of serum cortisol of 9 μg/dL or greater (≥248.3 nmol/L) is used as a diagnostic criterion, regardless of the baseline level. While the increment may confer some prognostic value, it is of questionable clinical significance in this setting and should not be used to diagnose relative adrenal dysfunction. Indeed, most patients who have a postcosyntropin increment less than 9 μg/dL have hypoproteinemia and it can be a normal variant in up to 20% of healthy persons.

An important, but often overlooked, limitation in testing for adrenal insufficiency in the context of significant illness is the influence of hypoproteinemia on serum cortisol levels. More than 90% of serum cortisol is bound to either cortisol-binding globulin (transcortin) or albumin, while the free fraction is the biologically active form. As is often the case, this patient who has had major surgery with a subsequent pneumonia has significant hypoalbuminemia, which will influence interpretation of serum cortisol levels and could erroneously lead to a diagnosis of relative adrenal insufficiency.

When serum-binding proteins are near normal (albumin >2.5 g/dL), a random measurement of serum cortisol can provide an accurate assessment of adrenal function. In such a setting, a serum cortisol concentration of 15 μg/dL or greater (≥413.8 nmol/L) would be satisfactory. In patients with hypoproteinemia (albumin <2.5 g/dL), a random serum cortisol concentration would be expected to be 11 μg/dL or greater (≥303.5 nmol/L). There is generally no need to perform an ACTH-stimulation test in the setting of critical illness, as this rarely provides meaningful information and often leads to confusion and unnecessary corticosteroid treatment.

Thus, the patient in this vignette has no clinical evidence to support adrenal insufficiency and has a satisfactory random serum cortisol level in the context of hypoproteinemia. Therefore, hydrocortisone replacement (Answer C) is not required and no further evaluation of the hypothalamic-pituitary-adrenal axis is needed (thus, Answers A, B, and D are incorrect).

Educational Objective
Identify the best strategy to recognize and treat adrenal insufficiency in acute illness.

UpToDate Topic Review(s)
Diagnosis of adrenal insufficiency in adults

Reference(s)

Hamrahian AH, Oseni TS, Arafah BM. Measurements of serum free cortisol in critically ill patients. *J Clin Endocrinol Metab*. 2004;350(16):1629-1638. PMID: 15084695

Arafah BM. Hypothalamic pituitary adrenal function during critical illness: limitations of current assessment methods. *J Clin Endocrinol Metab*. 2006;91(10): 3725-3745. PMID: 16882746

Annane D, Sébille V, Troché G, Raphaël JC, Gajdos P, Bellissant E. A 3-level prognostic classification in septic shock based on cortisol levels and cortisol response to corticotropin. *JAMA*. 2000;283(8):1038-1045. PMID: 10697064

Venkatesh B, Finfer S, Cohen J, et al; ADRENAL Trial Investigators and the Australian-New Zealand Intensive Care Society Clinical Trials Group. Adjunctive glucocorticoid therapy in patients with septic shock. *N Engl J Med*. 2018;378(9):797-808. PMID: 29347874

Annane D, Renault A, Brun-Buisson C, et al; CRICS-TRIGGERSEP Network. Hydrocortisone plus fludrocortisone for adults with septic shock. *N Engl J Med*. 2018;378(9):809-818. PMID: 29490185

56 ANSWER: A) Intrauterine device

Obesity is associated with reduced fertility secondary to anovulatory cycles. Rapid weight loss after bariatric surgery occurs in the first 6 to 18 months, which results in improved ovulation and higher fertility rates. Women of reproductive age who undergo bariatric surgery are counseled to avoid pregnancy for 12 to 18 months postoperatively, as pregnancy within 2 years of surgery increases the risk for adverse health outcomes. During the initial postoperative period, it can be difficult to meet the additional nutritional requirements of the developing fetus because maternal intake is markedly reduced.

When choosing the most appropriate contraceptive method, the type of bariatric surgery must be considered in addition to effectiveness and safety. A behavior-based method or sole use of a barrier method for contraception is not an ideal choice for this patient population due to higher failure rate (22% and 19%, respectively). After either a restrictive or malabsorptive procedure, the following are acceptable contraceptive options: (1) intrauterine device (Answer A), (2) progestin-only implant or injection, (3) combined hormonal patch, or (4) combined vaginal ring. Ninety percent of oral estrogen is absorbed in the stomach and the upper intestine, which are bypassed after malabsorptive surgeries. Given the concern of decreased absorption of oral hormonal preparations after malabsorptive surgery, patients should be counseled to avoid use of combined oral contraceptives or progestin-only pills unless other more appropriate methods are not available (thus, Answer A is correct and Answers B, C, D, and E are incorrect). Patients who undergo restrictive procedures are able to use oral contraceptive therapies.

Educational Objective

Counsel female patients regarding contraceptive options after bariatric surgery.

UpToDate Topic Review(s)

Fertility and pregnancy after bariatric surgery

Reference(s)

Curtis KM, Tepper NK, Jatlaoui TC, et al. U.S. Medical Eligibility Criteria for Contraceptive Use, 2016. *MMWR Recomm Rep*. 2016;65(3):1-103. PMID: 27467196

Kominiarek MA, Jungheim ES, Hoeger KM, Rogers AM, Kahan S, Kim JJ. American Society for Metabolic and Bariatric Surgery position statement on the impact of obesity and obesity treatment on fertility and fertility therapy Endorsed by the American College of Obstetricians and Gynecologists and the Obesity Society. *Surg Obes Relat Dis*. 2017;13(5):750-757. PMID: 28416185

Edelman AB, Cherala G, Stanczyk FZ. Metabolism and pharmacokinetics of contraceptive steroids in obese women: a review. *Contraception*. 2010;82(4): 314-323. PMID: 20851224

57 ANSWER: C) Order a continuous glucose monitor

This patient's hemoglobin A_{1c} level is in a reasonable range given her age. The variable glucose levels in the morning and fasting state, occasional late-afternoon hypoglycemia, and slight discordance between hemoglobin A_{1c} and mean glucose values throughout the day raise the possibility of unrecognized nocturnal hypoglycemia. The main issue is to determine whether this is due to excessive basal or bolus insulin. Her regimen demonstrates an imbalance in distribution of her insulin weighted more heavily towards basal insulin (70 units) than prandial insulin (45 units over the course of the day).

Reducing prandial insulin (Answer D) or discontinuing prandial insulin and adding a GLP-1 receptor agonist such as albiglutide (Answer E) would not be the best management steps. Although U300 glargine (Answer A) and U100 degludec (Answer B) offer some beneficial pharmacologic characteristics over U100 glargine, such as more reliable 24-hour coverage and less peak, this does not address the main issue of whether there is nocturnal hypoglycemia driving the hemoglobin A_{1c} down. Furthermore, because U100 degludec may be more potent than U100 glargine, most clinicians suggest that the starting dosage of degludec be reduced by 10% to 20% if fasting glucose values are at or near target range.

Continuous glucose monitoring (CGM) (Answer C), either intermittent or real-time, would help identify nocturnal hypoglycemia. Several studies have shown that use of CGM is associated with less time spent in hypoglycemia. A recent international consensus conference suggested that when there is a discrepancy between measured hemoglobin A_{1c} and estimated hemoglobin A_{1c} based on self-monitoring of blood glucose, alternative measures of glycemic control should be considered. Furthermore, assessment of glucose variability and hypoglycemia should be done with a CGM. While most studies demonstrating a beneficial effect of CGM have been conducted in patients with type 1 diabetes who use insulin pumps, 2 recent studies may be used to infer that this patient would benefit from CGM. In one study of patients with type 2 diabetes, use of intermittent CGM was associated with less hypoglycemia, but not lower hemoglobin A_{1c}. In a second study of patients with type 1 diabetes on a multiple daily insulin injection regimen, there was a significant reduction in hemoglobin A_{1c} and less biochemical hypoglycemia than that observed in the control group.

In this particular case, CGM may help in shared decision-making with the patient who is otherwise reluctant to change her regimen.

Educational Objective
Recommend continuous glucose monitoring to help identify nocturnal hypoglycemia in patients whose glycemic control seems good based on hemoglobin A_{1c} levels.

UpToDate Topic Review(s)
Self-monitoring of blood glucose in management of adults with diabetes mellitus

Reference(s)

Danne T, Nimri R, Battelino T, et al. International consensus on use of continuous glucose monitoring. *Diabetes Care.* 2017;40(12):1631-1640. PMID: 29162583

Beck RW, Riddlesworth T, Ruedy K, et al; DIAMOND Study Group. Effect of continuous glucose monitoring on glycemic control in adults with type 1 diabetes using insulin injections: the DIAMOND Randomized Clinical Trial. *JAMA.* 2017;317(4):371-378. PMID: 28118453

Beck RW, Riddlesworth TD, Ruedy K, et al; DIAMOND Study Group. Continuous glucose monitoring versus usual care in patients with type 2 diabetes receiving multiple daily insulin injections: a randomized trial. *Ann Intern Med.* 2017;167(6):365-374. PMID: 28828487

58 ANSWER: E) Start cholecalciferol, 2000 IU daily, and follow-up in 8 weeks

This patient presents with hypercalcemia and an inappropriately high-normal intact PTH level. This serum biochemical profile necessarily limits the differential diagnosis to PTH-mediated hypercalcemia (primary hyperparathyroidism due most often to a single or, less commonly, multiple parathyroid adenomas or very rare ectopic secretion of intact PTH) and familial hypocalciuric hypercalcemia (FHH) (due to an inactivating pathogenic variant in the gene encoding the calcium-sensing receptor [*CASR*] or in genes encoding downstream effector molecules that reduce the sensitivity of the receptor to extracellular calcium). It is critical to make the distinction between primary hyperparathyroidism and FHH due to the fact that the latter is almost universally a benign condition in which patients are neither cured nor clinically benefit from parathyroidectomy. FHH is generally suspected in patients who present with hypercalcemia and a high-normal or mildly elevated intact PTH level, as well as evidence of hypocalciuria (ie, calcium-to-creatinine ratio less than 0.01 based on the following formula:

$$\frac{\text{urine calcium (mg) x serum creatinine (mg)}}{\text{serum calcium (mg) x urine creatinine (mg)}}$$

This patient's calcium-to-creatinine ratio is 0.004 and is thus consistent with a possible diagnosis of FHH. However, her low-normal magnesium level argues against the presence of FHH, given that pathogenic variants in *CASR* also result in enhanced renal magnesium reabsorption and concomitant high-normal serum magnesium levels. Most importantly, she has evidence of true vitamin D deficiency, which is associated with a reduction in urinary calcium excretion, possibly due to an additional secondary increase in PTH secretion with an attendant increase in urinary calcium reabsorption. Additionally, a reduction in intestinal calcium absorption most likely results in a lowered filtered renal calcium load that is available for reabsorption. The presence of vitamin D deficiency reduces the sensitivity of the calcium-to-creatinine ratio in the diagnosis of primary hyperparathyroidism, rendering a result that appears to be more consistent with FHH. In contrast, the presence of higher 25-hydroxyvitamin D values (>10 ng/mL [>25 nmol/L]) generally does not confound interpretation of the calcium-to-creatinine ratio in patients with suspected primary hyperparathyroidism. Thus, the correct answer is to treat with cholecalciferol and retest once the patient is no longer deficient in 25-hydroxyvitamin D (Answer E). Overwhelming evidence suggests that vitamin replacement is safe in patients with primary hyperparathyroidism.

Although there is an initial clinical suspicion for FHH in this vignette, biochemical testing of first-degree relatives (Answer A) in an attempt to corroborate the diagnosis is premature given the patient's vitamin D deficiency. Based on earlier (and the most recent) National Institutes of Health consensus panel guidelines, this patient meets the criteria for surgical referral based on the presence of hypercalcemia and her age younger than 50 years (thus, Answer B is incorrect). The combination of hypercalcemia and an inappropriately normal or elevated intact PTH level, as is the case in this woman, essentially rules out the presence of humoral hypercalcemia due to PTHrP (Answer C), given that endogenous PTH secretion would be expected to be in the lower range of normal if not fully suppressed in such individuals. Finally, while cinacalcet (Answer D) is a pharmacologic approach to reducing PTH levels that are inappropriately elevated, it is not approved for patients with primary hyperparathyroidism who are candidates for surgical intervention.

Educational Objective
Describe the confounding influence of vitamin D deficiency in distinguishing between primary hyperparathyroidism and familial hypocalciuric hypercalcemia.

UpToDate Topic Review(s)
Primary hyperparathyroidism: diagnosis, differential diagnosis, and evaluation

Reference(s)

Jayasena CN, Mahmud M, Palazzo F, Donaldson M, Meeran K, Dhillo WS. Utility of the urine calcium-to-creatinine ratio to diagnose primary hyperparathyroidism in asymptomatic hypercalcaemic patients with vitamin D deficiency. *Ann Clin Biochem*. 2011;48(Pt 2):126-129. PMID: 21303875

Shah VN, Shah CS, Bhadada SK, Rao DS. Effect of 25 (OH) D replacements in patients with primary hyperparathyroidism (PHPT) and coexistent vitamin D deficiency on serum 25(OH) D, calcium and PTH levels: a meta-analysis and review of literature. *Clin Endocrinol (Oxf)*. 2014;80(6):797-803. PMID: 24382124

59 ANSWER: E) Muscle infarction

Diabetic muscle infarction (Answer E) is a rare occurrence, and it usually affects persons with longstanding diabetes and advanced microvascular complications. The cause of this condition is unknown, but it is thought to be a rare manifestation of microvascular disease. The typical presentation of diabetic muscle infarction is localized pain with a palpable mass in the thigh. Associated findings are swelling and limited range of motion. The thigh is the most commonly affected muscle, followed by the calf. The best technique to make the diagnosis is MRI of the affected limb. In this case, the T2-weighted images reveal an increased signal in the intramuscular and perimuscular tissues. Muscle biopsy is typically not necessary unless there is a suspicious area of fluid collection suggestive of an abscess. The characteristic findings on muscle biopsy are focal areas of necrosis with loss of the normal muscle architecture. Creatine kinase levels are often normal. The clinical course is gradual improvement of pain and swelling over several weeks. Treatment consists of pain control, bed rest, and diabetes control.

Normal findings on Doppler ultrasonography exclude deep venous thrombosis (Answer A). The absence of bone signal enhancement or fluid collection on the MRI image excludes osteomyelitis (Answer D) and muscle abscess (Answer B), respectively. Polymyositis (Answer C) is typically bilateral, painless, and associated with profound weakness. Polymyositis characteristically presents with elevated creatinine kinase levels.

Educational Objective
Diagnose diabetic muscle infarction.

UpToDate Topic Review(s)
Diabetic muscle infarction

Reference(s)

Umpierrez GE, Stiles RG, Klenbart J, Krendel DA, Watts NB. Diabetic muscle infarction. *Am J Med*. 1996;101(3):245-250. PMID: 8873484

60

ANSWER: C) Evolocumab

The patient in this vignette has a significant dyslipidemia in the setting of a moderate to severe reduction in estimated glomerular filtration rate (stage 3 chronic kidney disease [CKD]). The lipid profile in CKD varies respective to the stages of kidney disease, the presence and amount of proteinuria, and the type of dialysis. Hypertriglyceridemia with low HDL cholesterol is the hallmark of dyslipidemia and occurs in 40% to 50% of patients with CKD. Accumulation of highly atherogenic lipoproteins such as chylomicron remnants, intermediate-density lipoproteins, oxidized LDL, and small, dense LDL is characteristic. Lipoprotein (a) levels are increased in patients with CKD, most likely due to decreased clearance, and this is associated with increased cardiovascular risk. It is unclear whether the dyslipidemia of CKD contributes to or worsens kidney disease or whether it is simply a consequence of renal disease progression.

Cardiovascular disease is the most common cause of morbidity and mortality in patients with CKD. In these patients, cardiovascular disease mortality is 3- to 6-fold higher above age- and risk-adjusted mortality in the general population. The American Heart Association/American College of Cardiology cholesterol-lowering guidelines do not include CKD in the risk calculator, and no specific treatment recommendations are made for individuals with CKD. However, the patient in this vignette is at very high cardiovascular risk, and therapies to reduce this risk are essential. LDL-cholesterol reduction is the primary goal in CKD stage 3 and 4. Statins are the mainstay of cardiovascular risk reduction in CKD (statins have been shown to decrease cardiovascular disease in patients with CKD stages 1-4 and after transplant, but not in patients undergoing dialysis). However, in the setting of statin intolerance, as this patient has experienced, other therapies are necessary.

Evolocumab (Answer C) is a PCSK9 inhibitor antibody that is used to decrease LDL-cholesterol levels in patients with familial hypercholesterolemia and in those with atherosclerotic cardiovascular disease who need further risk reduction. There are no studies of PCSK9 inhibitors in individuals with CKD, and these agents are not currently indicated in statin-intolerant patients. The limited studies that have included individuals with an estimated glomerular filtration rate greater than 30 mL/min per 1.73 m^2 suggest that these antibodies are safe to use in this population. In this patient who is statin intolerant and is at very high cardiovascular risk, it is appropriate to attempt PCSK9 inhibitor therapy with the goal of decreasing LDL-cholesterol levels. Hence, evolocumab is the best next step in this patient, but its use is currently off-label.

Colesevelam (Answer A) is a bile acid resin that acts by forming insoluble complexes with bile acids in the intestine, which are then excreted in the feces. It decreases LDL cholesterol by 15% to 20% and can be safely used in the setting of CKD. Use of colesevelam is limited by its tendency to raise triglycerides and to bind other drugs and reduce their absorption. Therefore, colesevelam is not the best option for this patient in whom triglycerides are elevated.

Fish oil (Answer B) can be beneficial in decreasing triglyceride levels. Although published data in patients with CKD are limited, omega-3 fatty acids do not have significant interactions with other drugs and do not require dosage reductions in the setting of impaired renal function. However, they do not have any effects on LDL-cholesterol lowering, which is the goal in this individual.

Fibrates, including gemfibrozil, fenofibrate (Answer D), bezafibrate, and ciprofibrate, are a class of drugs that are agonists of the peroxisome proliferator–activator α receptors. Their principal effects are to raise HDL cholesterol and lower triglyceride concentrations. Fenofibrate can also lower LDL cholesterol. They are widely used for the management of marked hypertriglyceridemia. These drugs are excreted by the kidney and hence must be used with caution. Fenofibrate can result in creatinine elevations, so its use in patients with CKD cannot be recommended. Gemfibrozil can be used with caution at half dosage.

Ezetimibe (Answer E) is an intestinal cholesterol absorption inhibitor. Given that ezetimibe is only circulated in the enterohepatic circulation and does not directly act on the kidneys, it may be an ideal candidate for use in patients with CKD. However, monotherapy with ezetimibe results in very modest LDL-cholesterol lowering and has additive effects in combination with statins. There is no cardiovascular benefit of monotherapy. Hence, it is highly unlikely that ezetimibe alone will provide enough LDL-cholesterol lowering in this patient.

Educational Objective
Recommend appropriate therapy of dyslipidemia in an individual with chronic kidney disease.

UpToDate Topic Review(s)
Chronic kidney disease and coronary heart disease

Reference(s)

Hager MR, Narla AD, Tannock LR. Dyslipidemia in patients with chronic kidney disease. *Rev Endocr Metab Disord*. 2017;18(1):29-40. PMID: 28000009

Harper CR, Jacobson TA. Managing dyslipidemia in chronic kidney disease. *J Am Coll Cardiol*. 2008;51(25):2375-2384. PMID: 18565393

61 ANSWER: E) Measurement of SHBG

Many biochemical parameters change in association with alterations in thyroid status. Because of these associations, such parameters can serve as biomarkers or indirect indices of thyroid function. Examples of these biochemical parameters include lipids such as cholesterol, SHBG, ACE, and ferritin. None of these parameters is specific for alterations in thyroid status, so they are not generally useful for assessing thyroid function. In addition, they may not be sensitive and may only change with significant perturbations in thyroid hormone levels. The patient described in this vignette has severe thyrotoxicosis secondary to Graves disease. Although thyroid-stimulating immunoglobulin was measured, this was not necessary to diagnose Graves disease, given his thyroid examination and other physical examination findings. Hyperthyroidism can be associated with reduced cholesterol concentrations and elevated levels of SHBG, ACE, and ferritin. Elevated SHBG can be associated with significant increases in total testosterone, as seen in this patient. Measuring SHBG (Answer E) is therefore the best choice. Free testosterone concentrations may be normal. Both SHBG and total testosterone levels decline with treatment of the hyperthyroidism. Such normalization occurred in the patient described here, whose total testosterone returned to the normal range after his hyperthyroidism was successfully treated.

When an individual has an altered concentration of sex steroids, one aspect of the diagnostic process is to determine whether the abnormality is associated with elevated or low gonadotropin levels. In this case of an extremely elevated testosterone concentration, the FSH and LH could be elevated if these hormones were causing the testosterone elevation, or low if there were autonomous production of testosterone. Measurement of FSH and LH would have been a good next step if the patient did not also have severe thyrotoxicosis. However, because severe hyperthyroidism is present, there is a more likely explanation for the patient's elevated testosterone, and measuring FSH and LH (Answer C) is not the best choice. FSH and LH could be measured if the investigation into a link between the patient's thyrotoxicosis and elevated testosterone did not suggest causation. In addition, although gonadotropin-producing pituitary adenomas do occur, they often produce relatively nonfunctional forms of FSH and LH and may not be associated with high testosterone levels. For these reasons, pituitary MRI (Answer B) to look for a gonadotropin-producing adenoma should not be the initial diagnostic step. If autonomous or tumoral production of testosterone is suspected, adrenal CT (Answer A) or testicular ultrasonography might be reasonable investigations. However, thyrotoxicosis should first be excluded as the cause.

TSH and hCG are both glycoprotein hormones with a common α subunit, but distinct β subunits. Elevated hCG levels may cause hyperthyroidism, especially when the hCG concentration is above 500,000 IU/L, via a stimulatory effect on the TSH receptor. hCG levels should be measured (Answer D) if a patient has hyperthyroidism and the physical examination and biochemical evaluation do not point to a direct thyroidal cause. In this case, both physical examination and biochemical evaluation are consistent with Graves disease, and investigation for the relatively rare entity of hCG-induced hyperthyroidism is not necessary.

Educational Objective
Describe the relationship between thyroid status and SHBG concentration.

UpToDate Topic Review(s)
Overview of the clinical manifestations of hyperthyroidism in adults

Reference(s)

Ford HC, Cooke RR, Keightley EA, Feek CM. Serum levels of free and bound testosterone in hyperthyroidism. *Clin Endocrinol (Oxf)*. 1992;36(2):187-192. PMID: 1568351

Thaler MA, Seifert-Klauss V, Luppa PB. The biomarker sex hormone-binding globulin - from established applications to emerging trends in clinical medicine. *Best Pract Res Clin Endocrinol Metab*. 2015;29(5):749-860. PMID: 265224459

Zahringer S, Tomova A, von Werder K, Brabant G, Kumanov P, Schopohl J. The influence of hyperthyroidism on the hypothalamic-pituitary-gonadal axis. *Exp Clin Endocrinol Diabetes*. 2000;108(4):282-289. PMID: 10961359

62 ANSWER: A) *COL1A1* or *COL1A2* (collagen alpha-1 chain or collagen alpha-2 chain)

This postmenopausal woman presents with a history of excess fractures as a child/adolescent, osteoporosis, short stature, scoliosis, and bone deformities—all of which are clinical manifestations of osteogenesis imperfecta (OI). Other manifestations of OI may include blue-gray discoloration of the sclerae and hearing loss. There are many different subtypes of OI based on genetic and clinical characteristics. This patient most likely has mild (type I) OI, which is most commonly caused by pathogenic variants in the genes encoding the α1 and α2 chains of type I collagen (Answer A). Although not approved for this indication, bisphosphonates are the mainstay of pharmacologic therapy for fracture prevention in most forms of OI.

The *LRP5* gene (Answer B) encodes LDL receptor-related protein 5, which acts in the Wnt signaling pathway. Loss-of-function pathogenic variants in this gene have been shown to cause osteoporosis–pseudoglioma, an autosomal recessive disorder characterized by bone fragility, ocular abnormalities, and blindness. Conversely, gain-of-function pathogenic variants in *LRP5* cause hereditary high bone mass.

Activating pathogenic variants in the *GNAS* gene (Answer C) lead to McCune-Albright syndrome, characterized by fibrous dysplasia, precocious puberty, and café-au-lait skin lesions. Other endocrine manifestations include thyrotoxicosis, gigantism or acromegaly, and Cushing syndrome.

The *PHEX* gene (Answer D) encodes an endopeptidase enzyme expressed predominantly in bone and teeth. Pathogenic variants in this gene lead to an increase in circulating FGF-23 and are responsible for the development of X-linked hypophosphatemia, which is characterized by hypophosphatemia, teeth defects, and rickets or osteomalacia.

Finally, the *DMP1* gene (Answer E) encodes dentin matrix acidic phosphoprotein 1. Inactivating pathogenic variants in this gene lead to autosomal recessive hypophosphatemic rickets, which has similar manifestations to that of X-linked hypophosphatemia, including hypophosphatemia and rickets or osteomalacia.

Educational Objective

Identify the clinical manifestations of type I osteogenesis imperfecta in a patient presenting for evaluation of low bone mineral density and recall the genetic pathogenic variant associated with this condition.

UpToDate Topic Review(s)

Osteogenesis imperfecta: Clinical features and diagnosis

Reference(s)

Forlino A, Marini JC. Osteogenesis imperfecta. *Lancet.* 2016;387(10028):1657-1671. PMID: 26542481

Balemans W1, Van Hul W. The genetics of low-density lipoprotein receptor-related protein 5 in bone: a story of extremes. *Endocrinology.* 2007;148(6): 2622-2629. PMID: 17395706

Razali NN, Hwu TT, Thilakavathy K. Phosphate homeostasis and genetic mutations of familial hypophosphatemic rickets. *J Pediatr Endocrinol Metab.* 2015; 28(9-10):1009-1017. PMID: 25894638

63 ANSWER: B) Spironolactone and levonorgestrel-releasing intrauterine device

This patient has polycystic ovary syndrome that was not diagnosed until age 32 years because she had been on combined oral contraceptives (COCs) from adolescence until trying to conceive in her late 20s. Symptoms did not develop until she was off COCs and after pregnancy and breastfeeding. To address this patient's primary concern of treating symptoms of androgen excess (hirsutism and acne), first-line therapy would be COCs due to the multiple effects of suppressing LH secretion and ovarian androgen production while also increasing hepatic production of SHBG, which lowers serum free androgen concentrations.

Before prescribing COCs (Answer C), care providers should screen for risk factors that might increase adverse events, including stroke and venous thrombosis. In addition to older age, cigarette smoking, hypertension, and migraine headaches with aura, other factors that further increase stroke risk in women taking COCs include obesity, dyslipidemia, and prothrombotic mutations. The Centers for Disease Control have published resources to guide prescribers of contraception for women with specific risk factors and medical conditions. COCs for a woman with migraine headaches without aura is in the category of "advantages generally outweigh theoretical or proven risks."

Only in the case of migraine headaches with aura is COC use considered an "unacceptable health risk (method not to be used)" because of the increased risk for stroke.

This patient also has a family history of venous thromboembolic disease. Her mother could be considered to have a provoked venous thrombotic event related to surgery. Her sister had an episode that is concerning because it is related to COC initiation. It would be appropriate to suggest that the sister be referred for testing of inherited and acquired risk factors for thrombophilia. Then the patient could have more focused testing based on any condition diagnosed in the sister. Even if the patient were diagnosed with an inherited or acquired risk factor for thrombophilia, prescribing COCs after referral for possible addition of anticoagulant prophylaxis would not be the best next step because her medical history does not suggest that pregnancy would be a greater risk than COCs to warrant combining COCs with anticoagulant prophylaxis. There are other treatment options to consider.

Spironolactone (Answer B) is an aldosterone antagonist that also acts as a competitive inhibitor of the androgen receptor. It is considered second-line therapy for the treatment of hirsutism or first-line therapy in a patient who cannot be prescribed COCs. It is also an appropriate addition to COCs when symptoms are not controlled with COCs alone. Spironolactone is the best next step in this patient's management as an effective treatment for both androgenic acne and hirsutism, given that there is a greater risk for adverse events with COCs. Both to prevent conception while on an antiandrogen and to prevent irregular uterine spotting or bleeding that might occur with spironolactone, it is usually recommended to use spironolactone in combination with COCs or, in this case, an intrauterine device that releases levonorgestrel as contraception and to prevent bleeding.

Although lowering insulin concentrations can improve hyperandrogenemia, metformin (Answer A) has not been shown to have a greater effect on hirsutism than COCs, antiandrogen therapy, or even an additive effect in combination with oral contraceptives.

Progestin-only oral contraceptives (Answer D) are often prescribed to women who are breastfeeding or when COCs might be considered to carry a higher risk for adverse events such as in women with migraine headaches with aura. However, progestin-only pills do not consistently suppress ovulation and would not lower circulating free androgens by increasing SHBG. The effects of progestin-only pills to promote cervical mucus thickening to prevent sperm from entering into the uterus and endometrial thinning are the key factors that prevent conception. Therefore, progestin-only pills are not likely to improve this patient's symptoms of acne and hirsutism.

Topical retinoids and clindamycin are effective medications to reduce inflammation and comedogenesis in patients with acne. This patient has the classic androgenic pattern of acne clustering along the jawline. She has no evidence of scarring or more severe cystic acne, so topical treatments would be reasonable before referring to dermatology for consideration of systemic therapy. Eflornithine is an inhibitor of hair growth available for the treatment of unwanted facial hair in women. This patient has severe hirsutism not just confined to the face. Thus, a topical retinoid, clindamycin, and eflornithine (Answer E) would not be the best options.

Educational Objective
Identify relative and absolute contraindications for combined oral contraceptives in a patient seeking treatment for hirsutism.

UpToDate Topic Review(s)
Overview of the use of combined estrogen-progestin oral contraceptives
Treatment of hirsutism

Reference(s)

Legro RS, Arslanian SA, Ehrmann DA, et al; Endocrine Society. Diagnosis and Treatment of Polycystic Ovary Syndrome: An Endocrine Society Clinical Practice Guideline. *J Clin Endocrinol Metab*. 2013;98(12):4565-4592. PMID: 24151290

Centers for Disease Control and Prevention. US Medical Eligibility Criteria (US MEC) for Contraceptive Use, 2016. Atlanta, GA. Centers for Disease Control, 2015. Available at: http://www.cdc.gov/reproductivehealth/unintendedpregnancy/usmec.htm. Accessed November 1, 2018.

Martin KA, Chang RJ, Ehrmann DA, et al. Evaluation and treatment of hirsutism in premenopausal women: an Endocrine Society clinical practice guideline. *J Clin Endocrinol Metab*. 2008;93(4):1105-1120. PMID: 18252793

64 ANSWER: A) Continue the same therapies
Pituitary apoplexy is a relatively rare event that occurs due to sudden hemorrhagic necrosis of a preexisting pituitary adenoma. Precipitating factors are sometimes identified (eg, increase in intracranial pressure, arterial

hypertension, major surgery, anticoagulant therapy, pituitary dynamic testing, diabetic ketoacidosis), but it is more often an isolated event. Pituitary apoplexy is most often the presenting symptom of a previously undiagnosed pituitary macroadenoma. Determining the risk of pituitary apoplexy in a patient with a macroadenoma is difficult, but it is generally thought to occur in less than 1% of cases. In this patient, the previously documented hypogonadism was most likely due to a macroadenoma.

The acute enlargement of the adenoma that occurs in the setting of apoplexy typically causes intense headache and vision changes. Signs of meningeal irritation or altered consciousness can be present and may complicate the diagnosis. While head CT may miss the diagnosis, MRI invariably shows a sellar mass. Cerebral spinal fluid analysis is not needed, but when it is done to rule out a subarachnoid bleed, it may show an increase in both red and white blood cells. The acute onset of adrenal insufficiency can be lethal if it is unrecognized and untreated. Therefore, the most important aspect of acute treatment is glucocorticoid replacement therapy (unless normal adrenal function is proven). The management of apoplexy is controversial in terms of surgical indication. Acute visual field abnormalities and changes in consciousness are obvious surgical indications, but ocular nerve palsy is not, as it typically resolves with time even without surgery. Some authors believe that surgery increases the chance that pituitary function will recover.

The mechanism by which apoplexy causes hypopituitarism is 2-fold: one is substitution and necrosis of normal pituitary tissue, and the other is an increase in intrasellar pressure. As the intrasellar pressure normalizes (as result of surgery or digestion of blood), some or all pituitary function may recover. The prolactin concentration is a predictor of residual pituitary function. In this patient, prolactin remains very low, making recovery of function unlikely. Therefore, the present replacement therapy should be continued (Answer A). It must be noted that in the presence of central hypothyroidism, hypoadrenalism, and hypogonadism, this patient's chance of being GH deficient approaches 100%. Thus, IGF-1 should be measured and the pros and cons of GH replacement therapy should be discussed if the patient considers daily injections needed for GH replacement therapy.

Given the high likelihood of persistent hypopituitarism, discontinuing testosterone (Answer B), levothyroxine (Answer C), or hydrocortisone (Answer D) would not be advisable. Furthermore, if levothyroxine is stopped, free T_4 should not be measured before 4 weeks. Finally, there is no proof that adding liothyronine therapy (Answer E) in patients with central hypothyroidism and normal free T_4 is beneficial, and iatrogenic hyperthyroidism in this age group increases the risk of atrial fibrillation.

Educational Objective
Explain the role of prolactin measurement as an indicator of residual pituitary mass after apoplexy and how a low prolactin level after apoplexy predicts permanent hypopituitarism.

UpToDate Topic Review(s)
Causes of hypopituitarism

Reference(s)

Briet C, Salenave S, Bonneville JF, Laws ER, Chanson P. Pituitary apoplexy. *Endocr Rev.* 2015;36(6):622-645. 26414232

Zayour DH, Selman WR, Arafah BM. Extreme elevation of intrasellar pressure in patients with pituitary tumor apoplexy: relation to pituitary function. *J Clin Endocrinol Metab.* 2004;89(11):5649-5654. PMID: 15531524

Toledano Y, Lubetsky A, Shimon I. Acquired prolactin deficiency in patients with disorders of the hypothalamic-pituitary axis. *J Endocrinol Invest.* 2007;30(4): 268-273. PMID: 17556861

65   ANSWER: E) Pregabalin

Only 11% to 26% of patients with type 2 diabetes develop painful neuropathy, and it is important to rule out causes of neuropathy other than diabetes in this population. In addition, distinguishing between peripheral vascular disease and distal neuropathy secondary to diabetes is important. In this vignette, the patient's symptoms are typical of peripheral neuropathic pain rather than pain due to peripheral vascular disease.

Optimizing glycemic control has been shown to delay onset and prevent progression of peripheral neuropathy in patients with type 1 diabetes (Diabetes Control and Complications trial and Epidemiology of Diabetes Interventions and Complications; DCCT/EDIC). However, the data are much less robust in patients with type 2 diabetes. Several large randomized controlled trials in patients with type 2 diabetes report only modest reduction or no change in neuropathy in patients treated with intensive glycemic therapy. The patient in this case has reasonable glucose control. In fact, given the number of comorbidities, his current glycemic control may be near optimal. Starting insulin (Answer C) would not likely improve the neuropathic pain in this case.

Pregabalin (Answer E) and gabapentin are alpha-2-delta ligands that act as presynaptic inhibitors of excitatory neurotransmitters, including glutamate and substance P. Pooled analysis of 7 randomized controlled trials with more than 1500 patients treated with pregabalin demonstrated a significant reduction in pain score and pain-related sleep interference compared with placebo in patients with diabetic polyneuropathy. Gabapentin has also been used to treat diabetic neuropathy pain. However, the data from controlled trials with gabapentin are not as compelling as those demonstrated with pregabalin. Pregabalin can be dosed less frequently than gabapentin and is thus the preferred medication. Pregabalin is a schedule V medication. There is an increased risk of suicidal thoughts or behavior with pregabalin treatment, so these behaviors must be monitored carefully in individual patients. Both gabapentin and pregabalin can contribute to ankle edema and weight gain. The dosages of pregabalin and gabapentin should be reduced in the setting of renal insufficiency.

Fluoxetine (Answer A) is a selective serotonin reuptake inhibitor antidepressant that has been shown to improve depression scores in patients with diabetes. However, fluoxetine has not been shown in controlled studies to be effective in the treatment of diabetic neuropathy pain. Venlafaxine and duloxetine are other serotonin reuptake inhibitors that have been shown to significantly improve symptom scores in patients with neuropathic pain due to diabetes. However, neither is listed as a treatment option in this case.

Opioid narcotics (Answer B) are an option for treatment of diabetic neuropathy pain. In controlled trials, tramadol and sustained-release oxycodone have been shown to effectively reduce neuropathic pain in patients with diabetes. However, given the risk for drug dependence, these agents should not be considered first- or second-line therapy.

Amitriptyline (Answer D) and other tricyclic antidepressants have been shown in double-blind, randomized controlled trials to effectively reduce pain associated with diabetic neuropathy. However, given the presence of cardiovascular disease in this patient, amitriptyline and nortriptyline are contraindicated and would not be considered first-line therapy. Doxepin has the least cardiotoxicity of any of the tricyclic antidepressants and would be a treatment option, but it is not listed as a choice in this vignette.

Tricyclic antidepressants, anticonvulsants, and opioid narcotics can cause anticholinergic adverse effects that include constipation, dry mouth and eyes, blurred vision, dizziness, sedation, and urinary retention. These potential complications should be discussed with each patient before treatment initiation.

Educational Objective
Recommend treatment of peripheral neuropathic pain in patients with diabetes mellitus.

UpToDate Topic Review(s)
Treatment of diabetic neuropathy

Reference(s)

Boulton AJ, Vinik AI, Arezzo JC, et al; American Diabetes Association. Diabetic neuropathies: a statement by the American Diabetes Association. *Diabetes Care.* 2005;28(4):956-962. PMID: 15793206

Freeman R, Durso-Decruz E, Emir B. Efficacy, safety, and tolerability of pregabalin treatment for painful diabetic peripheral neuropathy: findings from seven randomized, controlled trials across a range of doses. *Diabetes Care.* 2008;31(7):1448-1454. PMID: 18356405

Callaghan BC, Cheng HT, Stables CL. Smith AL, Feldman EL. Diabetic neuropathy: clinical manifestations and current treatments. *Lancet Neurol.* 2012;11(6): 521-534. PMID: 22608666

66 **ANSWER: E) Refer for urologic evaluation**
Men on testosterone replacement therapy should be regularly monitored to determine whether their serum testosterone concentrations are at goal and whether they have developed any adverse effects related to the therapy.

Our understanding of the relationship between testosterone therapy and prostate cancer is complex and limited due to a lack of adequately powered randomized controlled trials of long duration. Testosterone therapy given to men with metastatic prostatic cancer can worsen their clinical course and is therefore contraindicated. In fact, androgen deprivation therapy is a common treatment modality for men with prostate cancer. Nonetheless, there is no solid evidence that testosterone therapy causes new prostate cancer to develop. It is well established that men treated with testosterone typically experience an average rise in PSA of 0.3 to 0.5 ng/mL (0.3-0.5 µg/L). The Endocrine Society's clinical practice guideline has a strong recommendation based on very low-quality evidence that clinicians should assess prostate cancer risk in men for whom testosterone therapy is being considered. It recommends against testosterone therapy without further urologic evaluation in men with a palpable prostate nodule or PSA level greater than 4 ng/mL (>4 µg/L) or greater than 3 ng/mL (>3 µg/L) in men at high risk of prostate cancer. The authors of the guideline also recommend a urologic consultation if the PSA level rises more than 1.4 ng/mL (>1.4 µg/L) within any 1-year period after initiation of testosterone therapy. Thus, this patient's PSA level should be addressed (Answer E). Continuing therapy at the same dosage (Answer A) does not address the significant rise in the PSA level. Decreasing the testosterone dosage (Answer C) would be appropriate in an elderly man, but not in a middle-aged man. The patient in this case most likely has benign prostatic hypertrophy. It is important to assess men for lower urinary symptoms before starting testosterone therapy and while on therapy. The presence of lower urinary symptoms on therapy is not a contraindication to treatment. The man in this vignette should also be screened for obstructive sleep apnea, which is common in obese men with hypertension.

It is well established that testosterone therapy increases hemoglobin and hematocrit. This phenomenon occurs more frequently in older men and more commonly occurs with the intramuscular testosterone esters (enanthate, cypionate), as this formulation is associated with peak and trough levels of testosterone. According to the Endocrine Society's clinical practice guideline on androgen deficiency, a baseline hematocrit level greater than 50% is a relative contraindication to therapy and should prompt an evaluation for potential causes. The authors recommend that testosterone therapy be discontinued if the hematocrit level reaches 54%. When this occurs, management options include reducing the testosterone dosage, switching to a formulation with a lower risk of erythrocytosis, and/or performing phlebotomy. Addressing this patient's hematocrit level by lowering his testosterone dosage (Answer B) is incorrect, as his hematocrit remains at less than 54% while on testosterone therapy.

Increasing the testosterone dosage (Answer D) due to a lack of improvement in bone density would be inappropriate, as the testosterone dosage should be based primarily on serum levels of testosterone rather than on signs or symptoms that may not improve with testosterone therapy.

Educational Objective
In a patient on testosterone therapy, determine when a rise in prostate-specific antigen should prompt urologic evaluation.

UpToDate Topic Review(s)
Testosterone treatment of male hypogonadism

Reference(s)

Bhasin S, Brito JP, Cunningham GR, et al. Testosterone therapy in men with hypogonadism: an Endocrine Society clinical practice guideline. *J Clin Endocrinol Metab.* 2018;103(5):1715-1744. PMID: 29562364

Fink HA, Ewing SK, Ensrud KE, et al. Association of testosterone and estradiol deficiency with osteoporosis and rapid bone loss in older men. *J Clin Endocrinol Metab.* 2006;91(10):3908-3915. PMID: 16849417

67 ANSWER: C) Hypophosphatasia

While it is tempting for the busy clinician to approach all patients who present with low bone mineral density with or without fragility fractures as representing some form of osteoporosis, it is critical to recognize that there are a number of metabolic bone disorders in which skeletal fragility is due to undermineralization of bone (eg, osteomalacia). This patient presents with many of the hallmark signs of hypophosphatasia (Answer C), an osteomalacic disorder that is due to pathogenic variants in the tissue nonspecific alkaline phosphatase gene (*ALPL*). *ALPL* pathogenic variants result in defective catabolism of pyrophosphate molecules, which are natural inhibitors of mineralization within the bone matrix. Abnormal dental mineralization with excessive primary tooth loss is also common. The disease has a variable presentation that confers disproportionate morbidity and mortality in neonates and infants due to respiratory failure (rib hypomineralization), whereas older children, and particularly adults, have a milder skeletal phenotype. In fact, many adults with *ALPL* pathogenic variants are asymptomatic. Affected adults with hypophosphatasia most commonly present with stress fractures of the lower extremities (metatarsal, proximal femur). This patient's history of right proximal femur pain and multiple previous metatarsal fractures, family history of femoral fracture in her mother, and frankly low alkaline phosphatase level are highly suggestive of hypophosphatasia.

The low bone density that is disparately lower in the lower extremity most likely represents hypomineralization instead of low bone density, particularly given her relatively young age and expected regional differences in bone mineral density decline at specific skeletal sites with aging (typically later declines in bone mineral density in the proximal femur compared with the spine). At present, there is no specific US FDA-approved therapy for adults with hypophosphatasia, although a recombinant form of alkaline phosphatase (asfotase alfa) is approved for treatment of hypophosphatasia of infantile and childhood onset. At least intuitively, bisphosphonates should be avoided because they may inhibit mineralization and exacerbate an underlying osteomalacic disorder. Indeed, previous reports have identified patients with hypophosphatasia who present with a femoral stress fracture that mimics atypical femoral fractures seen rarely in patients on long-term bisphosphonate therapy.

Although patients with type 1 osteogenesis imperfecta (Answer A) have increased skeletal fragility, the more diffuse pattern of early-life fractures, normal or higher alkaline phosphatase levels (reflective of higher skeletal turnover), and absence of reported physical examination characteristics (blue sclerae) make this diagnosis unlikely.

Paget disease of bone (Answer B) could be associated with bone pain, although it is characteristically associated with elevated alkaline phosphatase levels.

Patients with X-linked hypophosphatemic rickets (Answer D), which is due to pathogenic variants in the *PHEX* gene, have disordered metabolism of phosphate (low) and 1,25-dihydroxyvitamin D (low) due to excessive effect of a circulating phosphaturic factor called fibroblast growth factor 23. While patients with this osteomalacia disorder may develop stress fractures, as has this patient, the frankly normal phosphate level rules out this condition.

Finally, although celiac disease (Answer E) is an intestinal malabsorptive disorder that can result in osteoporosis, osteomalacia, and fractures, the presence of normal 25-hydroxyvitamin D, intact PTH, and 24-hour urinary calcium (commonly low in malabsorptive disease) and low alkaline phosphatase (typically elevated in patients with celiac-associated osteomalacia) makes this condition much less likely.

Educational Objective
Identify the clinical signs and laboratory findings that are characteristic of hypophosphatasia.

UpToDate Topic Review(s)
Skeletal dysplasias: specific disorders

Reference(s)

Mornet E. Hypophosphatasia. *Metabolism*. 2018;82:142-155. PMID: 28939177

Sutton RA, Mumm S, Coburn SP, Ericson KL, Whyte MP. "Atypical femoral fractures" during bisphosphonate exposure in adult hypophosphatasia. *J Bone Miner Res*. 2012;27(5):987-994. PMID: 22322541

68 **ANSWER: A) Start methimazole and continue breastfeeding**

Thyroid dysfunction is relatively common in the postpartum period. In patients presenting with thyrotoxicosis in the first 12 months following delivery, a differential diagnosis between Graves disease and postpartum thyroiditis must be established. The patient in this vignette has a history of Graves disease that remitted during pregnancy. She now presents with clinical and biochemical findings consistent with relapsed Graves thyrotoxicosis, including signs of ophthalmopathy and elevated TSH-receptor antibody (TRAb) concentrations. A few studies have indicated that maternal hyperthyroidism impairs lactation, although the evidence is not consistent and guidelines do not currently recommend treatment of maternal hyperthyroidism be warranted on the grounds of improving lactation. The decision to treat hyperthyroidism in lactating women is governed by the same principles that apply to nonpregnant women. Because the findings in this vignette indicate relapsed Graves hyperthyroidism, antithyroid treatment is warranted and symptomatic control with β-adrenergic–blocking agents only (Answer C) is not sufficient.

Both methimazole and propylthiouracil can be detected in the breast milk of treated hyperthyroid women. This finding initially raised concerns that maternal ingestion of these medications would have detrimental effects on the health of the baby. Studies evaluating the amount of propylthiouracil secreted into breast milk indicated that only 0.007% to 0.077% of the ingested dose was detected. Studies of methimazole confirm a 4- to 7-fold higher proportion of the medication transferred into breast milk compared with propylthiouracil, and approximately 0.1% to 0.2% of an orally administered methimazole dose is excreted into breast milk. A large study of methimazole use during breastfeeding assessed neonatal thyroid function in the breastfeeding offspring, as well as intellectual development and physical growth in a subset of infants, and no difference was observed in IQ or physical development of the breastfeeding children compared with the control children. Overall, experts have confirmed the safety of low to moderate dosages of both propylthiouracil (up to 450 mg daily) and methimazole (up to 20 mg daily) in breastfeeding mothers. Given the small but detectable amount of both propylthiouracil and methimazole transferred into breast milk, the lowest effective dosages of these medications should be administered. The patient in this vignette has previously experienced adverse effects when taking propylthiouracil (Answer B) and it would seem more appropriate to start methimazole (Answer A). Breastfed children of women who are treated with antithyroid drugs should be monitored for appropriate growth and development during routine pediatric health and wellness evaluations. Routine assessment of serum thyroid function in the child is not recommended as long as moderate dosages of antithyroid drugs are used.

Fetal Graves disease is caused by transplacental transfer of TRAb. While it is possible that this patient's baby was affected by the presence of these antibodies during pregnancy, there is no evidence that the high levels of TRAb in the mother are transferred in breast milk, thereby adversely affecting the baby. Similarly, the amount of T_4 and T_3 that is transferred in breast milk is minimal, and maternal Graves hyperthyroidism is not a contraindication for breastfeeding (thus, Answer E is incorrect).

Total thyroidectomy (Answer D) is a suitable therapeutic option for patients with relapsed Graves hyperthyroidism. However, this patient has severe thyrotoxicosis and is likely to require pretreatment with antithyroid drugs before surgery becomes a feasible option. The use of ^{131}I is contraindicated during lactation because of its relatively long half-life (8 days). If required for diagnostic purposes, ^{123}I can be used if breast milk is pumped and discarded for 3 to 4 days before breastfeeding is resumed. Similarly, ^{99m}Tc pertechnetate administration requires breast milk to be pumped and discarded during the day of testing.

Educational Objective
Counsel a breastfeeding patient regarding the safety of antithyroid drugs.

UpToDate Topic Review(s)
Graves hyperthyroidism in nonpregnant adults: Overview of treatment

Reference(s)

Azizi F, Khoshniat M, Bahrainian M, Hedayati M. Thyroid function and intellectual development of infants nursed by mothers taking methimazole. *J Clin Endocrinol Metab.* 2000;85(9):3233-3238. PMID: 10999814

Alexander EK, Pearce EN, Brent GA, et al. 2017 Guidelines of the American Thyroid Association for the Diagnosis and Management of Thyroid Disease During Pregnancy and the Postpartum. *Thyroid.* 2017;27(3):315-389. PMID: 28056690

69   ANSWER: A) Infuse 1000 mL 0.9% NaCl with 40 mEq of KCl over 1 hour

Appropriate fluid and electrolyte management is crucial in the treatment of diabetic ketoacidosis. This vignette focuses on fluid and potassium replacement in this setting. If there is no evidence of cardiac compromise, the initial fluid choice should be 0.9% NaCl to correct hypovolemia and hyperosmolality. An initial rate of fluid administration of 15 to 20 mL/kg is recommended for the first hour. Following this, if serum sodium is normal or high, fluid replacement can be switched to 0.45% NaCl. If serum sodium is low, 0.9% NaCl should be continued. This patient weighs 121 lb (55 kg), so 1000 mL replacement in first hour is a reasonable volume. The answer options that suggest initial fluid replacement should be 100 cc/h (Answers D and E) are incorrect because the replacement is not fast enough. NaCl 0.45% (Answer C) would not be the initial choice.

The serum potassium level at admission determines the timing of insulin use and the extent of potassium replacement. If the potassium value is less than 3.3 mEq/L, 20 to 40 mEq of KCl is added to each liter of fluid and replaced in the first hour. In addition, insulin administration is delayed until the potassium rises above 3.3 mEq/L. Since the patient's serum potassium is less than 3.3 mEq/L, insulin should not be administered now (Answer B).

The best choice is Answer A because no insulin is started, 0.9% NaCl is used with adequate KCl (40 mEq), and it is infused at an aggressive rate of 1000 mL over the first hour.

Educational Objective
Recommend appropriate fluid and electrolyte management in the setting of diabetic ketoacidosis.

UpToDate Topic Review(s)
Diabetic ketoacidosis and hyperosmolar hyperglycemic state in adults: Treatment

Reference(s)

Fayfman M, Pasquel FJ, Umpierrez GE. Management of hyperglycemic crises: diabetic ketoacidosis and hyperglycemic hyperosmolar state. *Med Clin North Am.* 2017;101(3):587-606. PMID: 28372715

Savage MW, Dhatariya KK, Kivert A, et al; Joint British Diabetes Societies. Joint British Diabetes Societies guideline for the management of diabetic ketoacidosis. *Diabet Med.* 2011;28 (5)508-515. PMID: 21255074

70 ANSWER: C) Free T_4, decreased; TSH, increased; total cholesterol, increased; hyperthyroid symptoms, no change; heart rate, no change

Daily administration of levothyroxine produces relatively steady levels of TSH, free T_4, and T_3. T_4 levels do increase by about 15% after a patient has just taken their levothyroxine dose and may be elevated for about 4 hours after dosing. However, in general, daily oral levothyroxine produces stable indices of thyroid status. Adherence to levothyroxine therapy is critical, as hypothyroidism is usually a lifelong condition. Most patients being treated for hypothyroidism are able to adhere to once-daily therapy. Optimal timing of levothyroxine administration is in a fasting state, but bedtime dosing is an option. In addition, absorption problems associated with alternate timing regimens may often be ameliorated by dosage adjustments. Unfortunately, some patients, such as the one described in this vignette, find it difficult to maintain once-daily dosing of levothyroxine. Full discussion with the patient regarding the benefits of optimally treated hypothyroidism, exploration of measures to aid in adherence, and incorporation of levothyroxine ingestion into the daily routine can be helpful. If such measures, and also addressing any coexistent depression or other psychiatric disorders, do not improve adherence, observed daily or weekly therapy could be considered. If malabsorption of levothyroxine is documented, which is not the case here, liquid formulations of levothyroxine or parenteral administration of levothyroxine may restore euthyroidism.

Several reports of successful management of levothyroxine nonadherence with observed weekly therapy exist in the literature. In addition, a randomized crossover trial of daily vs weekly oral levothyroxine therapy conducted by Grebe et al examined a weekly dose that was 7 times higher than the daily dose. This study's findings provide reassurance regarding potential toxicities of this weekly dosing approach. In this study, 12 patients were crossed over from one therapy to the other and TSH, free T_4, and free T_3 profiles were assessed at the end of a 6-week period on each therapy. When comparing trough levels of these hormones (before administering the next levothyroxine dose), the investigators documented that weekly levothyroxine administration was associated with higher serum TSH values and lower free T_4 and free T_3 values compared with that observed on the daily administration regimen. This pattern of elevated TSH trough levels and lowered free T_4 trough levels is presented only in Answers B and C (thus, Answers A, D, and E are incorrect). However, this study did show that postdosing levels of free T_4 and free T_3 were higher with the weekly regimen and that TSH values were higher at all time points with the weekly regimen.

Despite the generally higher free T_4 and free T_3 levels and the higher TSH levels during the weekly therapy, other indices of thyroid status were similar between the 2 groups. There were no differences in symptoms of either hypothyroidism or hyperthyroidism or measurement of well-being between the groups. Mean SHBG concentrations, bone marker measurements, and cardiac parameters such as heart rate also did not differ between the 2 groups. Total cholesterol was significantly higher in the group receiving weekly therapy at the trough sampling point, but not at either 8 or 24 hours after dose administration. Given all of these factors, the pattern in Answer C is the best reflection of the change from once-daily to once-weekly therapy. Since there is a more satisfactory achievement of normal thyroid function with daily therapy than with weekly therapy, weekly therapy should not be considered as first-line option, but should be recommended only if daily therapy is unsuccessful in achieving a normal serum TSH level.

Educational Objective
Identify the clinical and biochemical profile observed with once-weekly levothyroxine therapy.

UpToDate topic review(s)
Treatment of primary hypothyroidism in adults

Reference(s)

Grebe SK, Cooke RR, Ford HC, et al. Treatment of hypothyroidism with once weekly thyroxine. *J Clin Endocrinol Metab*. 1997;82(3):870-875. PMID: 9062499

Rangan S, Tahrani AA, Macleod AF, Moulik PK. Once weekly thyroxine treatment as a strategy to treat non-compliance. *Postgrad Med J*. 2007;83(984):e3. PMID: 17916865

Van Wilder N, Bravenboer B, Herremans S, Vanderbruggen N, Velkeniers B. Pseudomalabsorption of levothyroxine: a challenge for the endocrinologist in the treatment of hypothyroidism. *Eur Thyroid J*. 2017;6(1):52-56. PMID: 28611949

71 **ANSWER: C) Results cannot be interpreted; stop amiloride for a few weeks and repeat testing**
This patient's long history of hypertension that started at a young age, hypokalemia, and the need for 5 antihypertensive medications should all raise concern for a syndrome of mineralocorticoid excess. Primary aldosteronism is certainly the most common of the mineralocorticoid excess states with prevalence estimates of 5% to 10% in the general hypertension population and 10% to 20% in the resistant hypertension population. Other potential considerations for mineralocorticoid excess states include hypercortisolism (due to endogenous or exogenous glucocorticoids), licorice ingestion, or loss-of-function mutations in the 11β-hydroxysteroid dehydrogenase gene, or, rarely, certain forms of congenital adrenal hyperplasia or gain-of-function mutations in the genes encoding the epithelial sodium channel or mineralocorticoid receptor.

This patient meets the screening indications for primary aldosteronism, which include the following:

- Blood pressure greater than 150/100 mm Hg on 3 occasions
- Blood pressure greater than 140/90 mm Hg while on 3 or more medications
- Controlled blood pressure requiring 4 or more medications
- Spontaneous or drug-induced hypokalemia
- Hypertension with an adrenal mass
- Hypertension with sleep apnea
- Hypertension and a potential family history of primary aldosteronism

When attempting to diagnose primary aldosteronism, the objective is to determine whether a patient has *renin-independent aldosterone secretion* that is inappropriate and resulting in excessive mineralocorticoid receptor activation. Therefore, the physiologic expectation of a positive screening study involves suppression of renin (and angiotensin II, although this is rarely measured), and in the context of this renin suppression, an inappropriately elevated aldosterone level such that the aldosterone-to-renin ratio is consequently high. The exact cutoffs for renin suppression, inappropriate aldosterone elevation, and aldosterone-to-renin ratio elevation are debated. The most widely accepted standards are as follows:

- Suppression of renin <0.6 ng/mL per h (with some accepting even <1.0 ng/mL per h)
- Serum aldosterone >15 ng/dL (with some accepting even >10 ng/dL)
- Aldosterone-to-renin ratio >30 (with some accepting even >25 [with aldosterone in ng/dL and renin activity in ng/mL per h])

Of course, the variability in these cutoffs, which are relatively arbitrary, modifies the disease prevalence. Therefore, the most important aspect in interpreting biochemical testing for primary aldosteronism is to be convinced that there is a syndrome of excess mineralocorticoid receptor activation and renin-independent aldosterone secretion.

This patient has an aldosterone-to-renin ratio of 23 and a nonsuppressed renin activity of 1.7 ng/mL per h, values that are not physiologically consistent with renin-independent aldosteronism and a positive screen for primary aldosteronism (thus, Answer A is incorrect). The most common reason for a false-negative screen is the use of medications that block the effect of aldosterone on the distal nephron and decrease sodium reabsorption, limit volume expansion, and potentially induce volume contraction, which consequently results in a rise in renin that also lowers the aldosterone-to-renin ratio. The 2 most common culprit medications are mineralocorticoid receptor antagonists (such as spironolactone and eplerenone) and epithelial sodium channel inhibitors (such as amiloride and triamterene). This patient's laboratory results could imply a negative screen for primary aldosteronism (Answer B) or could represent the effect of treatment with high-dosage amiloride, which has potentially resulted in a rise in renin (Answer C). Since the pretest probability for primary aldosteronism was very high for this patient, a false-negative result due to amiloride use should be considered. If this patient has primary aldosteronism, the removal of amiloride for a few weeks should increase sodium reabsorption, volume expansion, and suppression of renin and most likely worsen hypokalemia and hypertension. This would allow confirmation of renin-independent aldosteronism. Medication washouts should proceed with caution, with careful blood pressure and potassium monitoring and the use of renin-aldosterone neutral antihypertensive agents such as α-antagonists, nondihydropyridine calcium channel blockers, and hydralazine.

Other notable antihypertensive medications that can influence the aldosterone-to-renin ratio by raising renin include ACE inhibitors and angiotensin receptor blockers, both of which either inhibit or block the action of angiotensin II on stimulating adrenal aldosterone release. However, the long-term use of these medications in primary aldosteronism rarely results in meaningful rises in renin because autonomous aldosterone secretion in primary aldosteronism is mostly independent of renin and angiotensin II, and therefore false-negative results due to ACE inhibitors and angiotensin receptor blockers are uncommon and washout is generally not necessary (thus, Answer E is incorrect). Hydrochlorothiazide does not typically result in meaningful alterations of renin or aldosterone that would lead to diagnostic uncertainty (thus, Answer D is incorrect).

This patient was instructed to stop taking amiloride and was given doxazosin for blood pressure control during the washout, which was monitored using an automated home sphygmomanometer. Potassium supplementation was increased and serum potassium was monitored during this time. After 2 weeks without amiloride, the patient's repeat laboratory tests showed a serum aldosterone concentration of 29 ng/dL (804 pmol/L), a renin activity less than 0.6 ng/mL per h, and an aldosterone-to-renin ratio of at least 48, thus indicating a positive screening test that also implies a confirmed diagnosis of primary aldosteronism.

Educational Objective
Identify medications that can result in a false-negative screening study for primary aldosteronism.

UpToDate Topic Review(s)
Diagnosis of primary aldosteronism

Reference(s)

Funder JW, Carey RM, Mantero F, et al. The management of primary aldosteronism: case detection, diagnosis, and treatment: an Endocrine Society clinical practice guideline. *J Clin Endocrinol Metab.* 2016;101(5):1889-1916. PMID: 26934393

Vaidya A, Malchoff CD, Auchus RJ; AACE Adrenal Scientific Committee. An individualized approach to the evaluation and management of primary aldosteronism. *Endocr Pract.* 2017;23(6):680-689. PMID: 28332881

72 ANSWER: E) Measurement of TRAb

Postpartum thyroiditis is the occurrence of thyroid dysfunction, excluding Graves disease, in the first postpartum year in women who were euthyroid before pregnancy. This is an inflammatory autoimmune disorder associated with the presence of thyroid autoantibodies (TPO and thyroglobulin antibodies), lymphocyte abnormalities, complement activation, increased levels of IgG1, increased natural killer cell activity, and specific HLA haplotypes. In the classic form, transient thyrotoxicosis is followed by transient hypothyroidism with a return to the euthyroid state by the end of the initial postpartum year. One-quarter of patients have isolated thyrotoxicosis and one-half have isolated hypothyroidism. Twenty to fifty percent of patients who present with the classic form develop permanent hypothyroidism. Women who have detectable levels of thyroid antibodies in the first trimester are at high risk of developing postpartum thyroiditis, which reflects the rebound of the immune system in the postpartum period after the relative immune suppression of pregnancy.

The prevalence of postpartum thyroiditis is approximately 5% and reported rates range between 1% and 16%. Patients with other autoimmune diseases such as type 1 diabetes mellitus or systemic lupus erythematosus and women with a history of autoimmune thyroid disease are more likely to develop postpartum thyroiditis. Women with a history of postpartum thyroiditis have a 50% to 70% chance of relapse in each subsequent pregnancy. This is a painless form of thyroiditis and often women have few or no symptoms of thyrotoxicosis. The levels of circulating thyroid hormones are usually only modestly raised. The hypothyroid phase is often more symptomatic. A link between postpartum thyroiditis and depression has been suggested, and patients with postpartum depression should be screened for thyroid dysfunction.

The major diagnostic challenge is to distinguish thyrotoxicosis caused by postpartum thyroiditis from that caused by Graves disease. The 2 disease entities require different treatments and have markedly different clinical courses. The patient in this vignette has typical symptoms and signs of thyrotoxicosis, which is confirmed biochemically on the laboratory tests. One of the most useful tests to establish the differential diagnosis is measurement of TRAb (Answer E).

Radioactive isotope scans with ^{99m}Tc pertechnetate or ^{123}I demonstrate diffuse increased uptake in Graves disease and reduced uptake in the hyperthyroid phase of postpartum thyroiditis, but the use of radioactive diagnostic procedures is rarely needed in lactating women such as the patient described in this vignette. These isotopes may be used during breastfeeding, as they have a short half-life. However, breast milk should be pumped and discarded for several days after the scan. The use of ^{131}I for diagnostic (Answer B) or therapeutic purposes is contraindicated.

The circulating free T_3 concentration (Answer D) is most likely to be elevated both in postpartum thyroiditis and Graves disease, and while an elevated T_4 to T_3 ratio is more likely to be associated with postpartum thyroiditis, this is less informative than measurement of TRAb.

Thyroid ultrasonography (Answer A) is likely to indicate the presence of a hypoechoic, enlarged thyroid gland in thyrotoxicosis caused by Graves disease and postpartum thyroiditis. Color-flow Doppler ultrasonography can help distinguish between the 2 conditions and will be increased in Graves disease and reduced in postpartum thyroiditis, but this is a less specific tool requiring a reasonable degree of expertise when compared with TRAb measurement. TPO antibodies (Answer C) are usually elevated in both forms of thyrotoxicosis and are therefore not helpful in distinguishing between the etiologies.

The thyrotoxic phase of postpartum thyroiditis may require treatment with β-adrenergic blockade to alleviate symptoms, and drugs including metoprolol and propranolol are safe during breastfeeding. It is advisable to use the lowest effective dosage. Antithyroid drugs are not effective in postpartum thyroiditis because this is a destructive thyroiditis in which thyroid hormone synthesis is not increased.

Educational Objective
Diagnose postpartum thyroiditis.

UpToDate Topic Review(s)
Postpartum thyroiditis

Reference(s)

Ide A, Amino N, Kang S, et al. Differentiation of postpartum Graves' thyrotoxicosis from postpartum destructive thyrotoxicosis using antithyrotropin receptor antibodies and thyroid blood flow. *Thyroid*. 2014;24(6):1027-1031. PMID: 24400892

Alexander EK, Pearce EN, Brent GA, et al. 2017 Guidelines of the American Thyroid Association for the Diagnosis and Management of Thyroid Disease During Pregnancy and the Postpartum. *Thyroid*. 2017;27(3):315-389. PMID: 28056690

73 **ANSWER: B) Surgery to remove the primary tumor and debulk liver metastases**

This patient has a metastatic gastrointestinal neuroendocrine tumor (NET) that is causing classic carcinoid syndrome with flushing and diarrhea. Carcinoid syndrome comprises a variety of symptoms caused by humoral factors produced by well-differentiated NETs of the gastrointestinal tract and lungs, which synthesize, store, and release a variety of polypeptides, biogenic amines, and prostaglandins. The liver inactivates most bioactive products secreted into the portal circulation, so this may explain why patients with gastrointestinal NETs most often develop carcinoid syndrome if they have hepatic metastases. While as many as 40 secretory products have been identified in various gastroenteropancreatic NETs, the most prominent of these are serotonin, histamine, and tachykinins. Altered metabolism of tryptophan with increased conversion to serotonin occurs in almost all patients with carcinoid syndrome. Serotonin is then metabolized to 5-hydroxyindole acetic acid (5-HIAA), which is usually measured in urine.

Therapy options for NETs are expanding and include peptide receptor radionuclide therapy; pharmacologic, hormonal, and liver-directed treatments; and surgery. Somatostatin analogues, including octreotide and lanreotide, are highly effective in controlling symptoms associated with carcinoid syndrome and should be the initial management strategy in these circumstances. Most early studies showed complete or partial relief of flushing and/or diarrhea in up to 90% of patients, as well as significant reduction in 5-HIAA levels. More recently, it has also been demonstrated that both octreotide and lanreotide can slow tumor progression and control symptoms.

In this scenario, use of a somatostatin analogue, while beneficial in terms of symptom control and possibly reducing tumor progression, is unlikely to be sufficient given the considerable tumor burden. Numerous retrospective studies suggest that removal of the primary NET (Answer B), even in the context of metastatic disease, significantly improves the time to progression and overall survival. The UKINETs study attempted to identify favorable and adverse prognostic factors for liver metastatic midgut carcinoid tumors such as in this vignette. They demonstrated, using univariate analysis, that older age at diagnosis, increasing urinary hydroxyindole acetic acid levels, increasing plasma chromogranin A levels, high Ki67, high tumor volume, and treatment with chemotherapy were factors associated with a significantly poorer outcome. In contrast, resection of liver metastases, resection of small-bowel primary, treatment with somatostatin analogue therapy, and treatment with peptide receptor therapy were associated with improved prognosis. Moreover, multivariate analysis revealed that age at diagnosis ($P = .014$), Ki67 level ($P = .039$), and resection of primary ($P = .015$) were independent predictors of survival. Of the 360 patients included in this study, 209 underwent resection of the primary tumor. Median survival was 9.92 years (confidence interval, 7.45-12.4 years) in this group compared with 4.68 years (confidence interval, 2.65-6.71 years) in the conservatively treated group. Surgery should therefore be the next course of action for this patient who has no significant comorbidity, and this would be more appropriate than surveillance only (Answer A), particularly if the patient is symptomatic.

Other therapeutic options such as liver ablation (Answer C) and peptide receptor radionuclide therapy (Answer D) are feasible for future management of this patient after initial debulking surgery, but they are less appropriate now. Radiolabeled somatostatin analogue therapy (or peptide receptor radionuclide therapy) has always shown promise for the treatment of advanced NET, most of which express high levels of somatostatin receptors. This targeted form of systemic radiotherapy allows the delivery of radionuclides directly to tumor cells. Very recently, the NETTER-1 trial showed that treatment with ^{177}Lu-DOTATATE (a radiolabeled somatostatin analogue) in patients with metastatic midgut NET resulted in markedly longer progression-free survival than high-dosage octreotide LAR alone and was approved for this use by the US FDA in early 2018.

Evidence of benefit of the mTOR inhibitor everolimus (Answer E) has only been shown in the context of progressive, advanced pancreatic NETs. The RADIANT-3 trial demonstrated that everolimus compared with placebo resulted in a significant prolongation of progression-free survival (11 months vs 4.6 months) in patients with progressive, advanced pancreatic NETs. More recently, the RADIANT-4 study in patients with advanced gastrointestinal or lung NETs also demonstrated significantly improved progression-free survival (11 months vs 3.4 months) with everolimus vs placebo.

Educational Objective
Manage symptomatic, metastatic gastroenteropancreatic neuroendocrine tumors.

UpToDate Topic Review(s)
Metastatic gastroenteropancreatic neuroendocrine tumors: Local options to control tumor growth and symptoms of hormone hypersecretion

Reference(s)

Modlin IM, Oberg K, Chung DC, et al. Gastroenteropancreatic tumours. *Lancet Oncol.* 2008;9(1):61-72. PMID: 18177818

Rinke A, Müller HH, Schade-Brittinger C, et al; PROMID Study Group. Placebo-controlled, double-blind, prospective, randomized study on the effect of octreotide LAR in the control of tumor growth in patients with metastatic neuroendocrine midgut tumors: a report from the PROMID Study Group. *J Clin Oncol.* 2009;27(28):4656-4663. PMID: 19704057

Caplin ME, Pavel M, Cwikla JB, et al; CLARINET Investigators. Lanreotide in metastatic enteropancreatic neuroendocrine tumors. *N Engl J Med.* 2014;371(3): 224-233. PMID: 25014687

Yao JC, Shah MH, Ito T et al; RAD001 in Advanced Neuroendocrine Tumors, Third Trial (RADIANT-3) Study Group. Everolimus for advanced pancreatic neuroendocrine tumors. *N Engl J Med*. 2011;364(6):514-523. PMID: 21306238

Yao JC, Fazio N, Singh S, et al; RAD001 in Advanced Neuroendocrine Tumours, Fourth Trial (RADIANT-4) Study Group. Everolimus for the treatment of advanced, non-functional neuroendocrine tumours of the lung or gastrointestinal tract (RADIANT-4): a randomised, placebo-controlled, phase 3 study. *Lancet*. 2016;387(10022):968-977. PMID: 26703889

Strosberg J, El-Haddad G, Wolin E, et al; NETTER-1 Trial Investigators. Phase 3 trial of 177Lu-dotatate for midgut neuroendocrine tumors. *N Engl J Med*. 2017;376(2):125-135. PMID: 28076709

Ahmed A, Turner G, King B, et al. Midgut neuroendocrine tumours with liver metastases: results of the UKINETS study. *Endocr Relat Cancer*. 2009;16(3): 885-894. PMID: 19458024

74 ANSWER: B) Stress radionuclide myocardial perfusion imaging with positron emission tomography

This patient has multiple risk factors for coronary artery disease (type 2 diabetes, hypercholesterolemia, obesity, positive family history of heart disease) and presents with exertional angina. Patients such as this who have symptoms of stable angina and a high pretest probability for coronary artery disease are good candidates for stress testing.

Factors that influence the choice of noninvasive cardiac testing include body habitus and lack of ability to exercise. This patient's severe arthritis will not allow her to achieve an adequate exercise level; therefore, she would benefit from a pharmacologic stress test and not from exercise testing (thus, Answers D and E are incorrect). Regarding body habitus, each imaging modality has a limit based on the patient's weight. The weight limit for the exercise treadmill ranges from 225 to 500 lb (102-227 kg). The table weight limit is 400 lb (182 kg) for positron emission tomography and 450 lb (205 kg) for CT.

Stress radionuclide myocardial perfusion imaging enables evaluation of myocardial perfusion and viability using a radioisotope and a camera system (either single-photon emission computed tomography [SPECT] or positron emission tomography [PET]). Decreased or absent radioactive tracer count is the hallmark of ischemic myocardium in this type of imaging test. In obese individuals (BMI ≥ 30 kg/m^2), the excess adipose tissue on the body wall attenuates the radioactivity when using SPECT, which can lead to the appearance of a myocardial perfusion defect when one does not actually exist. Stress radionuclide myocardial perfusion imaging with PET (Answer B) provides images with increased attenuation correction, leading to fewer artifacts and false-positive results and thus making it the test of choice in obese patients.

Echocardiography (Answer A) is a safe, cheap, and widely available test with the additional advantage that patients are not exposed to ionizing radiation. However, in patients with severe obesity, it provides suboptimal acoustic windows, poor endocardial visualization, and technically limited studies (due to increased distance between the heart and the ultrasound probe), resulting in inconclusive findings. Therefore, it is not considered a good imaging modality for the assessment of coronary artery disease in such patients. However, if stress radionuclide myocardial perfusion imaging with PET is not available, echocardiography can be considered.

CT coronary artery calcium scoring (Answer C) aids in predicting coronary artery disease events in asymptomatic patients, particularly in those with intermediate Framingham risk and in those with low cardiovascular risk with a family history of premature heart disease. However, this patient presents with exertional angina and she is at high cardiovascular risk.

Educational Objective
Order the correct cardiac testing during the evaluation of a patient with a body mass index greater than 30 kg/m^2.

UpToDate Topic Review(s)
Selecting the optimal cardiac stress test

Reference(s)
Shah BN, Senior R. Stress echocardiography in patients with morbid obesity. *Echo Res Pract*. 2016;3(2):R13-R18. PMID: 27249552

Bigvava T, Zamani SM, Pieske-Kraigher E, Gebker R, Pieske B, Kelle S. Prognostic value of non-invasive stress testing for coronary artery disease in obese patients. *Expert Rev Cardiovasc Ther*. 2015;13(12):1325-1332. PMID: 26536394

Lim SP, Arasaratnam P, Chow BJ, Beanlands RS, Hessian RC. Obesity and the challenges of noninvasive imaging for the detection of coronary artery disease. *Can J Cardiol*. 2015;31(2):223-226. PMID: 25661558

Gugliotti D, Grant P, Jaber W, et al. Challenges in cardiac risk assessment in bariatric surgery patients. *Obes Surg*. 2008;18(1):129-133. PMID: 18066696

75 ANSWER: A) 5-Hour mixed-meal test

Hypoglycemia is one of the most common problems seen by endocrinologists. The primary concern, to rule out insulinoma, is important, but such tumors are rare. This patient's symptoms are more typical of non–insulinoma-related postprandial syndrome. It remains to be established whether his symptoms are mediated by hypoglycemia. The approach to this patient is to first obtain a detailed history, including medications and over-the-counter or Internet-purchased products, recent consumption of ackee fruit, and alcohol intake. Obtaining a detailed dietary history is crucial to estimate his total carbohydrate intake. Does he crave sweets? What is his intake of soda and fruit juice?

The next step is to document his symptoms—adrenergic (shakiness, tremor, palpitations, nervousness) or neuroglycopenic (confusion, memory problems, black outs, syncope). Any evidence of severe hypoglycemia, defined as requiring the assistance of another person to help the patient, or the presence of severe neuroglycopenic symptoms, merits a full hypoglycemia evaluation, including a 48-hour fast (Answer C). If severe hypoglycemia is not evident, then the above patient has postprandial syndrome vs postprandial hypoglycemia. To distinguish between these 2 diagnoses, the patient will need laboratory glucose testing in a setting similar to the circumstances that precipitate his symptoms. Some physicians might order an oral glucose tolerance test (Answer B), but this test can precipitate hypoglycemia in persons with no disease. Charles et al found that patients who had glucose levels less than 60 mg/dL (<3.3 mmol/L) during an oral glucose tolerance test also had postprandial symptoms when challenged with a mixed-meal test (Answer A) but were normoglycemic. These authors advocate that the mixed-meal test is preferred over the oral glucose tolerance test. If hypoglycemia is not found, then the appropriate diagnosis is idiopathic postprandial syndrome.

To perform the mixed-meal test, the patient should ingest a meal of solid and liquid composition that is similar to that of a meal that induces symptoms. Blood samples are collected for plasma glucose, insulin, C-peptide, and proinsulin while fasting before the test and then every 30 minutes for 5 hours after the meal is consumed. Glucose should be analyzed at each time interval. To reduce costs, the other tests can be run only on the samples for which glucose is 60 mg/dL or lower (≤3.3 mmol/L). If the patient has a glucose value less than 55 mg/dL (<3.1 mmol/L) in addition to neuroglycopenic symptoms, the patient should be treated with glucose and observed. If the symptoms correct, the patient fulfills the Whipple triad and needs further evaluation.

Patients who have mild hypoglycemia (55-60 mg/dL [3.1-3.3 mmol/L]) or do not have hypoglycemia with the mixed-meal test can be treated conservatively by diet modification. Avoiding ethanol, simple carbohydrates, and sugars and ingesting 3 spaced meals and snacks consisting of mixed protein, complex carbohydrates, and healthful fats often resolve symptoms. Acarbose has been used as off-label treatment of postprandial hypoglycemia, but no formal clinical trials have been conducted.

Given that this patient does not have documented neuroglycopenic symptoms and does not meet the criteria for severe hypoglycemia, the 48-hour fast (Answer C) and testing for insulin autoantibodies (Answer E) are not necessary. The selective arterial calcium stimulation test (Answer D) is performed only in patients with documented insulin-mediated hypoglycemia and is done as a localization test before pancreas surgery.

Educational Objective
Guide the outpatient evaluation of postprandial hypoglycemia.

UpToDate Topic Review(s)
Hypoglycemia in adults without diabetes mellitus: Diagnostic approach

Reference(s)

Cryer PE, Axelrod L, Grossman AB, et al; Endocrine Society. Evaluation and management of adult hypoglycemic disorders: an Endocrine Society clinical practice guideline. *J Clin Endocrinol Metab.* 2009;94(3):709-728. PMID: 19088155

Charles MA, Hofeldt F, Shackelford A, et al. Comparison of oral glucose tolerance tests and mixed meals in patients with apparent idiopathic postabsorptive hypoglycemia: absence of hypoglycemia after meals. *Diabetes.* 1981;30(6):465-470. PMID: 7227659

Galati SJ, Rayfield EJ. Approach to the patient with postprandial hypoglycemia. *Endocr Pract.* 2014;20(4):331-340. PMID: 24246338

Golden KD, Williams OJ, Bailey-Shaw Y. High-performance liquid chromatographic analysis of amino acids in ackee fruit with emphasis on the toxic amino acid hypoglycin A. *J Chromatogr Sci.* 2002;40(8):441-446. PMID: 12387335

76 ANSWER: A) Secondary hypothyroidism

Immune checkpoint inhibitors that are being used to treat malignancies such as melanoma, lung cancer, and renal cancer have a whole host of endocrine adverse effects, exerted via an autoimmune mechanism. These endocrinopathies include hypophysitis with secondary adrenal insufficiency and secondary hypothyroidism, primary adrenal insufficiency, primary hypothyroidism, thyroiditis, and diabetes mellitus. The likelihood of the various endocrinopathies seems to vary depending on the specific agents being used. Anticytotoxic T-lymphocyte–associated antigen 4 (anti-CTLA-4) agents such as ipilimumab are associated with higher rates of hypophysitis, whereas antiprogrammed cell death 1 (anti-PD-1) agents such as nivolumab have higher risks of thyroid dysfunction. However, a range of effects can be seen because these agents are frequently given in combination.

The use of high-dosage glucocorticoid therapy, as was initially used in this patient, is not a uniformly used protocol. When it is used for the hypophysitis, it is initially effective, but there can be adverse effects and relapse. However, all patients with central adrenal insufficiency require glucocorticoid replacement. The patient's initial presentation with weakness, dizziness, and nausea is highly suggestive of adrenal insufficiency. Furthermore, the combination of low ACTH and low cortisol and the absence of hyperpigmentation are compatible with secondary adrenal insufficiency. This is also supported by the MRI findings of the diffuse pituitary enlargement that can be seen with hypophysitis.

The patient in this vignette felt better after receiving glucocorticoid therapy, but she still had some remaining symptoms, raising the possibility of a second endocrinopathy. Most of the answer choices have been reported with ipilimumab and nivolumab, with the exception of primary hypogonadism (Answer B). Reports of diabetes insipidus are extremely rare. A diagnosis of diabetes insipidus (Answer D) is not supported by the fact that the patient does not describe excessive thirst. Primary adrenal insufficiency has been reported in about 2.6% of patients receiving combined ipilimumab and nivolumab. If this patient has both primary and secondary adrenal insufficiency concurrently, her symptoms of glucocorticoid deficiency would have been treated by her hydrocortisone therapy, but she would remain mineralocorticoid deficient. A high serum potassium level would support this diagnosis. Her serum potassium level was 4.1 mEq/L, which is not characteristic of primary adrenal insufficiency. The fact that the patient now has fatigue and malaise, rather than more classic symptoms of volume depletion due to lack of mineralocorticoids, such as orthostasis, dizziness, syncope, etc, points away from primary adrenal insufficiency (Answer C).

Her symptoms are best explained by secondary hypothyroidism (Answer A) accompanying her secondary adrenal insufficiency. Combined ACTH and TSH deficiency are quite common with checkpoint inhibitor–induced hypophysitis. Thyroid disorders, including primary hypothyroidism, and hypophysitis, with varying numbers of pituitary hormones being affected, are the most frequent endocrine disorders seen with ipilimumab and nivolumab. Corticotroph deficiency often does not recover, whereas thyrotroph and gonadotroph function may recover. Primary hypothyroidism is not offered as a choice here, and it would be hard to diagnose with coexistent secondary hypothyroidism. However, both disorders would be treated with levothyroxine therapy, which should be initiated in this patient.

Diabetes mellitus (Answer E) is rare with the combination of ipilimumab and nivolumab (0.3% of cases). The absence of polydipsia and polyuria are also not consistent with the development of diabetes mellitus.

Although central hypogonadism has been reported with ipilimumab and nivolumab therapy, primary hypogonadism (Answer B) has not been observed.

Educational Objective
Diagnose the concomitant presentation of both secondary adrenal insufficiency and secondary hypothyroidism in a patient treated with immune checkpoint inhibitors.

UpToDate Topic Review(s)
Patient selection criteria and toxicities associated with checkpoint inhibitor immunotherapy

Reference(s)

Albarel F, Gaudy C, Castinetti F, et al. Long-term follow-up of ipilimumab-induced hypophysitis, a common adverse event of the anti-CTLA-4 antibody in melanoma. *Eur J Endocrinol.* 2015;172(2)195-204. PMID: 25416723

Ryder M, Callahan M, Postow MA, Wolchok J, Fagin JA. Endocrine-related adverse events following ipilimumab in patients with advanced melanoma: a comprehensive retrospective review from a single institution. *Endocr Relat Cancer.* 2014;21(2):371-381. PMID: 24610577

Sznol M, Postow MA, Davies MJ, et al. Endocrine-related adverse events associated with immune checkpoint blockade and expert insights on their management. *Cancer Treat Rev.* 2017;58:70-76. PMID: 28689073

Torino F, Corsello SM, Salvatori R. Endocrinological side-effects of immune checkpoint inhibitors. *Curr Opin Oncol.* 2016;28(4):278-287. PMID: 27136136

77 ANSWER: E) CT of the chest, abdomen, and pelvis

The patient described in this vignette has hypercalcemia associated with a low-normal PTH level and an inappropriately elevated 1,25-dihydroxyvitamin D level. In this scenario, one must consider extra-renal production of 1,25-dihydroxyvitamin D such as in granulomatous diseases or lymphoma. Given her clinical presentation and normal chest x-ray, it is unlikely that sarcoidosis or tuberculosis is the cause of her hypercalcemia. Thus, a tuberculin skin test (Answer A) would not be the best next step in the evaluation of this patient's hypercalcemia. This elderly woman's history of weight loss and cervical lymphadenopathy on exam should raise suspicion for lymphoma. In fact, CT of the patient's chest, abdomen, and pelvis (Answer E) revealed extensive multifocal lymphadenopathy, consistent with lymphoma. An inguinal lymph node biopsy confirmed the diagnosis of diffuse large B-cell lymphoma.

PTHrP (Answer B) is the principal mediator of hypercalcemia associated with solid tumors and is the most common cause of hypercalcemia in malignancy. Humoral hypercalcemia of malignancy should be suspected in cases when hypercalcemia is of relatively recent onset, particularly in someone with a known malignancy. Unlike in this case, 1,25-dihydroxyvitamin D levels are typically appropriately suppressed in these patients.

Serum protein electrophoresis (Answer C) for possible multiple myeloma would be indicated in the presence of low or low-normal serum levels of PTH and PTHrP and low or normal vitamin D metabolites, suggesting some other source for the hypercalcemia. Since this patient had an elevated 1,25-dihydroxyvitamin D level, this would not be the best next step in her evaluation. Similarly, a bone scan (Answer D) to detect possible skeletal metastases would not be indicated in this patient, since typical biochemical findings in patients with bone metastases include low or low-normal serum 1,25-dihydroxyvitamin D levels in the setting of low or low-normal PTH and PTHrP levels.

Educational Objective
Diagnose lymphoma as a cause of non–PTH-mediated hypercalcemia.

UpToDate Topic Review(s)
Diagnostic approach to hypercalcemia

Reference(s)

Lafferty FW. Differential diagnosis of hypercalcemia. *J Bone Miner Res*. 1991;6(Suppl 2):S51-S59. PMID: 1763670

Schilling T, Pecherstorfer M, Blind E, Leidig G, Ziegler R, Raue F. Parathyroid hormone-related protein (PTHrP) does not regulate 1,25-dihydroxyvitamin D serum levels in hypercalcemia of malignancy. *J Clin Endocrinol Metab*. 1993;76(3):801-803. PMID: 8445039

78 ANSWER: C) Request consultation with a mental health care provider

This young man with type 1 diabetes has had a clear drop-off in the level of self-care coincident with a rising hemoglobin A_{1c} level. Both registry and cohort data suggest that in older adolescence and young adulthood, glycemic control deteriorates with rising mean hemoglobin A_{1c} levels and higher odds of having a hemoglobin A_{1c} level greater than 9.5% (>80 mmol/mol). Patients in this age group are less likely to receive screening tests recommended by the American Diabetes Association. Further, adults with diabetes have a higher prevalence of both depression and anxiety than adults without diabetes. Survey data suggest a 19.5% lifetime prevalence of anxiety among persons with either type 1 or type 2 diabetes. Similarly, cross-sectional studies suggest that there is an increased prevalence of depression symptoms (up to 23%) in patients with type 1 diabetes. Diabetes-specific issues include fears related to hypoglycemia, insulin injections, or infusions and anxiety about glycemic targets and the onset of complications. Recent American Diabetes Association guidelines suggest that clinicians should consider screening patients annually for anxiety and depression in cases where there is reasonable suspicion for these disorders. Therefore, in this vignette, either screening for depression and anxiety or referring the patient to a psychologist (Answer C) is the best next step.

This patient has most likely previously received nutritional counseling (Answer B) and diabetes education (Answer D), and neither of these strategies will address the recent behavior changes. While advice on rotating pump insertion sites (Answer E) is a wise thing to do, it does not address the root cause of why this patient may not be taking care of himself. Finally, hypoglycemia or hypoglycemia unawareness was not described in the vignette, so a continuous glucose monitor (Answer A) is not likely to provide much clinical benefit.

Educational Objective

In adult patients with type 1 diabetes mellitus, follow the American Diabetes Association guidelines that suggest screening for depression and referral to a mental health care provider if indicated.

UpToDate Topic Review(s)

Overview of medical care in adults with diabetes mellitus

Reference(s)

de Groot M, Golden SH, Wagner J. Psychological conditions in adults with diabetes. *Am Psychol*. 2016;71(7):552-562. PMID: 27690484

Petitti DB, Klingensmith GJ, Bell RA, et al; SEARCH for Diabetes in Youth Study Group. *J Pediatr*. 2009;155(5):668-672. PMID: 19643434

Miller KM, Foster NC, Beck RW, et al; T1D exchange Clinic Network. Current state of type 1 diabetes treatment in the U.S.: update data from the T1D Exchange clinic registry. *Diabetes Care*. 2015;38(6):971-978. PMID: 25998289

Standards of medical care in diabetes-2018. *Diabetes Care*. 2018;41(Suppl 1):S1-S153.

79 ANSWER: E) Plasma renin activity, 5.5 ng/mL per h; serum aldosterone, <4 ng/dL

This patient had primary aldosteronism due to a left-sided aldosterone-producing adenoma, and following surgical removal of the adenoma, there was resolution of hypertension, then development of hypotension, hyperkalemia, and acute kidney injury—all likely due to intravascular volume depletion and hypoaldosteronism.

The adrenal venous sampling data provide important insights. The aldosterone-to-cortisol ratio in the left adrenal vein was 7, whereas in the right adrenal vein it was 0.27, suggesting a more than 25-fold lateralization of aldosterone to the left adrenal vein. Perhaps just as important is the fact that the aldosterone-to-cortisol ratio in the right adrenal vein (0.27) was even lower than that of the inferior vena cava (1.6), and the aldosterone level in the right adrenal vein (6.5 ng/dL) was even lower than that circulating in the inferior vena cava (15.0 ng/dL). Together, these data suggest that the left adrenal adenoma is producing all the systemic aldosterone, resulting in volume expansion and consequent suppression of endogenous renin and angiotensin II and complete suppression of right adrenal aldosterone secretion.

Understanding this pathophysiology explains the postoperative events. Immediately following resection of the left-sided aldosterone-producing adenoma, the patient would have had undetectable or severely suppressed levels of renin, angiotensin II, and aldosterone; however, because she still had an expanded intravascular state, her blood pressure did not become frankly low. Given the severity and duration of her primary aldosteronism, right-sided aldosterone secretion remained suppressed, even as intravascular volume and blood pressure decreased over the subsequent days, resulting in physiologic stimulation of renin and angiotensin II. Thus, the expected manifestations of hypoaldosteronism were observed 7 days later: with hypotension and intravascular volume contraction, renin and angiotensin II are stimulated, but given the prolonged suppression of right-adrenal aldosterone secretion, there was relative hypoaldosteronism resulting in persistent intravascular volume depletion (potential pre-renal acute kidney injury) and hyperkalemia (thus, Answer E is correct and Answers A, B, C, and D are incorrect).

This degree of prolonged hypoaldosteronism is uncommon and seen only after unilateral adrenalectomy in severe cases of primary aldosteronism. However, milder forms of transient hypoaldosteronism can occur in the first few days following surgery for a unilateral aldosterone-producing adenoma and should be suspected when there is a precipitous decline in blood pressure and/or rise in potassium or creatinine. Temporary treatment with fludrocortisone can be considered in severe cases, and this type of contralateral hypoaldosteronism usually resolves within a few days to a couple of weeks following surgery.

Educational Objective

Explain how transient hypoaldosteronism can occur after surgical resection of a unilateral aldosterone-producing adenoma.

UpToDate Topic Review(s)

Treatment of primary aldosteronism

Reference(s)

Funder JW, Carey RM, Mantero F, et al. The management of primary aldosteronism: case detection, diagnosis, and treatment: an Endocrine Society clinical practice guideline. *J Clin Endocrinol Metab.* 2016;101(5):1889-1916. PMID: 26934393

Fischer E, Hanslik G, Pallauf A, et al. Prolonged zona glomerulosa insufficiency causing hyperkalemia in primary aldosteronism after adrenalectomy. *J Clin Endocrinol Metab.* 2012;97(11):3965-3973. PMID: 22893716

Williams TA, Lenders JWM, Mulatero P, et al; Primary Aldosteronism Surgery Outcome (PASO) Investigators. Outcomes after adrenalectomy for unilateral primary aldosteronism: an international consensus on outcome measures and analysis of remission rates in an international cohort. *Lancet Diabetes Endocrinol.* 2017;5(9):689-699. PMID: 28576687

80 ANSWER: A) Cycling

Clinicians should be aware that men who participate in certain types of athletic activities have been found to have lower levels of serum testosterone. Prospective and cross-sectional studies have shown that men who participate in chronic intense exercise have similar or lower testosterone levels than men in control groups. These results have been primarily documented in endurance athletes.

Maimoun et al examined hormone profiles in 11 cyclists, 14 triathletes, 13 swimmers, and 10 control participants. The athletes had been training for an average of 7 to 8 years with a minimum of 10 hours per week. The age-matched controls did not participate in regular or vigorous activity in the past 2 years (>2 hours per week). Fasting morning hormone levels were measured and participants had not exercised in the preceding 48 hours. The total testosterone levels were as follows:

Controls:	608.1 ± 175.8 ng/dL (21.1 ± 6.1 nmol/L)
Swimmers:	547.6 ± 164.3 ng/dL (19.0 ± 5.7 nmol/L)
Triathletes:	472.6 ± 106.6 ng/dL (16.4 ± 3.7 nmol/L)
Cyclists:	429.4 ± 103.7 ng/dL (14.9 ± 3.6 nmol/L)

The testosterone concentrations were statistically lower for triathletes and cyclists. No differences were seen in serum levels of estradiol, LH, SHBG, or cortisol. There also were no differences in bone mineral density adjusted by lean body weight between any of the groups at the lumbar spine, femoral neck, and radius.

Cycling (Answer A) is the correct answer, as men who participate in this endurance sport have been found to have lower serum testosterone levels in some studies. Playing soccer (Answer B), powerlifting (Answer C), swimming (Answer D), and wrestling (Answer E) are not endurance sports and are less likely to be associated with lower testosterone levels. Although the patient in this vignette had a specific concern, he should be aware that none of the sports listed is contraindicated for health reasons. Although mean levels of total testosterone are lower in certain types of athletes, most athletes still have normal testosterone levels.

Educational Objective
Counsel patients that athletes of certain endurance sports may have lower levels of serum testosterone.

UpToDate Topic Review(s)
Clinical features and diagnosis of male hypogonadism

Reference(s)

Bennell KL, Brukner PD, Malcolm SA. Effect of altered reproductive function and lowered testosterone levels on bone density in male endurance athletes. *Br J Sports Med.* 1996;30(3):205-208. PMID: 8889111

Maïmoun L, Lumbroso S, Manetta J, Paris F, Leroux JL, Sultan C. Testosterone is significantly reduced in endurance athletes without impact on bone mineral density. *Horm Res.* 2003;59(6):285-292. PMID: 12784093

81 ANSWER: B) Measurement of TPO antibody titer

The diagnosis and management of subclinical hypothyroidism in pregnancy remains controversial. Current American Thyroid Association guidelines recommend that gestational thyroid dysfunction is best defined according to pregnancy-specific reference ranges calculated in a population of pregnant women free from major factors that interfere with thyroid function. Factors that may affect the determination of reference ranges include the presence of preexisting thyroid disease, thyroid autoimmunity, the use of thyroid-interfering drugs, twin pregnancies, a history of in vitro fertilization, and iodine deficiency. If pregnancy-specific reference ranges are not available, the use of population-based reference ranges that have been determined using the same assays and in a population with similar characteristics is recommended. Finally, if this is not feasible, the use of a fixed upper limit for the TSH concentration (ie, 4.0 mIU/L) is recommended.

Subclinical hypothyroidism, defined as an elevated serum TSH concentration with normal circulating thyroid hormone concentrations, is associated with a higher risk of pregnancy loss, placental abruption, premature delivery, preeclampsia, and neonatal death. Because thyroid hormones are crucial to fetal development and in particular fetal brain development, several studies have evaluated the effects of subclinical hypothyroidism in pregnancy on fetal developmental outcomes. Prospective cohort studies have not demonstrated an association between subclinical hypothyroidism and adverse neurobehavioral outcomes in the offspring. Importantly, 2 recent randomized controlled intervention trials did not find differences in offspring IQ when maternal subclinical hypothyroidism was treated during pregnancy.

Thyroid autoimmunity is a major risk factor for subclinical hypothyroidism, and approximately one-third of women with subclinical hypothyroidism have elevated circulating TPO antibodies. Regardless of the presence of subclinical hypothyroidism, the combination of high TSH concentrations and TPO-antibody positivity synergistically increases the risk of adverse pregnancy outcomes compared with the presence of only high TSH concentrations or TPO-antibody positivity. Current American Thyroid Association guidelines recommend that the upper normal limit for serum TSH in women with positive TPO antibodies is 2.5 mIU/L, and that levothyroxine replacement should be considered if serum TSH measurements exceed this threshold. The patient in this vignette has a serum TSH concentration of 3.8 mIU/L in the first trimester of pregnancy. Since the cut-off to recommend levothyroxine replacement is different depending on the presence or absence of TPO antibodies, their measurement (Answer B) is indicated.

Shifts between hypothyroidism and hyperthyroidism, often with a period of euthyroidism in between, have been described in patients with thyroid autoimmunity. This may be caused by fluctuating concentrations of thyrotropin receptor–blocking antibodies and thyrotropin receptor–stimulating antibodies. There is no history of thyroid dysfunction in this patient and it seems unlikely that thyrotropin receptor–blocking antibodies (Answer C) are responsible for the relative rise in serum TSH. While repeated measurement of TSH (Answer A) and free T_4 after 4 weeks is appropriate, the determination of TPO antibody status will best guide further management. Measurement of serum free T_3 (Answer D) is not informative in patients with hypothyroidism either during or outside pregnancy. Thyroid ultrasonography (Answer E) may demonstrate evidence of thyroiditis, but it would not inform treatment decisions.

Educational Objective
Diagnose subclinical hypothyroidism in pregnancy.

UpToDate Topic Review(s)
Hypothyroidism during pregnancy: Clinical manifestations, diagnosis, and treatment

Reference(s)

Korevaar TIM, Medici M, Visser TJ, Peeters RP. Thyroid disease in pregnancy: new insights in diagnosis and clinical management. *Nat Rev Endocrinol*. 2017;13 (10):610-622. PMID: 28776582

Alexander EK, Pearce EN, Brent GA, et al. 2017 Guidelines of the American Thyroid Association for the Diagnosis and Management of Thyroid Disease During Pregnancy and the Postpartum. *Thyroid*. 2017;27(3):315-389. PMID: 28056690

Lazarus JH, Bestwick JP, Channon S, et al. Antenatal thyroid screening and childhood cognitive function [published correction appears in *N Engl J Med*. 2012; 366(17):1650]. *N Engl J Med* 2012 366(6):493-501. PMID: 22316443

Casey BM, Thom EA, Peaceman AM, et al; Eunice Kennedy Shriver National Institute of Child Health and Human Development Maternal-Fetal Medicine Units Network. Treatment of subclinical hypothyroidism or hypothyroxinemia in pregnancy. *N Engl J Med*. 2017;376(9):815-825. PMID: 28249134

82   ANSWER: D) Change meal ratio for breakfast and lunch to 1 unit per 20 g carbohydrate

Control of blood glucose during exercise is often challenging in patients with type 1 diabetes mellitus. Type, duration, and intensity of exercise can all affect glycemic status. Exercise that involves continuous, repeated large muscle activity for more than 10 minutes is considered aerobic. This type of activity usually results in reduction of blood glucose. Anaerobic activity can be either muscle activity against resistance or bursts of high-intensity activity for short periods and can result in hyperglycemia. Longer duration and higher-intensity exercise can also cause hypoglycemia.

When blood glucose drops with exercise in persons without diabetes, the first response is a drop in insulin levels, followed by an increase in counterregulatory hormones that increase glycolysis from breakdown of glycogen. In patients with type 1 diabetes, regulation of insulin availability is difficult unless the patient preemptively adjusts the injected insulin dose. Counterregulatory mechanisms can also be blunted in some patients. Those with a history of hypoglycemia may be particularly prone to recurrent hypoglycemia. In addition to changes in insulin and carbohydrate needs during activity, insulin sensitivity is often increased for hours after exercise.

Blood glucose must be measured before exercise. If the blood glucose is low (<90 mg/dL [<5.0 mmol/L]), consumption of carbohydrate is recommended. If the blood glucose is moderately elevated (150-250 mg/dL [8.3-13.9 mmol/L]), it could be managed with exercise alone. In this situation, the patient would not need to eat or adjust insulin. If the blood glucose is between 250 and 350 mg/dL (13.9-19.4 mmol/L), insulin can be given (lower than the usual dose, possibly 50%) and the patient should wait until blood glucose normalizes before starting exercise. If the blood glucose is greater than 350 mg/dL (>19.4 mmol/L), ketones should be checked and, if present, hyperglycemia should be treated and exercise should be avoided. If exercise is to last more than 60 minutes, the patient should be counseled to lower short-acting insulin before the exercise session and to eat a carbohydrate snack at the start and possibly during exercise.

Review of this patient's exercise pattern and blood glucose reveals that he is involved in high-intensity, prolonged exercise most days of the week. He exercises after breakfast and is fairly consistent with this timing. His blood glucose values are low after breakfast, before lunch, and after lunch, especially on the days that he exercises. Although a continuous glucose monitor (Answer A) and insulin pump (Answer E) may help titrate insulin more readily, these strategies should not be the first steps in management. This patient needs immediate adjustment of insulin and counseling on nutrition intake. Starting a conversation about insulin pump therapy and a continuous glucose monitor is important. In the long-term, use of these devices would likely be the safest and most effective way of controlling blood glucose in this physically active patient.

Insulin glargine is a long-acting insulin that is not particularly amenable to daily alterations in dosage. In this patient, morning blood glucose values are high, and the bedtime snack size should be reviewed. On the basis of this patient's history, consideration may need to be given to either bedtime bolus or a slight increase in the basal dose once the daytime hypoglycemia is addressed. Thus, lowering the insulin glargine dose to 6 units on the days that he plans to exercise (Answer C) is incorrect. Because the bedtime blood glucose values are well controlled, his dinner bolus ratio does not need adjustment (Answer B).

This patient's breakfast and lunch-time meal ratios should be adjusted (Answer D) to avoid mid-morning and early afternoon low blood glucose values. He should also be counseled on exercise and risk of hypoglycemia, the complications of which can include seizures and death. The prolonged effect of exercise on blood glucose should also be reviewed. The detailed strategy described above should be reviewed with the patient. Availability of glucagon and use of an alert bracelet/necklace should be encouraged.

Education Objective
Adjust insulin therapy to accommodate exercise in patients with type 1 diabetes mellitus.

UpToDate Topic Review(s)
Cases illustrating the effects of exercise in intensive insulin therapy for diabetes mellitus

Reference(s)
Riddell MC, Gallen IW, Smart CE, et al. Exercise management in type 1 diabetes: a consensus statement. *Lancet Diabetes Endocrinol.* 2017;5(5):377-390. PMID: 28126459

Mallad A, Hinshaw L, Schiavon M, et al. Exercise effects on postprandial glucose metabolism in type 1 diabetes: a triple-tracer approach. *Am J Physiol Endocrinol Metab.* 2015;308(12):E1106-E1115. PMID: 25898950

83 ANSWER: B) Fibrous dysplasia
This patient presents with a painful left humeral lesion of uncertain etiology. The markedly elevated alkaline phosphatase in the presence of otherwise normal liver function studies is consistent with a bone-specific source. While an increase in bone alkaline phosphatase is observed in a number of diseases that affect the skeleton,

specific clinical factors in this patient confirm a diagnosis of fibrous dysplasia/McCune-Albright syndrome (Answer B). This condition is due to mosaic, somatic activating pathogenic variants in the *GNAS* gene that encodes the cAMP pathway-associated G-protein, $G_s\alpha$. Affected patients present with skeletal lesions (monostotic or polyostotic), pigmented skin macules, and endocrinopathies. The displayed humeral shaft lesion has a "ground-glass" appearance that is characteristic of fibrous dysplasia/McCune-Albright syndrome. The presence of headaches suggests that he may well have

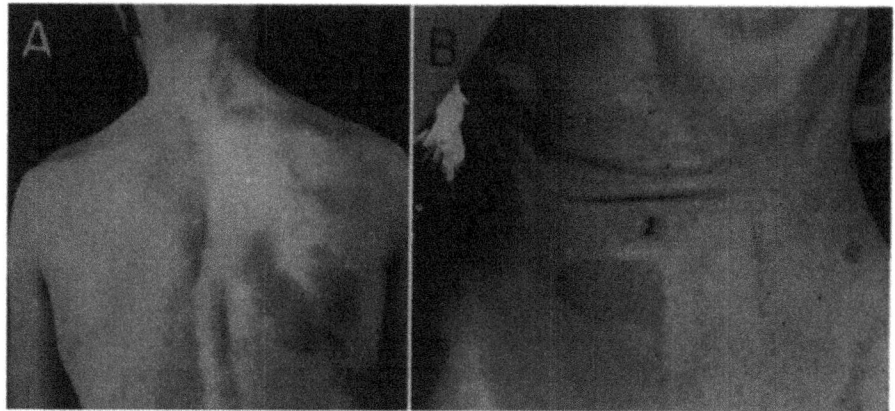

Pigmentation in neurofibromatosis compared to that in Syndrome X. Note "coast-of-Maine" contour of areas of pigmentation in A as opposed to "coast-of-California" contours in B. Incidentally, note subcutaneous nodules in B and their absence in A. (A.—A.K. with Syndrome X; B.—E.G. with neurofibromatosis.)

Reprinted from Albright F. Polyostotic fibrous dysplasia; a defense of the entity. *J Clin Endocrinol Metab.* 1947;7 (5):307-324. PMID: 20251641.

skull involvement, which is common in this syndrome. Additionally, his unilateral skin finding is consistent with a café-au-lait lesion that is pathognomonic for the disease. The irregular border of the lesion is commonly referred to as mimicking the coast of Maine, as opposed to smooth-bordered café-au-lait lesions (coast of California) that are seen in neurofibromatosis type 1.

Finally, the patient's weight loss, thyromegaly, and thyroid biochemical findings are consistent with fibrous dysplasia/McCune-Albright syndrome, in which hyperthyroidism is present in approximately one-third of patients. Other common endocrinopathies include precocious puberty in females and macro-orchidism in males, although less common endocrine disorders also occur (eg, hypercortisolism and GH excess). While there is no specific therapy for this syndrome, parenteral bisphosphonates may decrease bone pain at sites of skeletal involvement. Additionally, regular surveillance for skeletal and endocrine manifestations and targeted management of such disorders is recommended.

While Paget disease of bone (Answer D) is a diagnostic consideration for this patient, the specific radiographic appearance of the lesion, young age of onset, and absence of associated endocrinopathies in patients with Paget disease make this very unlikely.

Tumor-induced osteomalacia (Answer E), which is most commonly due to benign mesenchymal tumors that overproduce the phosphaturic factor fibroblast growth factor 23, can also present with bone pain and an elevated alkaline phosphatase level. However, this patient's normal serum phosphate level essentially rules out this disorder.

Graves disease (Answer C) can sometimes be associated with an elevated alkaline phosphatase level due to an increase in bone remodeling that is induced by elevated levels of thyroid hormone. However, autoimmune thyroid disease is not associated with localized skeletal lesions.

Finally, although celiac disease (Answer A) can present with signs and symptoms of osteomalacia that may mimic those seen in this patient (bone pain and high alkaline phosphatase), it does not cause focal lesions.

Educational Objective
Diagnose McCune-Albright syndrome and fibrous dysplasia.

UpToDate Topic Review(s)
Congenital and inherited hyperpigmentation disorders

Reference(s)
Wong SC, Zacharin M. Long-term health outcomes of adults with McCune-Albright syndrome. *Clin Endocrinol (Oxf).* 2017;87(5):627-634. PMID: 28699175

Robinson C, Collins MT, Boyce AM. Fibrous dysplasia/McCune-Albright syndrome: clinical and translational perspectives. *Curr Osteoporos Rep.* 2016;14(5): 178-186. PMID: 27492469

Albright F. Polyostotic fibrous dysplasia; a defense of the entity. *J Clin Endocrinol Metab.* 1947;7(5):307-324. PMID: 20251641

84 ANSWER: E) Defer treatment until after the baby is delivered

On the basis of this patient's clinical features, family history, and laboratory values, she has familial hypercholesterolemia (FH), a genetic disorder characterized by very high blood LDL-cholesterol levels. FH is an autosomal dominant disorder caused by pathogenic variants in the genes involved in LDL-receptor–mediated cholesterol uptake pathways. The severity of the phenotype depends on residual LDL-receptor activity. FH is diagnosed on the basis of clinical findings (if present), family history, and lipid levels. A pathognomonic clinical finding in FH, as observed in this patient, is the presence of tendon xanthomas on the extensor tendons of the hands or in the Achilles tendons; such xanthomas can also occur in the triceps and patellar tendons. Genetic testing is not widely used for diagnosis in the United States, in part because of lack of insurance coverage.

Cholesterol levels rise by up to 50% during pregnancy in women, regardless of whether they have FH. Although the relative increase in cholesterol levels is comparable in those with FH and unaffected individuals, the absolute plasma concentrations are usually much greater in those with FH. The rise in cholesterol levels in pregnancy can be attributed to several factors—an estrogen-dependent increase in liver cholesterol synthesis and the need to maintain adequate nutrition for the mother and fetus. It has been hypothesized that maternal hyperlipidemia may induce acute atherosclerosis in the uteroplacental spiral arteries that could result in local thrombosis and placental infarctions, leading to placental insufficiency and fetal compromise. However, no differences in pregnancy outcomes have been reported in women with FH. Measurement of cholesterol levels is not routinely recommended in pregnancy.

Treatment of FH typically involves starting lipid-lowering therapy as early as possible given the increased lifetime risk of premature cardiovascular disease. Statins are the most effective therapy and they increase the functional activity of residual LDL receptors. Treatment of FH in women of childbearing age presents a challenge, as use of statins is contraindicated during pregnancy and lactation (category X). Some animal studies have demonstrated evidence of the teratogenicity of statins during pregnancy. Structural birth defects have been reported following maternal use of statins, while some observational studies do not show an increase in congenital anomalies. Thus, starting a statin (Answer A) is incorrect.

Ezetimibe (Answer B), an intestinal cholesterol absorption inhibitor, has modest LDL-cholesterol–lowering effects as a single agent. It has been associated with teratogenic effects in animals. Adverse events have been observed in some animal reproduction studies; therefore, ezetimibe should not be recommended in pregnancy (pregnancy category C).

Nicotinic acid or niacin (Answer C) is water-soluble vitamin B_3 that lowers LDL cholesterol and raises HDL cholesterol. Addition of niacin can decrease LDL cholesterol up to 25%. However, in this patient, niacin would not provide sufficient LDL-cholesterol lowering. In general, current use of niacin for lipid-lowering is limited to specific situations. Fetal effects of niacin at dosages used for lipid-lowering are unknown (pregnancy category C). Hence, use of niacin should be avoided.

Lipoprotein apheresis (Answer D) is an extracorporeal method of removing apolipoprotein B–containing lipoproteins from the circulation. Criteria for lipoprotein apheresis in patients receiving maximally tolerated lipid-lowering therapy include an LDL-cholesterol level greater than 500 mg/dL (>12.95 mmol/L) in patients with homozygous FH; an LDL-cholesterol level greater than 300 mg/dL (>7.77 mmol/L) in patients with heterozygous FH; and an LDL-cholesterol level greater than 200 mg/dL (>5.18 mmol/L) in patients with heterozygous FH and atherosclerotic cardiovascular disease. Treatments are given every 1 to 2 weeks and each session takes 3 to 4 hours. This patient does not meet the criteria for LDL apheresis, as she has no history of atherosclerotic cardiovascular disease.

At this time, the best option is to defer treatment until pregnancy and lactation are complete (Answer E). There is a hypothetical risk of possible progression of atherosclerosis due to no treatment, but this is unclear.

Educational Objective
Describe the effects of pregnancy on lipid levels in a woman with genetic hypercholesterolemia.

UpToDate Topic Review(s)
Familial hypercholesterolemia in adults: Treatment

Reference(s)

Amundsen AL, Khoury J, Iversen PO, et al. Marked changes in plasma lipids and lipoproteins during pregnancy in women with familial hypercholesterolemia. *Atherosclerosis*. 2006;189(2):451-457. PMID: 16466729

Kusters DM, Homsma SJ, Hutten BA, et al. Dilemmas in treatment of women with familial hypercholesterolaemia during pregnancy. *Neth J Med*. 2010;68(1): 299-303. PMID: 20739726

85 ANSWER: E) Monitoring the patient's TSH without further therapy now

The patient described here presented with subclinical hyperthyroidism. Given the homogenous uptake throughout his thyroid gland, radioactive iodine therapy could have been administered, were it not for the presence of the nonfunctioning nodule, which appropriately was targeted for FNA biopsy. Given both the hyperthyroidism and the indeterminate cytology, a total thyroidectomy would have been a reasonable treatment approach for the patient's hyperthyroidism and establishing the histopathology of the left-sided nodule. Because the patient underwent a left lobectomy, the issues to consider are whether he has had sufficient treatment for his papillary microcarcinoma and whether he will now be euthyroid or continue to have subclinical hyperthyroidism.

With respect to his diagnosis of papillary microcarcinoma, the patient needs no further treatment. In fact, it is highly likely that the removal of his microscopic thyroid cancer has not altered his life expectancy. Neither completion thyroidectomy (Answer A) nor radioactive iodine therapy following completion thyroidectomy will improve his prognosis. Similarly, TSH suppression (Answer B) is not indicated for a papillary microcarcinoma.

With his hyperfunctioning right thyroid lobe remaining in place, it is not clear what the patient's thyroid status will be. He could now be (1) euthyroid, (2) hyperthyroid, or (3) currently euthyroid, but trend back into hyperthyroidism over time. Starting methimazole (Answer D) is not needed now, as it is not yet known what the patient's thyroid status will be following his lobectomy. It is possible his subclinical hyperthyroidism will be either permanently or transiently resolved. Radioactive iodine therapy (Answer C) could be used to treat hyperthyroidism in this patient. However, it has not yet been established that he is hyperthyroid after his lobectomy. Given this uncertainty, monitoring his serum TSH (Answer E) is the best approach. Although no trials of treatment of subclinical hyperthyroidism directly address this, it would be anticipated that treatment to resolve his hyperthyroidism, if he continues to exhibit subclinical hyperthyroidism, would be more likely to decrease adverse outcomes than treatment of his papillary microcarcinoma.

Educational Objective

Determine the appropriate management of microscopic papillary thyroid cancers.

UpToDate Topic Review(s)
Papillary thyroid cancer

Reference(s)

Carle A, Andersen SL, Boelaert K, Laurberg P. Management of endocrine disease: subclinical thyrotoxicosis: prevalence, causes and choice of therapy. *Eur J Endocrinol*. 2017;176(6):R325-R337. PMID: 28274949

Cecoli F, Ceresola EM, Altrinetti V, et al. Therapeutic strategies and clinical outcome in papillary thyroid microcarcinoma: a multicenter observational study. *Eur Thyroid J*. 2016;5(3):180-186. PMID: 27843808

Haugen BR, Alexander EK, Bible KC, et al. 2015 American Thyroid Association Management Guidelines for Adult Patients with Thyroid Nodules and Differentiated Thyroid Cancer: The American Thyroid Association Guidelines Task Force on Thyroid Nodules and Differentiated Thyroid Cancer. *Thyroid*. 2016;26(1):1-133. PMID: 26462967

Ross DS, Burch HB, Cooper DS, et al. 2016 American Thyroid Association Guidelines for Diagnosis and Management of Hyperthyroidism and Other Causes of Thyrotoxicosis. *Thyroid*. 2016;26(10):1343-1421. PMID: 27521067

86 ANSWER: A) Cancel surgery, no further routine imaging required

Adrenal imaging abnormalities are common; most adrenal masses identified incidentally are benign and nonsecretory. Overall, approximately 3% to 4% of adults have an incidentally discovered adrenal nodule on imaging and the incidence increases with age. Radiologic factors associated with benign adrenal masses include small size

(<4 cm), homogeneous appearance with a smooth contour, low unenhanced CT attenuation values (<−10 Hounsfield units), and rapid washout of contrast medium (usually >50% 10 minutes after contrast administration).

Although the adrenal mass in this case is larger than the 4-cm threshold, it has an extremely low attenuation value (−44 Hounsfield units). This means that the lesion is composed of mostly fat and this is diagnostic of an adrenal myelolipoma. These lesions are easy to identify by low Hounsfield units (usually much less than −10, as is seen here). Adrenal myelolipomas are benign neoplasms composed of both mature adipose and hematopoietic tissue. Although these lesions may grow over time, this is unusual. Therefore, this patient who has an asymptomatic myelolipoma can be reassured that surgery is not indicated and further imaging would only be required if she developed abdominal or loin pain (thus, Answer A is correct and Answer B is incorrect). However, when a myelolipoma is larger than 6 cm in diameter or when it causes local mass-effect symptoms, surgical removal can be considered.

Given that this lesion is clearly a myelolipoma, the history of lung cancer is not relevant in this case and adrenal biopsy (Answer C) is unnecessary. Almost any solid organ tumor can metastasize to the adrenal but, in practice, this is most commonly seen in primary tumors of lung, breast, and kidney. Adrenal biopsy can be helpful in cases of a known extra-adrenal malignancy where there is an adrenal lesion with indeterminate or overtly malignant imaging characteristics to distinguish between a primary adrenocortical carcinoma and metastatic disease. Before adrenal biopsy is performed, however, catecholamine excess must first be excluded.

PET scanning with fluorodeoxyglucose (FDG) (Answer D) is not routinely required in the evaluation of adrenal masses. However, it may be helpful in identifying potentially malignant lesions if the adrenal mass looks suspicious on cross-sectional imaging, particularly if there is already a known malignancy. It is not required in this case of definite myelolipoma.

This patient failed to fully suppress plasma cortisol after an overnight dexamethasone suppression test. Up to 5% of adrenal incidentalomas overproduce cortisol and this can be an indication for adrenalectomy. Under these circumstances, the function of the contralateral adrenal gland is suppressed. Therefore, such patients routinely require perioperative steroid coverage that can be tapered and withdrawn once adrenal function has recovered. At least 75% of circulating cortisol is bound to cortisol-binding globulin and only free cortisol is biologically active. Cortisol-binding globulin production by the liver is often increased by oral estrogen, which leads to an increase in total plasma cortisol and is likely to be the case in this patient with no clinical features of cortisol excess and normal 24-hour urinary cortisol excretion. Therefore, the elevated plasma cortisol in this case is not of any clinical significance and perioperative steroids (Answer E) would not be necessary if this patient were to undergo adrenalectomy. To provide definitive evidence, either free plasma cortisol could be measured or the overnight dexamethasone suppression test could be repeated after the patient has discontinued estrogen. However, neither of these options is offered and measurement of free plasma cortisol is not routinely available in most centers.

Educational Objective
Identify the characteristic imaging features of adrenal myelolipoma, recommend appropriate management, and describe the effect of oral hormone therapy on plasma cortisol levels.

UpToDate Topic Review(s)
The adrenal incidentaloma

Reference(s)
Nieman LK. Approach to the patient with an incidental adrenal adenoma. *J Clin Endocrinol Metab*. 2010;95(9):4106-4113. PMID: 20823463

Fassnacht M, Arlt W, Bancos I, et al. Management of adrenal incidentalomas: European Society of Endocrinology Clinical Practice Guideline in collaboration with the European Network for the Study of Adrenal Tumors. *Eur J Endocrinol*. 2016;175(2):G1-G34. PMID: 27390021

87 **ANSWER: C) Perform electrocardiography**
The recognition of atypical chest pain or subtle new symptoms without chest pain in a high-risk patient with type 1 diabetes can be lifesaving. This patient is middle-aged and has type 1 diabetes. Although the vignette does not specify the duration of diabetes, the lack of this information should not deter the clinician from ordering the correct test. Nesto et al reported the high prevalence of silent ischemia in patients with diabetes vs patients without diabetes. The authors studied 50 consecutive patients with diabetes and 50 consecutive patients without diabetes, all with cardiac ischemia, using exercise thallium scintigraphy. The authors found only 7 of 50 patients with diabetes had angina during

ischemia compared with 17 of 50 patients without diabetes. The authors concluded that angina is an unreliable index for myocardial ischemia in diabetic patients with coronary artery disease. The reason for lack of chest pain in patients with diabetes and coronary artery disease is unclear. Marchant et al found that patients with diabetes and silent exertional ischemia have evidence of autonomic impairment. The autonomic impairment was not observed in patients without diabetes, suggesting that subclinical neuropathy may be the cause of the silent ischemia in those with diabetes.

This vignette describes a patient with sudden fatigue that does not resolve with rest. The patient typically has no problems with exercise. The absence of chest pain should not deter the clinician from having a high index of suspicion for cardiac ischemia as the cause of the patient's symptoms. The best test to perform now is a 12-lead electrocardiogram (Answer C). Even if findings on electrocardiography are normal, the patient should be referred to a hospital and have serial troponin measurements done, as well as echocardiography.

While this patient with type 1 diabetes is at increased risk for development of other autoimmune diseases compared with general population risk, he does not have symptoms suggestive of hyperthyroidism, hypothyroidism, or adrenal insufficiency. Thus, measuring TSH and free T_4 (Answer B) or performing an ACTH-stimulation test (Answer E) is not presently indicated. Similarly, he has no nausea, vomiting, or abdominal pain to suggest ketoacidosis, so checking urine for ketones (Answer D) is not the best next step. Checking core body temperature (Answer A) is useful, but a simple oral temperature can screen for hyperthermia and it does not directly address the most important objective of ruling out cardiac ischemia.

Educational Objective
Evaluate for cardiac ischemia in a patient with diabetes mellitus, even in the absence of chest pain.

UpToDate Topic Review(s)
Prevalence of and risk factors for coronary heart disease in diabetes mellitus

Reference(s)

Nesto RW, Phillips RT, Kett KG, et al. Angina and exertional myocardial ischemia in diabetic and nondiabetic patients: assessment by exercise thallium scintigraphy [published correction appears in *Ann Intern Med*. 1988;108(4):646]. *Ann Intern Med*. 1998;108(2):170-175. PMID: 3341650

Marchant B, Umachandran V, Stevenson R, Kopelman PG, Timmis AD. Silent myocardial ischemia: role of subclinical neuropathy in patients with and without diabetes. *J Am Coll Cardiol*. 1993;22(5):1433-1437. PMID: 8227802

88 ANSWER: D) Pituitary TSH-producing adenoma

This patient presents with clinical symptoms and signs of thyrotoxicosis. The biochemical findings, however, are unusual with significantly elevated concentrations of circulating thyroid hormones and a normal serum TSH level. When discordant biochemical findings are present, potential confounding factors should first be considered, including alterations in normal physiology (eg, pregnancy), intercurrent illness (nonthyroidal), and medication usage (eg, levothyroxine, amiodarone, heparin). Once these have been excluded, laboratory artifacts in commonly used TSH or thyroid hormone immunoassays, as well as the presence of heterophilic antibodies and familial dysalbuminemic hyperthyroxinemia, should be screened for, thus avoiding unnecessary further investigation and/or treatment in cases where there is assay interference. Following exclusion of these diagnoses, the main challenge is to distinguish between a TSH-secreting pituitary adenoma and resistance to thyroid hormone, most commonly caused by a pathogenic variant in the *THRB* gene.

Thyrotropinomas account for 0.5% to 3% of all pituitary tumors, and their prevalence is approximately 1 case per million per year. These adenomas are seen in all age groups, but they occur most often during the fifth and sixth decades of life. Tumor prevalence is similar in males and females. Thyrotroph cells represent less than 5% of all pituitary cells and are widely distributed in the pituitary, but they are most concentrated in the anteromedian area. This might explain why most invasive macroadenomas are medially located. Thyrotropinomas share many characteristics with other pituitary hormone-secreting adenomas. They usually appear chromophobic and polymorphous under light microscopy and are characterized by large nuclei and prominent nucleoli. Malignant transformation is rare. Most benign tumors secrete TSH alone. However, cosecretion of GH or prolactin exists in 16% and 10% of cases, respectively.

Older series report a higher prevalence of macroadenomas among thyrotropinomas, whereas more recent series indicate a significant number of microadenomas. Most thyrotroph adenomas are large and invasive at diagnosis, and they present with signs and symptoms of an expanding mass, including temporal visual field defects. The severity of hyperthyroidism is often milder than expected on the basis of circulating thyroid hormone levels. The presence of a goiter is common, even in previously thyroidectomized patients, because residual thyroid tissue may grow due to TSH hyperstimulation.

Disproportionate hypersecretion of free α-glycoprotein and an elevated α-glycoprotein-to-TSH molar ratio is usually present. In postmenopausal women, an elevated α-glycoprotein-to-FSH molar ratio may be of diagnostic value. Increased bone and liver markers as a consequence of increased thyroid hormone action are often found, including SHBG and carboxy-terminal cross-linked telopeptide of type 1 collagen. These are usually elevated in patients with thyrotropinoma, but not in those with resistance to thyroid hormone. The biochemical findings of an inappropriately normal serum TSH level with high circulating thyroid hormones, elevated α-glycoprotein, and elevated SHBG concentration make a pituitary TSH-producing adenoma (Answer D) the most likely diagnosis. Resistance to thyroid hormone (Answer B) is less likely.

Interference in the laboratory TSH assay (Answer E) is possible, but this would not explain the other biochemical findings. In patients with Graves disease (Answer A), the serum TSH concentration would be undetectable, and in Hashimoto thyroiditis (Answer C) the serum free T_3 and free T_4 concentrations are likely to be low and the TSH elevated.

Dynamic tests such as a thyrotropin-releasing hormone stimulation test may be useful. The results of this test, during which 200 mcg of thyrotropin-releasing hormone was administered intravenously to this patient at 0 minutes, are displayed (*see table*). A blunted TSH response to thyrotropin-releasing hormone is seen in most persons with thyrotropinoma, including this patient. Patients with resistance to thyroid hormone generally show a slow rise in TSH levels after thyrotropin-releasing hormone administration.

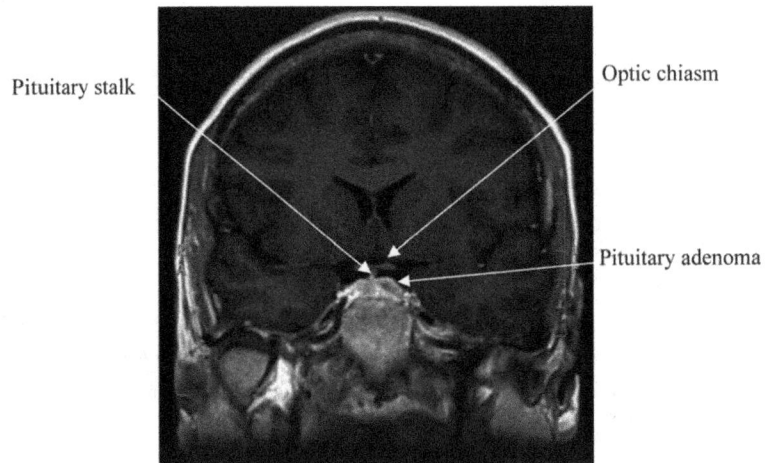

Pituitary stalk

Optic chiasm

Pituitary adenoma

Time Point	TSH	Free T_4	Free T_3
0 minutes	1.87 mIU/L	5.8 ng/dL (SI: 74.7 pmol/L)	12.9 pg/mL (SI: 19.8 pmol/L)
20 minutes	2.29 mIU/L	5.7 ng/dL (SI: 73.4 pmol/L)	13.1 pg/mL (SI: 20.1 pmol/L)
60 minutes	1.88 mIU/L	6.2 ng/dL (SI: 79.8 pmol/L)	13.1 pg/mL (SI: 20.1 pmol/L)

Pituitary MRI identified a left-sided pituitary adenoma causing deviation of the stalk to the right (*see image*).

Transsphenoidal resection of thyrotropinoma remains the treatment modality of choice for most patients. Other treatment options include somatostatin analogues, since many tumors express somatostatin receptors (mainly SSTR2 and SSTR5). Dopamine receptors can also be present, and dopamine agonists have been used with various success rates. Radiation therapy, including fractioned conventional radiotherapy or radiosurgery, has been used when surgery is inadvisable or not chosen. More often it is used as postoperative therapy in patients with residual or recurrent thyrotropinomas. The patient in this vignette underwent transsphenoidal surgery, which normalized her thyroid function tests, resolved her symptoms, and resulted in the disappearance of the adenoma on pituitary MRI (*see image*).

Educational Objective
Diagnose a pituitary TSH-producing adenoma.

UpToDate Topic Review(s)
TSH-secreting pituitary adenomas

Reference(s)

Amlashi FG, Tritos NA. Thyrotropin-secreting pituitary adenomas: epidemiology, diagnosis, and management. *Endocrine*. 2016;52(3):427-440. PMID: 26792794

Koulouri O, Moran C, Halsall D, Chatterjee K, Gurnell M. Pitfalls in the measurement and interpretation of thyroid function tests. *Best Pract Res Clin Endocrinol Metab*. 2013;27(6):745-762. PMID: 24275187

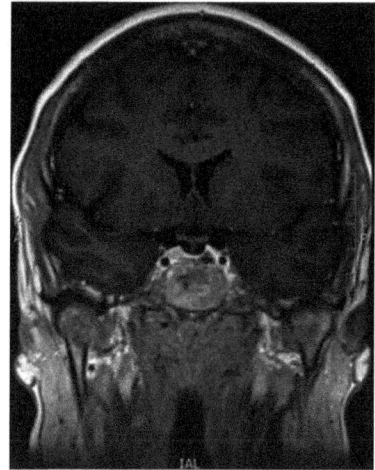

89 ANSWER: A) At an andrology laboratory 2 to 3 days after abstinence with or without an isotonic lubricant

Semen analysis is an important part of an evaluation of male infertility and certain cases of hypogonadism. Semen contains spermatozoa, which are stored in the epididymides, as well as fluid secretions from the prostate and seminal vesicles. During ejaculation, the first portion contains more sperm-rich prostatic fluid than the later portions, which contain more seminal vesicular fluid. The 3 common parameters measured in semen analysis are concentration, motility, and morphology.

It is important that patients are counseled and given information on how to provide a semen sample, so that the collected specimen is suitable for analysis. Men may use approved isotonic lubricants that do not affect motility, viability, membrane integrity, or percentage of DNA damage. Patients should be aware that many common lubricants, although often labeled "nonspermicidal," adversely affect motility and viability. According to the World Health Organization laboratory manual, men should be advised to collect the sample after 2 to 6 days of sexual abstinence. The sample should be collected in a private room near the andrology laboratory to limit exposure of the sample to fluctuations in ambient temperature and to ensure that the analysis is performed within the appropriate window (thus, Answer A is correct). In rare circumstances, a sample may be collected at home with or without a special nontoxic condom. Such samples should be delivered to the andrology lab for analysis within an hour of collection (thus, Answer E is incorrect). Collecting the sample 7 to 8 days after sexual abstinence and/or at home is not recommended (thus, Answers B, C, and D are incorrect).

Educational Objective
Counsel a man regarding the appropriate timing and conditions to obtain an optimal sample for semen analysis.

UpToDate Topic Review(s)
Approach to the male with infertility

Reference(s)

Agarwal A, Malvezzi H, Sharma R. Effect of an isotonic lubricant on sperm collection and sperm quality. *Fertil Steril*. 2013;99(6):1581-1586. PMID: 23490168

World Health Organization, Department of Reproductive Health and Research. *WHO laboratory manual for the examination and processing of human semen*. 5th ed. Geneva, Switzerland: World Health Organization; 2010.

90 ANSWER: D) Start hydrochlorothiazide

This patient has osteoporosis with worsening bone mineral density despite taking appropriate bisphosphonate therapy. In such a scenario, potential factors contributing to low bone mineral density should be considered. Secondary contributors to low bone mineral density are common and must be identified and corrected to treat osteoporosis effectively. Many conditions and medications can contribute to bone loss and increased fracture risk; some examples are provided in the table. While Z-scores that are –2.0 or lower (ie, below expected range for age) may indicate an underlying cause of secondary osteoporosis, studies show that Z-score diagnostic thresholds have only limited value in discriminating between primary and secondary osteoporosis.

Examples of Conditions Associated With Secondary Osteoporosis	Examples of Drugs Associated With Secondary Osteoporosis
Hyperthyroidism, hyperparathyroidism, hypercortisolism, hypogonadism, diabetes mellitus, vitamin D deficiency, malnutrition/malabsorption, idiopathic hypercalciuria, rheumatoid arthritis, multiple myeloma, chronic obstructive pulmonary disease, osteogenesis imperfecta	Glucocorticoids, depot medroxyprogesterone acetate, androgen deprivation therapy, aromatase inhibitors, excess thyroid hormone, anticonvulsant drugs, proton-pump inhibitors, selective serotonin reuptake inhibitors, thiazolidinediones, heparin

Assessment of urinary calcium is helpful to identify idiopathic hypercalciuria as a cause of secondary osteoporosis, especially in this woman with a history of kidney stones. Idiopathic hypercalciuria, defined as a 24-hour urinary calcium excretion greater than 300 mg or more than 4 mg/kg, is associated with an increased risk of nephrolithiasis, as well as decreased bone mineral density likely related to a negative calcium balance. In this case, treatment with a thiazide diuretic (Answer D) should be considered because this appears to be associated with improved bone mineral density and decreased fracture risk.

Switching from alendronate to a more potent osteoporosis medication (Answers A, B, and C) may be considered when the decrease in bone mineral density truly reflects a treatment failure in the absence of discernible contributing factors, which is not the case here. Furthermore, anabolic agents such as PTH/PTHrP analogues (Answer C) should probably be avoided in individuals with a history of kidney stones or persistent hypercalcuria because hypercalcemia and hypercalciuria are common adverse effects of such treatment.

Finally, it would not be appropriate to only monitor this patient (Answer E) when her workup revealed a condition most likely contributing to her bone loss. Treatment of this patient's hypercalciuria would be an important aspect in the management of her osteoporosis.

Educational Objective
Identify idiopathic hypercalciuria as a cause of bone loss and recommend appropriate treatment.

UpToDate Topic Review(s)
Clinical manifestations, diagnosis, and evaluation of osteoporosis in postmenopausal women

Reference(s)

Hudec SM, Camacho PM. Secondary causes of osteoporosis. *Endocr Pract*. 2013;19(1):120-128. PMID: 23186949

McKiernan FE, Berg RL, Linneman JG. The utility of BMD Z-score diagnostic thresholds for secondary causes of osteoporosis. *Osteoporos Int*. 2011;22(4): 1069-1077. PMID: 20533026

Bolland MJ, Ames RW, Horne AM, Orr-Walker BJ, Gamble GD, Reid IR. The effect of treatment with a thiazide diuretic for 4 years on bone density in normal postmenopausal women. *Osteoporos Int*. 2007;18(4):479-486. PMID: 17120180

Rejnmark L, Vestergaard P, Mosekilde L. Reduced fracture risk in users of thiazide diuretics. *Calcif Tissue Int*. 2005;76(3):167-175. PMID: 15719207

Aung K, Htay T. Thiazide diuretics and the risk of hip fracture. *Cochrane Database Syst Rev*. 2011;10:CD005185. PMID: 21975748

91 **ANSWER: D) Switch insulin regimen to U500 insulin only, 160 units twice daily**
Requirement for 200 to 300 units or more of insulin per day is considered severe insulin resistance. Although this dosage is somewhat arbitrary, it is known that the insulin dose response is reduced as the dosage requirement increases. While use of higher dosages of U100 insulins have additional benefit, the volume of insulin required to reach a therapeutic target becomes very challenging. Higher-volume injections are associated with leakage of insulin from the site and poor adherence. For example, in a patient using 300 units per day, the volume of injection would be 3 mL over the course of the day. In contrast, U500 regular insulin, which is 5 times concentrated, could be used to administer the same dose of insulin with only 0.6 mL.

For these reasons, neither use of a continuous subcutaneous insulin infusion pump (Answer A) nor increasing the dosage of U100 glargine (Answer B) is an appropriate choice. While U200 degludec (Answer E) offers advantages over U100 glargine in terms of a flatter, more consistent insulin action profile and longer duration of action, it does not address the issue of postprandial hyperglycemia that most likely exists for this patient.

Studies of U500 insulin are small and retrospective, but most show a reduction in hemoglobin A_{1c} (decrease by 1.7% to 3.5%), variable weight gain, an increase in total insulin dosage, and possibly increased number of hypoglycemic events (although study results on this are mixed). At least one study suggests that the improvements in hemoglobin A_{1c} are sustainable over 3 years. Thus, it is reasonable to conclude that U500 insulin would allow the increase in dosage needed to achieve glycemic targets.

U500 regular insulin is 5 times as concentrated as U100 regular insulin. Studies suggest that the pharmacokinetic profile of U500 regular insulin resembles that of NPH insulin. A study in obese patients suggests that the time to onset is 45 minutes, time to peak is 7 to 8.5 hours, and duration of action is approximately 11.5 hours. Compared with U100 regular insulin, the time to peak appears to be delayed, and the peak insulin concentration is blunted with U500 regular insulin. Given these factors, U500 insulin can be used as both a basal and bolus insulin. Often, therefore, patients on multiple daily insulin doses can be transitioned to a U500-only–based regimen.

Finally, this patient is already receiving 320 units of insulin and her hemoglobin A_{1c} is still elevated. Most studies show that substantial increases in insulin dosage after transitioning to U500 insulin are associated with reduced hemoglobin A_{1c} levels, which is the goal for this patient. Therefore, reduction in the total daily insulin dose is likely not required (Answer C). If the patient's hemoglobin A_{1c} level were close to or at target, reducing the insulin dosage might be reasonable, but not in this case. The best management option for this patient is to start U500 insulin, 160 units twice daily (Answer D).

Educational Objective
Explain the limitations of U100-based insulin regimens in the setting of severe insulin resistance and describe how to transition to a U500 regular insulin regimen.

UpToDate Topic Review(s)
General principles of insulin therapy in diabetes mellitus

Reference(s)
Dailey AM, Gibert JA, Tannock LR. Durability of glycemic control using U-500 insulin. *Diabetes Res Clin Pract*. 2012;95(3):340-344. PMID: 22088791

Cochran E, Musso C, Gorden P. The use of U-500 in patients with extreme insulin resistance. *Diabetes Care*. 2005;28(5):1240-1244. PMID: 15855601

Reutrakul S, Wroblewski K, Brown RL. Clinical use of U-500 regular insulin: review and meta-analysis. *J Diabetes Sci Technol*. 2012;6(2):412-420. PMID: 22538155

92 ANSWER: B) Cushing syndrome with fluticasone-induced secondary adrenal insufficiency

This patient presents with the clinical features of Cushing syndrome; however, her biochemical evaluation reveals a low morning cortisol level with an inappropriately low ACTH, as well as a suboptimal cortisol response to cosyntropin (an ideal stimulated cortisol would be >18 µg/dL). Collectively, this patient has clinical Cushing syndrome combined with chronic secondary adrenal insufficiency (secondary adrenal insufficiency that has resulted in prolonged ACTH suppression, consequent atrophy of the zona fasciculata, and suboptimal cortisol stimulation to cosyntropin).

The main culprit is the combination of ritonavir and fluticasone. Ritonavir is a unique protease inhibitor because it is a potent inhibitor of P450 CYP3A4. CYP3A4 is responsible for the hepatic metabolism of many medications, including glucocorticoids; therefore, ritonavir inhibits the metabolism of glucocorticoids and results in a potentiation of exogenous glucocorticoids. In fact, ritonavir is most commonly used to "boost" the effect of other protease inhibitors in HIV therapy. Since some protease inhibitors cause gastrointestinal adverse effects that limit their tolerability, administering them in smaller and less toxic doses in combination with ritonavir permits tolerability while maintaining adequate blood levels due to CYP3A4 inhibition. However, an undesired consequence of ritonavir use is that exogenous glucocorticoids, including inhaled, topical, and intraarticular glucocorticoids that have small systemic absorption, are potentiated. This patient's combination of fluticasone (Answer B) and ritonavir most likely resulted in high levels of systemic fluticasone circulation, resultant Cushing syndrome, and hypothalamic-pituitary-adrenal axis suppression. Fluticasone is a synthetic glucocorticoid and is not measured by the cortisol assay.

This patient's management is complex. While the fluticasone is most likely being potentiated at supratherapeutic levels and inducing Cushing syndrome and adrenal insufficiency, it is also treating adrenal insufficiency. Cessation of the medication could result in an adrenal crisis. Replacing fluticasone with an oral glucocorticoid taper is also challenging because the concomitant use of ritonavir will decrease glucocorticoid metabolism and result in unpredictable pharmacokinetics. A multidisciplinary discussion is recommended for these challenging cases. This patient's antiretroviral regimen was changed to avoid the use of ritonavir, her fluticasone was stopped, and she was treated with a gradual low-dosage prednisone taper until her hypothalamic-pituitary-adrenal axis normalized.

There is no evidence of primary adrenal insufficiency (Answer A), which would be characterized by very high ACTH and renin activity levels. There is no evidence of ectopic ACTH syndrome (Answer D), an ACTH-secreting pituitary adenoma (Answer E), or hypercortisolism, all of which would be characterized by a high cortisol level combined with an inappropriately high ACTH level. Hyperglycemia (Answer C) would not cause this pattern of Cushing syndrome.

Educational Objective
Diagnose secondary adrenal insufficiency in a patient taking ritonavir (a protease inhibitor that inhibits CYP3A4 activity) and glucocorticoids.

UpToDate Topic Review(s)
Pituitary and adrenal gland dysfunction in HIV-infected patients

Reference(s)
Bornstein SR, Allolio B, Arlt W, et al. Diagnosis and treatment of primary adrenal insufficiency: an Endocrine Society clinical practice guideline. *J Clin Endocrinol Metab.* 2016;101(2):364-389. PMID: 26760044

93 ANSWER: C) Liraglutide

To choose the best medication for each patient, one must consider, among other factors, the patient's comorbidities and the adverse effects and interactions of the new medication. Lorcaserin (Answer A) is a selective serotonin receptor agonist that reduces appetite and should be used with caution in patients who are taking a selective serotonin reuptake inhibitor, a serotonin norepinephrine reuptake inhibitor, or a monoamine oxidase inhibitor, as it may increase the risk of developing serotonin syndrome. Also, it should be avoided in patients with severe liver or renal disease. This patient is taking sertraline for his depression; thus, lorcaserin is not the best choice.

Orlistat (Answer B) is a lipase inhibitor that reduces dietary fat absorption. It is contraindicated in patients with oxalate nephrolithiasis, cholestasis, and chronic malabsorption syndrome. Orlistat decreases the absorption of fat-soluble vitamins, so patients taking this medication should also take a multivitamin. Patients who decide to take orlistat must follow a low-fat diet (<30% of calories from fat), as this results in fewer gastrointestinal adverse effects (fecal urgency, oily stool, flatus with discharge, and fecal incontinence). This patient has no contraindications for this medication. However, orlistat is not an appetite suppressant, so other weight-loss medications should be considered first.

Phentermine (Answer E), a norepinephrine-releasing agent that suppresses appetite, is the most prescribed antiobesity medication in the United States. Phentermine is a controlled substance (schedule IV) that is contraindicated in patients with a history of cardiovascular disease, hyperthyroidism, glaucoma, or drug abuse, as well as during or within 14 days following monoamine oxidase inhibitor therapy. Phentermine can increase heart rate and blood pressure, so it should be avoided in patients with uncontrolled hypertension. This patient has uncontrolled hypertension, so phentermine is not the best choice.

The combination of naltrexone and bupropion (Answer D) activates pro-opiomelanocortin neurons in the arcuate nucleus, which promotes the release of α-melanocyte–stimulating hormone, an anorectic hormone. This combination pill is a good option for patients who are trying to stop smoking or those with a history of depression. Given that bupropion lowers the seizure threshold, this medication would be contraindicated in this patient with a seizure disorder.

Liraglutide (Answer C) is a GLP-1 receptor agonist that was initially approved for the treatment of type 2 diabetes. The recommended dose for long-term weight management is 3 mg daily. It is contraindicated for patients with a personal or family history of medullary thyroid cancer or for patients with multiple endocrine neoplasia syndrome type 2. It should be used with caution in patients with a history of pancreatitis. This patient would be an excellent candidate for this medication, as he has type 2 diabetes with suboptimal glycemic control and thus would likely benefit from both weight loss and improved diabetes control.

Educational Objective
Prescribe an appropriate weight-loss medication for a patient with type 2 diabetes mellitus, bearing in mind various contraindications.

UptoDate Topic Review(s)
Obesity in adults: Drug therapy

Reference(s)

Igel LI, Kumar RB, Saunders KH, Aronne LJ. Practical use of pharmacotherapy for obesity. *Gastroenterology*. 2017;152(7):1765-1779. PMID: 28192104

Lee PC, Dixon J. Pharmacotherapy for obesity. *Aust Fam Physician*. 2017;46(7):472-477. PMID: 28697290

Apovian CM, Aronne LJ, Bessesen DH, et al; Endocrine Society. Pharmacological management of obesity: an Endocrine Society clinical practice guideline. *J Clin Endocrinol Metab*. 2015;100(2):342-362. PMID: 25590212

94 ANSWER: E) Tumor-induced osteomalacia

This woman presents with convincing clinical evidence of hypophosphatemic osteomalacia (skeletal pain, hypophosphatemia, and elevated alkaline phosphatase in the presence of otherwise normal liver function tests), which can be due to a number of specific disorders. The fact that her signs and symptoms were acquired late in life strongly suggests that she has tumor-induced osteomalacia (Answer E), instead of inherited conditions such as X-linked hypophosphatemic rickets, autosomal dominant hypophosphatemic rickets, or autosomal recessive hypophosphatemic rickets. These conditions are due to dysregulation of FGF-23 metabolism, which is a skeletal-derived factor that actively promotes renal phosphate excretion and downregulation of 1,25-dihydroxyvitamin D production. As a result, the serum 1,25-dihydroxyvitamin D level is often low as it is in this patient.

Tumor-induced osteomalacia is generally due to benign mesenchymal tumors that overproduce FGF-23, leading to hypophosphatemia, muscle weakness, and clinical osteomalacia with bone pain with or without stress fractures. The presence of bilateral foot pain and tenderness suggests that this patient has stress fractures. In addition, an increase in skeletal pain is not uncommon with bisphosphonate treatment in these patients, given that this drug class was initially developed to inhibit mineralization and was found serendipitously to increase mineralization and to reduce the risk of osteoporotic fracture. FGF-23 can be measured by commercial laboratories and is characteristically very elevated in patients with tumor-induced osteomalacia, whereas it is often high but inappropriately normal or mildly elevated in patients with inherited disorders of FGF-23 metabolism. Efforts should be directed towards localization and curative resection of the culprit tumor, and ^{111}indium-octreotide with single-photon emission CT is the most sensitive and specific means of localization.

Hypophosphatasia (Answer C) is due to pathogenic variants in the gene encoding tissue nonspecific alkaline phosphatase. This disorder can present with skeletal pain and stress fractures of the lower extremities, but it is characterized by an abnormally low (not elevated) alkaline phosphatase. In addition, serum phosphate is often high-normal to slightly elevated in patients with hypophosphatasia.

Primary hyperparathyroidism (Answer A) is associated with mild hypophosphatemia in approximately one-third of patients and it can occasionally present with an elevated alkaline phosphatase level and bone pain. However, this patient's frankly normal calcium and intact PTH level rule out the diagnosis.

Neither postmenopausal osteoporosis (Answer D) nor pseudogout (Answer B) is associated with hypophosphatemia, which is the defining clinical finding in this woman. Indeed, osteoporosis is often misdiagnosed and treated in patients with tumor-induced osteomalacia, as is the case in this vignette. Moreover, the diagnosis of tumor-induced osteomalacia is frequently delayed and not initially considered because phosphate levels are not routinely included in comprehensive chemistry panels.

Educational Objective
Diagnose tumor-induced osteomalacia as the cause of hypophosphatemia.

UpToDate Topic Review(s)
Causes of hypophosphatemia

Reference(s)

Minisola S, Peacock M, Fukumoto S, et al. Tumour-induced osteomalacia. *Nat Rev Dis Primers*. 2017;3:17044. PMID: 28703220

Chong WH, Andreopoulou P, Chen CC, et al. Tumor localization and biochemical response to cure in tumor-induced osteomalacia. *J Bone Miner Res*. 2013;28(6): 1386-1398. PMID: 23362135

95 ANSWER: E) Defer testing

Posttransplant hyperglycemia is quite common, with some estimates as high as 90% after kidney allograft. There is increasing recognition that this is often transient. High-dosage immunosuppressant drugs, infection, and other factors in the immediate postoperative period are thought to lead to hyperglycemia, which may not be sustained. Thus, relying on blood glucose values measured during the hospital stay (Answer A) is incorrect. A statement from the International Consensus Meeting on Post Transplantation Diabetes Mellitus recommends waiting to assess for diabetes until the immunosuppressant dosages are stable and the patient is stable clinically. Since this patient is being seen only 1 week after transplant, the dosages of his immunosuppressant medications will most likely be adjusted. It is unlikely that he will remain on prednisone, 20 mg daily, over the long term. Therefore, screening for posttransplant diabetes mellitus now is not recommended, and testing should be deferred (Answer E).

The new terminology adopted for posttransplant diabetes is new-onset diabetes after transplant (NODAT). The reported incidence rates for NODAT are variable (7%-46%). The rates are influenced by criteria used for diagnosis, follow-up duration, and immunosuppressive medications used. All of the current modalities for screening for type 2 diabetes can be used to screen transplant recipients for NODAT. Thus, measuring fasting blood glucose (Answer B) and performing an oral glucose tolerance test (Answer C) are only incorrect because the patient was just released from the hospital and has not achieved stable blood glucose. The oral glucose tolerance test is considered the gold standard for diagnosis of NODAT, although there are some specific considerations. Hemoglobin A_{1c} (Answer D) should not be used as the only method of diagnosis in the first year after transplant. Because of anemia, blood transfusion (as in this patient), and dynamic changes in renal function, hemoglobin A_{1c} may not be accurate in the first 12 months after surgery. The consensus statement guidance suggests that a hemoglobin A_{1c} value of 6.5% or greater ($\geq$48 mmol/mol) is most likely accurate, but a value between 5.7% and 6.4% (39-48 mmol/mol) may need to be followed more closely. Therefore, the recommendation is to use another test to corroborate the hemoglobin A_{1c} finding in the first year after transplant. The consensus does not indicate how frequently screening should be undertaken. Since one-third of patients have impaired glucose tolerance by 6 months, some authors suggest measuring fasting blood glucose weekly for a month after transplant. Suggested monitoring of fasting blood glucose is 3 months, 6 months, and 12 months after transplant, followed by annual screening.

In the immediate posttransplant period, hyperglycemia is treated with insulin. The insulin regimen should account for the patient's nutritional intake, immunosuppressive regimen, ongoing infection, etc. For instance, glucocorticoids would be more likely to cause postprandial hyperglycemia and necessitate use of higher prandial insulin doses. If a patient is diagnosed with NODAT, management should start with lifestyle modification, followed by consideration of oral agents and then insulin if necessary. Choice of oral agent must be patient specific. Potential interaction of glucose-lowering agents with immunosuppressive agents should be reviewed. For instance, use of sitagliptin with cyclosporin may cause prolongation of the QT interval. Renal and hepatic function should be reviewed, as this can also influence choice of oral agent.

Educational Objective
Diagnose diabetes mellitus after kidney transplant.

UpToDate Topic Review(s)

New-onset diabetes after transplant (NODAT) in renal transplant recipients

Reference(s)

Sharif A, Hecking M, de Vries AP, et al. Proceedings from an International Consensus Meeting on Posttransplantation Diabetes Mellitus: recommendations and future directions. *Am J Transplant.* 2014;14(9):1992-2000. PMID: 25307034

Shivaswamy V, Boerner B, Larsen J. Post-transplant diabetes mellitus: causes, treatment, and impact on outcomes. *Endocr Rev.* 2016;37(1):37-61. PMID: 26650437

96 ANSWER: E) Stop current therapy; do not routinely monitor IGF-1 during pregnancy

In pregnancy, the placenta produces a biologically active placental variant of GH, which is indistinguishable from pituitary GH on conventional assays. This GH variant stimulates IGF-1 production, which can result in increased levels, particularly in the second half of pregnancy, but it is counterbalanced by increased estrogen. Therefore, normal reference ranges for GH and IGF-1 levels cannot be applied in pregnancy. This patient had well-controlled acromegaly both biochemically and radiologically before her pregnancy. This, along with her lack of significant symptoms, means that the current higher GH and IGF-1 levels can be attributed to her pregnancy and not to disease progression. Similarly, serum prolactin rises significantly in pregnancy (probably due to rising estradiol levels), and it should not be routinely measured nor relied on to monitor a preexisting prolactinoma.

Somatostatin analogues such as lanreotide cross the placenta and their safety in pregnancy has not been established, although no apparent adverse effects have been confirmed (albeit in very small numbers). Similarly, safety data on the GH receptor antagonist pegvisomant are lacking. One global safety database describes 30 pregnancies exposed to pegvisomant and 3 pregnancies in which pegvisomant was used throughout; no adverse outcomes were described in either circumstance. However, it is recommended that, when possible, somatostatin analogues and pegvisomant be discontinued before conception and not taken during pregnancy.

This is a case of stable disease without evidence of optic chiasm compromise on a recent pituitary MRI. Therefore, the optimal and safest course of action is to stop all therapy and do not monitor IGF-1 (Answer E). This patient will require close monitoring during pregnancy with regular assessment for symptoms and visual field testing. Medical therapy of acromegaly may need to be reinstituted in the setting of tumor growth or worsening headaches. In this situation, cabergoline (Answer C) has been shown to be safe when used in the management of macroprolactinoma in pregnancy and could be an option in this case only if she had genuine evidence of disease progression.

Because GH and IGF-1 levels cannot be used to guide assessment of disease activity in pregnancy for reasons described above, stopping therapy and restarting if IGF-1 levels rise (Answer D) is incorrect. Continuation of current therapy (Answer A) is not required and it would potentially expose the fetus to unnecessary risk. There are no safety data that favor pegvisomant over somatostatin analogues, so it is not necessary to stop one drug and continue the other (Answer B).

MRI does not use ionizing radiation and relies on electromagnetic waves to generate radiologic images. There are no reports of harm through the use of noncontrast MRI during pregnancy and it should always be considered, irrespective of gestation, if clinically indicated (for instance, if women with known pituitary tumors develop significant visual field deficits). However, it would not be routinely required during this pregnancy if there are no vision symptoms. Contrast-enhanced MRI is not recommended, as the contrast crosses the placenta and there are reports of increased risk of neonatal morbidity and stillbirth.

Educational Objective

Manage acromegaly during pregnancy and counsel patients about the difficulty of monitoring GH status in this setting.

UpToDate Topic Review(s)

Treatment of acromegaly

Reference(s)

Katznelson L, Laws ER Jr, Melmed S, et al; Endocrine Society. Acromegaly: an Endocrine Society Clinical Practice Guideline. *J Clin Endocrinol Metab.* 2014;99 (11):3933-3951. PMID: 25356808

Neggers SJ, Franck SE, de Rooij FW, et al. Long-term efficacy and safety of pegvisomant in combination with long-acting somatostatin analogs in acromegaly. *J Clin Endocrinol Metab.* 2014;99(10):3644-3652. PMID: 24937542

Fleseriu M. Medical treatment of acromegaly in pregnancy, highlights on new reports. *Endocrine.* 2015;49(3):577-579. PMID: 25931411

97 ANSWER: B) Whole-body radiation exposure to the fetus

Radioactive iodine therapy with ^{131}I for hyperthyroidism is contraindicated during pregnancy because of fetal exposure to radiation. Before radioactive iodine administration, pregnancy should be excluded by measuring β-hCG. In addition, female patients should be asked if they could be pregnant and should be advised to delay pregnancy for 6 months after receiving radioactive iodine therapy, both to prevent radiation exposure to the fetus and also to establish a stable euthyroid state before conception. Serum β-hCG should be detectable 7 to 10 days after conception. False-negative results of β-hCG pregnancy testing are uncommon, but can occur when the measurement is performed soon after conception. Pregnancy tests are more sensitive for detecting pregnancy when performed after a missed period than at other times of the menstrual cycle. Because of these precautions, radioiodine exposure of a pregnant woman and her fetus has rarely been reported. In contrast, a survey conducted in 1976 (before routine testing) identified 237 cases of exposure. The rate of complications was not above the expected rates, but 55 patients had therapeutic abortions, 6 children had hypothyroidism, and 4 children had decreased mental capacity.

Should radioactive exposure inadvertently occur, the consequences depend on the gestational age of the fetus. Iodine readily crosses the placenta, and the concentration of iodine in the fetal blood increases throughout pregnancy. The fetal thyroid is able to accumulate iodine beginning at approximately 12 to 13 weeks' gestation. Before development of the fetal thyroid, radioactive iodine would be expected to cause exposure of the whole fetal body to radiation. Once the fetal thyroid is formed, the greatest exposure is to this gland, which would be damaged by the accumulation of the radiolabeled isotope.

Mathematical models based on iodine kinetics of patients treated with radioactive iodine have been developed to predict fetal exposure. In addition, iodine kinetics have been studied in cases of accidental exposure. In such analyses, the whole-body dose that the fetus was exposed to was estimated to be maximum at 1 to 2 months' gestation and was inversely related to the radioiodine uptake in the mother's thyroid gland. In cases where there was less radioactive iodine in the mother's thyroid, there was also more radiation accumulation in the mother's bladder. The photon energy emitted from activity in the bladder was then absorbed by the fetus, in addition to exposure through radioisotope in the bloodstream. The activity of administered radioactivity is measured in millicuries (mCi), where 1 mCi = 37 MBq, whereas the radiation dose that is delivered to the body is measured in grays, where 1 Gy = 100 rads. One estimate of fetal exposure is 0.083 mGy/MBq. Thus, if 10 mCi (370 MBq) of radioactive iodine were administered to the mother, the estimated absorbed dose to the fetus under modeling assumptions would be 0.031 Gy. The radiation dose to the fetal thyroid has been predicted to be maximum at 6 months gestation. One estimate of the dose absorbed by the fetal thyroid once it has formed was 1.2 Gy/MBq, or roughly 444 Gy after 10 mCi. This would be an "ablative" dose of radioactive iodine. In this vignette, the radioactive iodine activity was administered to the patient when she was about 2 weeks pregnant. Thus, the fetus would have received whole-body exposure (Answer B). However, the fetal thyroid would not yet have formed, so it would not have been damaged, and ultimately fibrosed, by the radioactive iodine (thus, Answer C is incorrect). Once the fetal thyroid has formed, radioactive iodine administration causes fibrosis of the gland and fetal hypothyroidism, but not fetal goiter (Answer A). Although radioactive iodine can cause brief hyperthyroidism associated with damage to the thyroid gland and release of thyroid hormone, this cannot occur before the thyroid gland has formed. Thus, fetal hyperthyroidism (Answer D) is incorrect.

There are scant and very variable data on the adverse effects to a fetus from radiation exposure. The risk of congenital effects is considered to be negligible at 0.05 Gy (5 rads) or less when compared with the rates in unexposed pregnancies, and the risk of malformations is significantly increased over that observed in control populations only at doses above 0.15 Gy (15 rads). The increased risk of childhood solid cancers and leukemias is not really known, but is thought to increase by about 0.3% per 100 mGy exposure. Risks of effects on the brain, such as impaired development or mental retardation are imperfectly understood, but a threshold effect has been proposed such that there is no negative consequence at less than 200-700 mGy. These threshold effects would be reached with administered activities of approximately 100 mCi (3700 MBq) to 200 mCi (7400 MBq). Fetal death (Answer E) is possible, but it would not be a foregone conclusion after radioactive iodine exposure.

Several case reports are available in the literature. A patient treated with 1 mCi (37 MBq) at 3 weeks' gestation delivered an infant without any apparent abnormalities. Following inadvertent treatment of a patient with 13.5 mCi (500 MBq) at 20 weeks' gestation, the fetus was calculated to have absorbed 600 Gy to the thyroid gland, 100 mGy to the whole body, and 40 mGy to the gonad. The dose delivered to the thyroid was an ablative dose, and the fetal hypothyroidism was treated by levothyroxine administration to the mother. The child reportedly had some cognitive deficits after birth. The thyroid gland of an aborted fetus whose mother was treated with radioactive iodine at both 2 and 22 weeks' gestation showed atrophy and fibrosis.

Educational Objective

For a pregnant patient, explain the differential impact of inadvertent radioactive therapy based on the gestational age of the fetus.

UpToDate Topic Review(s)

Radioiodine in the treatment of hyperthyroidism

Reference(s)

Berg GE, Nystrom EH, Jacobsson L, et al. Radioiodine treatment of hyperthyroidism in a pregnant women. *J Nucl Med*. 1998;39(2):357-361. PMID: 9476950

Gorman CA. Radioiodine and pregnancy. *Thyroid*. 1999;9(7):721-726. PMID: 10447020

Stabin MG, Watson EE, Marcus CS, Salk RD. Radiation dosimetry for the adult female and fetus from iodine-131 administration in hyperthyroidism. *J Nucl Med*. 1991;32(5):808-813. PMID: 2022987

Stoffer SS, Hamburger JI. Inadvertent 131I therapy for hyperthyroidism in the first trimester of pregnancy. *J Nucl Med*. 1976;17(02):146-149. PMID: 1245878

98 ANSWER: C) Posttransplant diabetes mellitus

Posttransplant diabetes mellitus (PTDM) is relatively common in patients following kidney and pancreas transplant. PTDM should only be diagnosed in patients who are on a maintenance immunosuppressive regimen, who have stable renal allograft function, and who do not have acute infection. Hyperglycemia must be persistent after transplant, and PTDM is diagnosed regardless of whether the patient had diabetes before undergoing transplant.

Most reports on the outcomes of pancreas transplant rely on registry data, and definitions of graft failure differ from center to center. The 5-year adjusted pancreas graft survival rate for simultaneous pancreas and kidney recipients in the United States is 73%. The national 5-year pancreas graft survival in the United Kingdom is 75% (reported as insulin-independence). The following factors increase the risk for development of PTDM: older age (>40 years), obesity, history of diabetes, family history of diabetes, and the type of immunosuppressant medications. The standard World Health Organization and American Diabetes Association definitions for the diagnosis of diabetes after transplant apply. An additional definition for new-onset diabetes after transplant is an absence of measured C-peptide.

PTDM has been reported with glucocorticoid immunosuppression since the early days of kidney transplant. Glucocorticoids lead to weight gain and increased risk of the metabolic syndrome. Glucocorticoids promote hepatic glucose output and impairment of glucose uptake by adipocytes. Calcineurin inhibitors such as cyclosporine and tacrolimus also adversely affect β-cell function. These drugs lead to impairment in insulin production and secretion. Patients on modern-day immunosuppressive regimens following transplant generally develop insulin resistance over time.

The patient in this vignette is 17 months out from kidney-pancreas transplant and is on a stable immunosuppressive regimen. There is mild renal impairment, which is typical following transplant. She has no signs of pancreas rejection (Answer A), as the amylase level is in the normal range. Transient hyperglycemia after transplant occurs in up to 90% of patients in the first 6 weeks after transplant. Hyperglycemia typically resolves and most patients revert to near normoglycemia during the first 6 months after surgery. This patient had evidence of impaired glucose tolerance 6 and 12 months after transplant, which is quite common, and this increases the risk for eventual development of overt diabetes. Due to the length of time since the transplant occurred, this does not represent transient hyperglycemia (Answer B).

Recurrence of type 1 diabetes (Answer D) is possible following kidney-pancreas transplant, but this is unlikely. In a recent study, only 8% of patients with a history of type 1 diabetes developed recurrence of type 1 diabetes in the pancreas allograft. In this vignette, the C-peptide is in the normal range and there has been no evidence of autoimmune destruction of the pancreas graft. Therefore, this is unlikely to be the cause of the hyperglycemia in this vignette.

This patient was treated for a sinus infection (Answer E) several weeks ago, but she has no signs of infection now.

The cause of the hyperglycemia in this case is PTDM (Answer C). Treatment of PTDM is similar to the approach in nontransplant patients with diabetes. She should be referred to a nutritionist to review a diet treatment plan, with recommendations on losing weight and exercising. A decrease in the prednisone and/or tacrolimus dosage could be considered, but this must be balanced against the increased risk of graft rejection. Oral antihyperglycemic agents, including metformin, insulin secretogogues, and DPP-4 inhibitors, can be used to treat PTDM. Unless the patient has marked hyperglycemia or requires hospitalization, insulin treatment can often be delayed as long as C-peptide is detectable.

Educational Objective
Diagnose posttransplant diabetes mellitus and summarize recommendations for appropriate treatment.

UpToDate Topic Review(s)
Overview of care of the adult kidney transplant recipient

Reference(s)

Sharif A, Hecking M, de Vries AP, et al. Proceedings from an international consensus meeting of posttranplantation diabetes mellitus: recommendations and future directions. *Am J Transplant.* 2014;14:1992-2000. PMID: 25307034

Dean PG, Kukla A, Stegall MD, Kudva YC. Pancreas transplantation. *BMJ.* 2017;357:j1321. PMID: 28373161

Vendrame F, Hopfner Y-Y, Diamantopoulos S, et al. Risk factors for type 1 diabetes recurrence in immunosuppressed recipients of simultaneous pancreas-kidney transplants. *Am J Transplant.* 2016;16(1):235-245. PMID: 26317167

Strom Halden TA, Asberg A, Vik K, Hartmann A, Jenssen T. Short-term efficacy and safety of sitagliptin treatment in long-term stable renal recipients with new-onset diabetes after transplantation. *Nephrol Dial Transplant.* 2014;29(4):926-933. PMID: 24452849

99 ANSWER: D) Increase the levothyroxine dosage

During management of hypopituitarism, the endocrinologist must pay attention to interactions that occur between different replacement therapies. The most obvious example is the acceleration of cortisol catabolism when thyroid hormone replacement is started, which poses a risk for adrenal crisis if hypothyroidism is treated before adrenal insufficiency.

GH has important effects on both levothyroxine and hydrocortisone therapy. GH increases the deiodination of T_4. Therefore, untreated GH deficiency may mask central hypothyroidism in a significant proportion of patients with hypopituitarism, and hypothyroidism may become evident only after GH replacement is initiated. In patients already on levothyroxine, free T_4 serum levels may decline after initiation of GH therapy (or after a dosage increase). This patient's free T_4 level is now at the low end of normal; it was most likely higher (mid- to high-normal) before GH was started. As one cannot rely on TSH, the goal in patients with hypopituitarism is generally a free T_4 level in the mid-upper half of the normal range. Furthermore, this patient reports symptoms that are consistent with hypothyroidism, so increasing the levothyroxine dosage (Answer D) is correct. No change in therapy (Answer E) would be inappropriate.

GH therapy does not significantly affect the testosterone level. This patient's serum testosterone is age-appropriate. Thus, increasing the testosterone dosage (Answer A) is incorrect.

Similar to what is observed in central hypothyroidism, untreated low GH and IGF-1 levels can reduce the severity of central hypoadrenalism, most likely by reducing the inactivating conversion of cortisol to cortisone. GH replacement (or GH dosage increase) may worsen adrenal insufficiency. Therefore, this patient may require an increase in his hydrocortisone dosage because GH therapy has been initiated, but certainly a reduction in the hydrocortisone dosage (Answer B) would not be warranted.

The patient's current GH dosage is appropriate, as demonstrated by the age-adjusted serum IGF-1 level. He has no signs or symptoms of GH overdosing, such as fluid retention. Therefore, the GH dosage does not need to be adjusted (Answer C).

Educational Objective

In a patient with panhypopituitarism, explain why GH replacement may cause an increase in the levothyroxine requirement by increasing T_4 to T_3 conversion.

UpToDate Topic Review(s)

Treatment of hypopituitarism

Reference(s)

Fleseriu M, Hashim IA, Karavitaki N, et al. Hormonal replacement in hypopituitarism in adults: an Endocrine Society Clinical Practice Guideline. *J Clin Endocrinol Metab*. 2016;101(11):3888-3921. PMID: 27736313

Agha A, Walker D, Perry L, et al. Unmasking of central hypothyroidism following growth hormone replacement in adult hypopituitary patients. *Clin Endocrinol (Oxf)*. 2007;66(1):72-77. PMID: 17201804

Giavoli C, Libé R, Corbetta S, et al. Effect of recombinant human growth hormone (GH) replacement on the hypothalamic-pituitary-adrenal axis in adult GH-deficient patients. *J Clin Endocrinol Metab*. 2004;89(11):5397-5401. PMID: 15531488

100 ANSWER: A) Ergocalciferol

On initial review of this patient's clinical data, she appears to have severe osteoporosis based on her bone mineral density assessment and would seem to be a good candidate for pharmacologic antifracture therapy. However, closer review of her clinical and biochemical data reveals information that should cause one to hesitate to use this approach. Her lower-extremity pain, while nonspecific, could suggest an alternative metabolic bone disorder (ie, osteomalacia). This suspicion is supported by the presence of tibial tenderness on examination, which in osteomalacia is thought to be due to expansion of the highly enervated periosteal lining by excess unmineralized osteoid. A diagnosis of osteomalacia is further supported biochemically by low-normal serum calcium and phosphate and elevated alkaline phosphatase. Most importantly and most likely the underlying etiology, this patient is frankly deficient in vitamin D with evidence of secondary hyperparathyroidism. Interestingly and not unexpectedly, this patient's serum 1,25-dihydroxyvitamin D level is slightly high, which is common in the setting of 25-hydroxyvitamin D deficiency and is due to PTH-mediated up-regulation of renal 1α-hydroxylase activity. Given that DXA cannot distinguish reduced bone mineral content from unmineralized osteoid, treatment with ergocalciferol (generally 50,000 IU weekly for 8 weeks) should be the initial treatment offered to this patient (Answer A). Additionally, existing evidence supports achievement of an adequate 25-hydroxyvitamin D status for optimal bone mineral density response and antifracture benefit.

For the reasons described above, bisphosphonate therapy (Answer B) would not be indicated until this patient's vitamin D deficiency and associated osteomalacia are addressed. Moreover, bisphosphonate therapy could potentially precipitate and aggravate underlying osteomalacia due to vitamin D deficiency. Given the patient's borderline-low calcium level and concomitant vitamin D deficiency, denosumab (Answer C) would also be contraindicated at this time because of concern over posttreatment hypocalcemia.

Calcium supplementation independent of vitamin D repletion (Answer D) would not address underlying osteomalacia if present, and it has also not been shown to independently reduce the risk of osteoporotic fracture.

Finally, calcitriol and phosphorus treatment (Answer E), which is prescribed to patients with hypophosphatemic osteomalacia due to disorders of fibroblast growth factor 23 excess, would not adequately address osteomalacia due to 25-hydroxyvitamin D deficiency.

Educational Objective

Identify subclinical osteomalacia due to vitamin D deficiency in a patient with osteoporosis and explain the importance of vitamin D repletion before bisphosphonate treatment.

UpToDate Topic Review(s)

Clinical manifestations, diagnosis, and treatment of osteomalacia

Reference(s)

Deane A, Constancio L, Fogelman I, Hampson G. The impact of vitamin D status on changes in bone mineral density during treatment with bisphosphonates and after discontinuation following long-term use in post-menopausal osteoporosis. *BMC Musculoskelet Disord*. 2007;8:3. PMID: 17214897

Prieto-Alhambra D, Pagès-Castellà A, Wallace G, et al. Predictors of fracture while on treatment with oral bisphosphonates: a population-based cohort study. *J Bone Miner Res.* 2014;29(1):268-274. PMID: 23761350

101 ANSWER: C) Prescribe progesterone treatment for 10 days

This patient presents with secondary amenorrhea after stopping oral contraceptives. Her laboratory evaluation reveals a mildly elevated prolactin concentration. She also has symptoms of androgen excess with cystic acne as an adult and a Ferriman-Gallwey score of 8, consistent with mild hirsutism, so the diagnosis of polycystic ovary syndrome is a possibility. Hyperprolactinemia from a pituitary tumor results in anovulatory cycles and secondary amenorrhea due to suppression of gonadotropin secretion. This leads to secondary hypogonadism and estrogen deficiency. Polycystic ovary syndrome causes anovulatory bleeding or amenorrhea with estrogen present. In the evaluation of menstrual irregularity and secondary amenorrhea, the progesterone withdrawal test (Answer C) is a useful tool to distinguish between estrogen-sufficient amenorrhea, which results in withdrawal bleeding of the endometrial lining, vs estrogen deficiency caused by secondary hypogonadism. At the same time, withdrawal bleeding is reassuring in that there is no anatomic abnormality interfering with menstrual bleeding or preventing the development of the endometrial lining.

Although pelvic ultrasonography (Answer A) could also be reassuring if the endometrial lining is thicker than 4 mm and it might show the presence of multiple follicles suggestive of polycystic ovary syndrome, the progesterone withdrawal test is more likely to give clinically useful information if the elevated prolactin is causing estrogen deficiency. Similarly, progesterone and estradiol levels (Answers D and E) might be helpful if they are both in the high end of normal for the luteal phase, but they will not be diagnostic if within the early follicular range in terms of determining whether the elevated prolactin is causing secondary hypogonadism.

The prolactin elevation is very mild in this patient and is not likely to be clinically significant. If a pituitary MRI (Answer B) demonstrated a possible small microadenoma, it would not necessarily indicate whether this elevation is symptomatic and requires treatment. With this prolactin level, a small microadenoma would not be expected to be visible. Although hyperprolactinemia might be seen with other features of polycystic ovary syndrome, a pathophysiologic link has not been identified to date. Therefore, further evaluation would be warranted, but the best next step would not necessarily be MRI. A repeated prolactin measurement should be considered first because hyperprolactinemia due to a microadenoma would not be expected to normalize but would continue to rise untreated.

In this case, the patient had withdrawal bleeding after 10 days of oral progesterone. A repeated prolactin measurement also normalized. Therefore, polycystic ovary syndrome was diagnosed and no additional imaging was required.

Educational Objective
Diagnose polycystic ovary syndrome in a woman with mildly elevated prolactin.

UpToDate Topic Review(s)
Diagnosis of polycystic ovary syndrome in adults

Reference(s)
Melmed S, Casanueva FF, Hoffman AR, et al; Endocrine Society. Diagnosis and treatment of hyperprolactinemia: an Endocrine Society Clinical Practice Guideline. *J Clin Endocrinol Metab.* 2011;96(2):273-288. PMID: 21296991

Practice Committee of the American Society for Reproductive Medicine. Current evaluation of amenorrhea. *Fertil Steril.* 2008;90(Suppl 5):S219-S225. PMID: 19007635

Robin G, Catteau-Jonard S, Young J, Dewailly D. Pathophysiological link between polycystic ovary syndrome and hyperprolactinemia: myth or reality? *Gynecol Obstet Fertil.* 2011;39(3):141-145. PMID: 21388855

102 ANSWER: A) Hydrochlorothiazide

A very low-calorie diet is defined as fewer than 800 kcal per day. This calorie restriction provides an average weight loss of 31 lb (14.2 kg) to 46.2 lb (21.0 kg) over 11 to 14 weeks. Participants follow a full replacement meal plan, consuming 0.8 to 1.5 g of protein per kilogram of ideal body weight. The most common adverse effects when following this plan are fatigue, constipation, hair loss, dry skin, volume depletion, dizziness, and cold intolerance. Other more significant adverse effects are gout and gallstones.

When starting a patient on a very low-calorie diet, it is important to review their medications, as some may need to be discontinued or their dosage may need to be reduced. Diuretics (Answer A) should be discontinued at the beginning to avoid enhancing the electrolyte and fluid shifts associated with starting this diet. Patients with type 2 diabetes who take antihyperglycemic agents or insulin must be counseled to monitor their glucose frequently after starting a very low-calorie diet because they are at risk for hypoglycemia. Also consider stopping sulfonylureas and short-acting insulin and decreasing the dosage of long-acting insulin by 50% when a very low-calorie diet is started. Insulin-sensitizing agents such as metformin (Answer C) are usually continued during this meal plan as they do not usually cause hypoglycemia. Antihypertensive agents (Answer D) are usually continued. There is no specific guideline for thyroid supplementation (Answer E), but the dosage will likely need to be reduced 6 to 8 weeks after starting this program. No dosage adjustment is necessary for statins (Answer B).

Patients on antihypertensive medication should be encouraged to monitor their blood pressure while following this program, as they may need a dosage adjustment. This type of diet should be conducted under close medical supervision in order to adjust the patient's medication and to monitor for electrolyte abnormalities. Close monitoring will minimize adverse outcomes. There is no standard protocol regarding laboratory testing before or during a very low-calorie diet. Most centers perform a basic chemistry panel before starting the diet and then reassess biweekly for the first month. If the patient has a history of gout, uric acid should be measured initially and monitored periodically. If the patient is started on supplements, follow-up laboratory work should be performed to make sure the patient is getting adequate supplementation. Very low-calorie diet formulations usually provide an adequate amount of vitamins and minerals, so serious insufficiencies are unusual.

Educational Objective
Manage medications for patients prescribed a very low-calorie diet.

UpToDate Topic Review(s)
Obesity in adults: Dietary therapy

Reference(s)

Jensen MD, Ryan DH, Apovian CM, et al; American College of Cardiology/American Heart Association Task Force on Practice Guidelines; Obesity Society. 2013 AHA/ACC/TOS guideline for the management of overweight and obesity in adults: a report of the American College of Cardiology/American Heart Association Task Force on Practice Guidelines and The Obesity Society [published correction appears in *J Am Coll Cardiol*. 2014;63(25 Pt B): 3029-3030]. *J Am Coll Cardiol*. 2014;63(25 Pt B):2985-3023. PMID: 244239920

Tsai AG, Wadden TA. The evolution of very-low-calorie diets: an update and meta-analysis. *Obesity (Silver Spring)*. 2006;14(8):1283-1293. PMID: 16988070

Very low-calorie diets. National Task Force on the Prevention and Treatment of Obesity, National Institutes of Health. *JAMA*. 1993;270(8):967-974. PMID: 8345648

103 ANSWER: D) Measure fasting glucose every 3 months

With improvement in antiretroviral therapies and excellent clinics and physicians available, patients with HIV can live a normal lifespan. However, the disease itself and various antiretroviral medications, in particular protease inhibitors, can predispose patients to diabetes. The cause of this increased risk appears to be via increased insulin resistance and possibly apoptosis of pancreatic β cells. Nucleoside reverse transcriptase inhibitors may also increase risk for diabetes by adversely affecting fat distribution. Because of this increased risk, the American Diabetes Association recommends that patients with HIV be screened for diabetes and prediabetes by measuring fasting glucose every 6 to 12 months before starting antiretroviral therapy and every 3 months after starting or changing antiretroviral therapy (Answer D). If initial screening results are normal, then checking fasting glucose every year is advised.

Screening this patient by measuring hemoglobin A_{1c} (Answer B) is not recommended because it underestimates glycemia in patients with HIV who are receiving antiretroviral therapy. Kim et al compared hemoglobin A_{1c} with fasting glucose levels in a cohort of patients with HIV vs in patients without HIV. The authors found that hemoglobin A_{1c} measurement underestimates fasting glucose by 29 mg/dL in patients with HIV. The discordance appears to be associated with the use of nucleoside reverse transcriptase inhibitors. A random glucose measurement (Answer C) is only useful if the value is <100 mg/dL or ≥200 mg/dL, so it is not the best test. Although oral glucose tolerance testing (Answer A) is the gold standard for defining glycemia, it requires multiple blood draws and the test may need to be repeated every 3 months, which would be cumbersome. The American Diabetes Association does not recognize a fingerstick glucose test from a glucometer (Answer E) as a method for diagnosing diabetes. The glucose value from a glucometer may be up to 20% higher or 20% lower than the laboratory value.

Educational Objective

Recommend appropriate screening for diabetes mellitus in a patient with HIV infection.

UpToDate Topic Review(s)

Management of cardiovascular risk (including dyslipidemia) in the HIV-infected patient

Reference(s)

American Diabetes Association. Comprehensive medical evaluation and assessment of comorbidities: standards of medical care in diabetes-2018. *Diabetes Care*. 41(Suppl 1):S28-S37. PMID: 29222374

Kim PS, Woods C, Georgoff P, et al. A1C underestimates glycemia in HIV infection. *Diabetes Care*. 2009;32(9):1591-1593. PMID: 19502538

104 ANSWER: D) Late-night salivary cortisol testing

This patient presents with weight gain and difficulty sleeping, but she does not have overt signs of Cushing syndrome on physical examination. The first step in evaluating Cushing syndrome is to convincingly confirm hypercortisolism. Once hypercortisolism is documented, subsequent steps involve determining whether the hypercortisolism is ACTH-dependent or ACTH-independent and localizing the source of the problem.

The most commonly recommended methods to confirm hypercortisolism include late-night salivary cortisol testing, 24-hour urinary free cortisol testing, and 1-mg dexamethasone suppression testing. This patient's 1-mg dexamethasone suppression test shows a relatively high serum cortisol level with unsuppressed ACTH. One interpretation of these results could be that this is ACTH-dependent hypercortisolism. However, caution should be taken in interpreting dexamethasone suppression tests in patients using estrogen-containing oral contraceptives. Estrogens can increase hepatic globulin synthesis, including that of cortisol-binding globulin. Higher cortisol-binding globulin levels result in higher total serum cortisol levels, and, therefore, a substantial proportion of these patients have a false-positive result on dexamethasone suppression testing. Further, without a dexamethasone level at the time of the morning blood testing, it may not be safe to assume that the testing conditions were appropriate.

The best options to test for hypercortisolism in this patient would be (1) late-night salivary cortisol testing (Answer D) (preferably on 2 separate occasions); (2) 24-hour urinary free cortisol testing (preferably on 2 separate occasions); or (3) withdrawal of oral contraception for 6 to 8 weeks followed by a 1-mg dexamethasone suppression test. Some clinicians prefer to also measure morning dexamethasone to ensure adequate levels were achieved and cortisol results are interpretable.

All the other choices involve a localizing method (Answers A and E) or treatment intervention (Answers B and C) that is not indicated since evidence for hypercortisolism has not yet been convincingly established.

This patient coincidentally elected to stop her oral contraception, and 8 weeks later results from a 1-mg dexamethasone suppression test and a late-night salivary cortisol test were normal. Her symptoms were ascribed to other factors and gradually resolved without intervention.

Educational Objective

Evaluate for Cushing syndrome by ensuring a confident biochemical confirmation of hypercortisolism and recognize when dexamethasone suppression testing may not be accurate or reliable.

UpToDate Topic Review(s)

Establishing the diagnosis of Cushing's syndrome

Reference(s)

Nieman LK, Biller BM, Findling JW, et al. The diagnosis of Cushing's syndrome: an Endocrine Society clinical practice guideline. *J Clin Endocrinol Metab*. 2008; 93(5):1526-1540. PMID: 18334580

105 ANSWER: B) Serum magnesium

The woman in this vignette has symptomatic hypocalcemia that is refractory to treatment with calcium and active vitamin D supplementation. Her laboratory workup reveals a low PTH level in the setting of hypocalcemia. Given these findings, one should consider hypomagnesemia (Answer B) as a cause of her refractory hypocalcemia. Low magnesium levels impair PTH release in response to hypocalcemia and may also cause hypocalcemia by impairing PTH action, leading to functional hypoparathyroidism. Despite this, most patients with hypomagnesemia have normal or even low phosphate levels, most likely due to poor intake. Identification of patients with low magnesium requires clinical suspicion because serum magnesium is not usually measured as part of routine blood tests. Risk factors for hypomagnesemia include diarrhea, malabsorption, proton-pump inhibitor therapy, diuretic use, alcoholism, malnutrition, and severe illness. Clinical manifestations of hypomagnesemia include refractory hypocalcemia or hypokalemia, neuromuscular disturbances, and cardiac arrhythmias. Patients with severe hypomagnesemia should receive intravenous magnesium, while oral repletion may be given to patients with mild symptoms. In addition, the underlying cause of low magnesium should be corrected if possible. This patient had a serum magnesium level of 0.9 mg/dL and was treated with both intravenous and oral magnesium therapy; her hypocalcemia resolved once her magnesium was replenished.

Measuring 24-hour urinary calcium excretion (Answer A) would be helpful in establishing the diagnosis of autosomal dominant hypocalcemia, which is a familial disorder caused by an activating pathogenic variant in the *CASR* gene. Most persons with autosomal dominant hypocalcemia are asymptomatic and are diagnosed incidentally on routine laboratory tests. While the biochemical findings presented in this case may be consistent with this condition, this patient is symptomatic and has no family history of calcium disorders.

Measuring 1,25-dihydroxyvitamin D (Answer C) would be appropriate if one suspected inherited disorders that result from the deficiency in the renal production of 1,25-dihydroxyvitamin D or a defect in the vitamin D receptor, both of which are rare conditions associated with secondary hyperparathyroidism, so this test would not be helpful in this clinical scenario. In addition, there is no concern for celiac disease since she has no evidence of chronic malabsorption with a normal 25-hydroxyvitamin level. Therefore, checking tissue transglutaminase antibodies (Answer D) is incorrect.

In the absence of hypomagnesemia, persistent hypocalcemia with a low or inappropriately normal PTH level would be consistent with a diagnosis of primary hypoparathyroidism. Most patients with hypoparathyroidism have an elevated phosphate level. Autoimmune hypoparathyroidism is typically suspected in patients with a personal or family history of autoimmune diseases and no history of neck surgery. This condition is a common feature of polyglandular autoimmune syndrome type I, which is a rare autosomal recessive disorder also characterized by chronic mucocutaneous candidiasis and adrenal insufficiency. Patients with this syndrome typically present in childhood or early adolescence. Measuring PTH antibodies (Answer E) may be useful to screen patients suspected of having autoimmune hypoparathyroidism, but it would not be the most appropriate next step in evaluating this patient's refractory hypocalcemia.

Educational Objective
Identify hypomagnesemia as a cause of refractory hypocalcemia and summarize the effect of magnesium on PTH.

UpToDate Topic Review(s)
Diagnostic approach to hypocalcemia
Evaluation and treatment of hypomagnesemia

Reference(s)

Fatemi S, Ryzen E, Flores J, Endres DB, Rude RK. Effect of experimental human magnesium depletion on parathyroid hormone secretion and 1,25-dihydroxyvitamin D metabolism. *J Clin Endocrinol Metab*. 1991;73(5):1067-1072. PMID: 1939521

Cooper MS, Gittoes NJ. Diagnosis and management of hypocalcaemia. *BMJ*. 2008;336(7656):1298-1302. PMID: 18535072

106 ANSWER: C) Benign thyroid cyst

This patient presents with a slowly enlarging neck swelling that is causing compressive symptoms. Clinical findings are unilateral thyroid enlargement without retrosternal extension. He has no clinical features of thyroid dysfunction. Because thyroid enlargement caused by thyroid dysfunction requires different management than euthyroid nodules and goiters, the first evaluation in patients presenting with thyroid swelling should be measurement of serum TSH (which is within normal limits in this patient). If serum TSH is subnormal, a radioisotope scan should be performed to assess for the presence of toxic nodules. To assess the size and nature of the thyroid nodule, high-resolution thyroid ultrasonography with survey of the cervical lymph nodes should be performed. The ultrasound report should convey nodule size (in 3 dimensions) and location, as well as a description of the nodule's sonographic features, including composition (solid, cystic proportion, or spongiform), echogenicity, margins, presence and type of calcifications, shape (eg, taller than wide), and vascularity. The pattern of sonographic features associated with a nodule confers a risk of malignancy, and combined with nodule size, this guides decision-making with regard to FNA biopsy.

In this patient, thyroid ultrasonography indicates the presence of a right-sided, large (32 x 38 x 51 mm), well-defined, thin-walled, predominantly cystic thyroid nodule with a minimal amount of isoechoic solid tissue causing a small degree of tracheal deviation. The nodule has regular margins, no microcalcifications, and no other suspicious features. The ultrasonographic findings are consistent with a benign thyroid cyst (Answer C).

While multiple thyroid nodules may be present in patients presenting with a visible and palpable dominant nodule, there is no evidence of multiple nodules either on clinical or radiologic grounds and the presence of a multinodular goiter (Answer D) is less likely.

Anaplastic thyroid cancer (Answer A) is the most aggressive and rarest form of thyroid cancer, often originating from a differentiated tumor following a process of dedifferentiation. Affected persons typically present with locally advanced disease, including tracheal and esophageal invasion, carotid artery involvement, and distant metastases. The clinical presentation and ultrasonographic findings of a large cystic mass with regular margins and not invading adjacent structures make a diagnosis of anaplastic thyroid cancer unlikely.

Differentiated thyroid cancers can undergo cystic degeneration (Answer B), but in the absence of suspicious ultrasound features such as an irregular nodule margin, presence of microcalcifications, and a large, less homogeneous solid component, this diagnosis is less likely.

A thyroglossal cyst (Answer E) is a fibrous cyst that originates from a persistent thyroglossal duct during developmental stages, and it usually presents as an irregular neck mass or a lump. Thyroglossal cysts are the most common cause of midline neck masses and are generally located caudal to the hyoid bone. These neck masses can occur anywhere along the path of the thyroglossal duct, from the base of the tongue to the suprasternal notch, but they are usually located in the midline. Typically, the cyst moves upwards on protrusion of the tongue, given its attachment to the embryonic duct. While the image in this vignette may represent a thyroglossal duct cyst, the thyroid swelling is not located in the midline and there is no suggestion that this moves with tongue protrusion.

Surgery is the long-established therapeutic option for benign thyroid nodules, which steadily grow and become symptomatic. The cost of thyroid surgery, the risk of temporary or permanent complications, and the effect on quality of life, however, remain relevant concerns. Therefore, various minimally invasive treatments have gained momentum in recent years. Ultrasound-guided percutaneous ethanol injection is a very effective treatment for relapsing thyroid cysts, and radiofrequency ablation of solid, nonfunctioning nodules usually results in a 50% volume decrease. Hyperfunctioning nodules remain best treated with radioactive iodine, which results in better control of hyperthyroidism and reduction in thyroid size. Newer minimally invasive approaches that are being investigated include high-intensity focused ultrasound and microwave or laser ablation.

Educational Objective
Identify ultrasound features of a large, benign thyroid cyst.

UpToDate Topic Review(s)
Cystic thyroid nodules

Reference(s)

Haugen BR, Alexander EK, Bible KC, et al. 2015 American Thyroid Association Management Guidelines for Adult Patients with Thyroid Nodules and Differentiated Thyroid Cancer: the American Thyroid Association Guidelines Task Force on Thyroid Nodules and Differentiated Thyroid Cancer. *Thyroid.* 2016;26(1):1-133. PMID: 26462967

Papini E, Gugliemi R, Pacella CM. Laser, radiofrequency, and ethanol ablation for the management of thyroid nodules. *Curr Opin Endocrinol Diabetes Obes.* 2016;23(5):400-406. PMID: 27504993

107 ANSWER: C) Add lisinopril

Diabetic retinopathy is estimated to be present in 35.4% of patients with diabetes mellitus. In those with diabetic retinopathy, 7.5% have proliferative changes in the retina. Development of diabetic retinopathy is associated with a number of risk factors, including younger age of onset, longer duration of disease, hypertension, and dyslipidemia. Improvement in the incidence and progression of diabetic retinopathy has been associated with good glycemic control, good blood pressure control, and possibly good control of dyslipidemia.

Every 10 mm Hg rise in blood pressure increases the risk of retinopathy by 30%. The patient in this vignette has a systolic blood pressure of 146 mm Hg, which is elevated. In addition to improving cardiovascular outcomes, control of systolic blood pressure to less than 140 mm Hg and diastolic blood pressure less than 90 mm Hg reduces the risk of diabetic retinopathy. Hence, the addition of lisinopril (Answer C) to his regimen is the best option now. Not addressing his hypertension (Answer E) is substandard care.

Although good glycemic control is beneficial, no specific pharmacologic agent has been associated with improved diabetic retinopathy outcomes. Pioglitazone (Answer A) reduces retinal angiogenesis and neovascularization in animal studies, but no human trials have replicated this. There is also inconsistent case report evidence of increased macular edema with use of thiazolidinediones. Similarly, topical GLP-1 receptor agonists (Answer B) have shown reduction in neurodegeneration in mice. In human trials, there is concern for worsening diabetic retinopathy. In Sustain-6, a study that evaluated the role of the GLP-1 receptor agonist semaglutide on cardiovascular outcomes, diabetic retinopathy progression was a secondary outcome. There was an increased risk of diabetic retinopathy progression in the group treated with semaglutide. The group that demonstrated progression of diabetic retinopathy had longer duration of diabetes, higher hemoglobin A_{1c} levels, and history of diabetic retinopathy that required intervention. Commentators have speculated that rapid reduction in blood glucose levels may have a role in progression of diabetic retinopathy. At this time, addition of a GLP-1 receptor agonist specifically for prevention of diabetic retinopathy is currently not supported.

Both fibrates (Answer D) and statins appear to reduce hard exudates. In the FIELD study, fenofibrate reduced the need for laser photocoagulation for either diabetic macular edema or proliferative diabetic retinopathy by 31% for patients on fenofibrate vs 4.9% for those on placebo ($P < .001$). In the ACCORD-EYE study, the combination of fenofibrate and simvastatin reduced the rate of progression of diabetic retinopathy by 40% compared with simvastatin alone. This effect was no longer seen when the fibrate was stopped. Although intriguing, the addition of a fibrate for prevention of diabetic retinopathy is not currently the standard of care. Further studies on the effect of fibrates on diabetic retinopathy risk as a primary outcome must be conducted. Therefore, the addition of a fibrate is incorrect at this time. Optimal combination of therapy with statins and fibrates in primary prevention and in patients with known diabetic retinopathy must be determined.

Educational Objective
Address the risk factors for development of diabetic retinopathy.

UpToDate Topic Review(s)
Diabetic retinopathy: prevention and treatment

Reference(s)

Solomon SD, Chew E, Duh EJ, et al. Diabetic retinopathy: a position statement by the American Diabetes Association. *Diabetes Care.* 2017;40(3):412-418. PMID: 28223445

Klein R, Klein BE, Moss SE, Davis MD, DeMets DL. The Wisconsin epidemiology study of diabetic retinopathy. III. Prevalence and risk of diabetic retinopathy when age at diagnosis is 30 or more years. *Arch Ophthalmol.* 1984;102(4):527-532. PMID: 6367725

Leske MC, Wu SY, Hennis A, et al; Barbados Eye Study Group. Hyperglycemia, blood pressure, and the 9-year incidence of diabetic retinopathy. *Ophthalmology.* 2005;112(5):799-805. PMID: 15878059

Marso SP, Bain SC, Consoli A, et al; SUSTAIN-6 Investigators. Semaglutide and cardiovascular outcomes in patients with type 2 diabetes. *N Engl J Med.* 2016; 375(19):1834-1844. PMID: 27633186

108 ANSWER: E) Recommend elective orchiectomy

The goal of hormone therapy for transgender women (male-to-female) is to achieve serum levels of sex steroids in the female range. The route of estrogen administration can be oral, sublingual, transdermal, or intramuscular. Which formulation to recommend to a particular patient should be personalized based on factors such as age, medical comorbidities, risk of venous thromboembolism, ease of monitoring, cost, and patient preference. Many patients request the intramuscular formulation due to the high levels of estrogen obtained a few days after an injection and due to advice from others in the community who believe that the levels of estrogen obtained with the intramuscular route promote greater feminization. The disadvantages of the intramuscular formulation are the peaks and troughs of serum estradiol levels, fear of needles for some patients, and stronger potential for abuse than with other formulations. Ethinyl estradiol is a semisynthetic estrogen given orally that should be avoided due to increased risk of venous thromboembolism. The nonoral formulations of estrogen are presumed to have a lower risk of venous thromboembolism, as they avoid the first-pass metabolism in the liver. A disadvantage of conjugated oral estrogens is that serum estradiol levels cannot be followed to allow for dosage titration. Options to lower the androgens include antiandrogens such as spironolactone and cyproterone acetate, as well as GnRH agonists given every 1 to 3 months. The Endocrine Society guidelines recommend achieving estradiol and testosterone levels in the normal female range (100-200 pg/mL and <50 ng/dL, respectively).

Some transgender women do not achieve target levels of sex hormones despite adequate or high dosages of estrogen and spironolactone. The most effective method to lower this patient's androgens is an elective orchiectomy (Answer E), which is a low-risk surgery. Further increasing the dosages of spironolactone and/or estrogen (Answers A and B) is incorrect, as this approach will most likely not adequately lower her testosterone and will increase the risk of greater adverse effects. While switching from oral to sublingual estradiol (Answer C) might increase the estrogen level, it would most likely not adequately lower her testosterone. It is also uncertain whether progesterone (Answer D) would adequately lower her testosterone level and this medication may carry adverse effects.

Educational Objective
Identify appropriate treatment strategies to normalize testosterone levels in transgender women.

UpToDate Topic Review(s)
Transgender women: Evaluation and management

Reference(s)

Hembree WC, Cohen-Kettenis PT, Gooren L, Hannema SE, Meyer WJ, Murad MH, Rosenthal SM, Safer JD, Tangpricha V, T'Sjoen GG. Endocrine treatment of gender-dysphoric/gender-incongruent persons: an Endocrine Society clinical practice guideline. *J Clin Endocrinol Metab.* 2017;102(11):3869-3903. PMID: 28945902

Tangpricha V, den Heijer M. Oestrogen and anti-androgen therapy for transgender women. *Lancet Diabetes Endocrinol.* 2017;5(4):291-300. PMID: 27916515

109 ANSWER: C) Reinitiate GH therapy

Increasing evidence suggests that treating GH deficiency in young adulthood increases the patient's chance of reaching optimal bone mineral density. Furthermore, GH deficiency in adulthood is associated with hypercholesterolemia and, in some studies, with reduced quality of life. Therefore, endocrinologists must discuss GH deficiency with young adults who were treated with GH therapy during childhood. Patients with childhood-onset GH deficiency may or may not have GH deficiency in adulthood. In some studies, up to 50% of children with isolated GH deficiency diagnosed in childhood (and a normal pituitary MRI) are no longer GH deficient when re-tested with GH stimulation as adults. It is unknown whether this is due to real "maturation" of the GH axis or to overdiagnosis of GH deficiency in childhood secondary to poor specificity of the GH stimulation tests. Therefore, in patients with a history of childhood isolated GH deficiency and a normal pituitary MRI, reinitiating GH therapy without a GH stimulation test would be inappropriate. However, this patient has a pituitary anatomic abnormality, central hypothyroidism, and a frankly low serum IGF-1 level. In this scenario, a GH stimulation test would be redundant, and reinitiating GH replacement therapy (at an adult dosage) would be appropriate (Answer C). Accordingly, the Endocrine Society guidelines state: "We recommend that because of the irreversible nature of the cause of the GHD in children with structural lesions with multiple hormone deficiencies and those with proven genetic causes, a low IGF-1 level at least 1 month off GH therapy is sufficient documentation of persistent GHD without additional provocative testing."

This patient's free T_4 level is mid-normal, so increasing his levothyroxine dosage (Answer A) is not necessary. An ACTH stimulation test (Answer B) does not seem to be needed, as his weight is stable and he has no symptoms that suggest adrenal insufficiency. Similarly, he has normal-sized testes and normal serum testosterone, and therefore testosterone therapy (Answer D) is not necessary (and it may reduce his future fertility). Measuring prolactin (Answer E) would not be informative in this case.

Educational Objective

Determine when to reinitiate GH therapy in a young adult who was previously treated for childhood-onset GH deficiency.

UpToDate Topic Review(s)
Growth hormone treatment during the transition period

Reference(s)

Conway GS, Szarras-Czapnik M, Racz K, et al; 1369 GHD to GHDA Transition Study Group. Treatment for 24 months with recombinant human GH has a beneficial effect on bone mineral density in young adults with childhood-onset GH deficiency. *Eur J Endocrinol.* 2009;160(6):899-907. PMID: 19324976

Radovick S, DiVall S. Approach to the growth hormone-deficient child during transition to adulthood. *J Clin Endocrinol Metab.* 2007;92(4):1195-1200. PMID: 17409338

Molitch ME, Clemmons DR, Malozowski S, Merriam GR, Vance ML; Endocrine Society. Evaluation and treatment of adult growth hormone deficiency: an Endocrine Society clinical practice guideline. *J Clin Endocrinol Metab.* 2011;96(6):1587-1609. PMID: 21602453

110 ANSWER: D) Start NPH insulin at bedtime and insulin aspart before the evening meal

Maturity-onset diabetes of the young (MODY) is a heterogeneous group of disorders that is typified by early onset (usually diagnosed before age 30 years), lack of autoimmune diabetes markers, and autosomal dominant inheritance. MODY is the most common form of monogenic diabetes and accounts for about 2% of all cases of diabetes. Each subtype of MODY is typified by a single gene pathogenic variant that affects β-cell development, function, or action.

The 2 most common forms of MODY are caused by pathogenic variants in the genes encoding hepatocyte nuclear factor 1α (*HNF1A*) (MODY 3) and glucokinase (*GCK*) (MODY 2). Pathogenic variants in the *HNF1A* gene on chromosome 12 lead to abnormal insulin secretion and lower the renal threshold for glucose, which results in lifelong glycosuria. Affected patients typically develop postprandial hyperglycemia before development of overt diabetes. Patients with *HNF1A* pathogenic variants are generally markedly sensitive to the hypoglycemic effects of sulfonylureas, and many patients can be initially treated with this class of medications. Eventually, many patients with MODY 3 require insulin treatment. Patients with MODY 3 develop microvascular and macrovascular complications, similarly to patients with type 1 and type 2 diabetes.

The woman in this vignette has MODY 3 and is late in the second trimester of pregnancy. Despite dietary treatment, she has developed fasting hyperglycemia, as well as hyperglycemia, after the evening meal. Appropriate glucose goals in pregnant women are more stringent than in nonpregnant women in order to reduce the risk of complications, including macrosomia, hyperbilirubinemia, and hypoglycemia in the neonate at birth. Both the American Diabetes Association and the American College of Obstetricians and Gynecologists recommend the following glucose goals during pregnancy in women with pregestational diabetes:

Fasting glucose ≤95 mg/dL (≤5.3 mmol/L)
Premeal glucose levels ≤100 mg/dL (≤5.6 mmol/L)
One-hour postprandial glucose levels ≤140 mg/dL (≤7.8 mmol/L)
Two-hour postprandial glucose levels ≤120 mg/dL (≤6.7 mmol/L)

Dietary treatment in this pregnant patient has been appropriate until now. However, the stress of pregnancy has led to elevated fasting and postprandial glucose levels and diet alone is inadequate to control glucose levels (thus, Answer E is incorrect). Of the options available, starting NPH insulin at bedtime and insulin aspart before the evening meal (Answer D) is the best treatment. Starting either NPH at bedtime alone (Answer A) or insulin aspart before the evening meal (Answer C) would not be adequate in this case. There are limited long-term data on the safety of insulin degludec (a newer long-acting basal insulin) in pregnancy. Therefore, starting insulin degludec (Answer B) is not the best choice.

Given that this patient has an *HNF1A* pathogenic variant, some clinicians would consider treatment with glyburide during pregnancy. However, glyburide was not listed as an option in this vignette.

Educational Objective

Describe the characteristics of the most common forms of monogenic diabetes and counsel women with diabetes about appropriate glucose treatment goals during pregnancy.

UpToDate Topic Review(s)

Classification of diabetes mellitus and genetic diabetic syndromes

Reference(s)

Thanabalasingham G, Owen KR. Diagnosis and management of maturity onset diabetes of the young (MODY). *BMJ*. 2011;343:d6044. PMID: 22012810

Naylor R, Philipson LH. Who should have genetic testing for maturity-onset diabetes of the young? *Clin Endocrinol (Oxf)*. 2011;75(4):422-426. PMID: 21521318

Management of Diabetes in Pregnancy. American Diabetes Association Standards of Medical Care in Diabetes-2017. American Diabetes Association. *Diabetes Care*. 2017;40(Suppl 1):S114-S119. PMID: 21521318

ACOG Committee on Practice Bulletins. ACOG Practice Bulletin. Clinical management guidelines for obstetrician-gynecologists. Number 60, March 2005. Pregestational diabetes mellitus. *Obstet Gynecol*. 2005;105(3):675-685. PMID: 15738045

111 ANSWER: A) Refer for medical nutrition therapy

The patient in this vignette presents for management of elevated triglyceride levels and cardiovascular risk. Elevated triglyceride levels are common and often occur in conjunction with other metabolic abnormalities associated with increased cardiovascular disease risk. On the basis of the triglyceride levels, hypertriglyceridemia can be classified as mild (triglycerides <200 mg/dL [<2.26 mmol/L]), moderate (200-999 mg/dL [2.26-11.29 mmol/L]), or severe (>1000 mg/dL [>11.30 mmol/L]). Hypertriglyceridemia of any degree results from a combination of genetic factors and secondary nongenetic factors, which determine the severity of the phenotype. In the presence of genetic susceptibility, secondary factors contributing to increases in serum triglycerides include weight gain, physical inactivity, excess alcohol intake, initiation of therapy with certain drugs (β-adrenergic blockers, thiazides, estrogen), and uncontrolled type 2 diabetes mellitus. The common forms of hypertriglyceridemia emerge as adults get older, become overweight and sedentary, and develop insulin resistance as commonly seen in the metabolic syndrome and type 2 diabetes. Recent genetic studies implicate elevated triglycerides as a causal factor for development of atherosclerosis; however, disentangling the involvement of low HDL cholesterol is difficult.

Lifestyle therapy, including dietary counseling to achieve appropriate diet composition, physical activity, and a program to achieve weight reduction in overweight and obese individuals is the initial treatment of mild to moderate hypertriglyceridemia. Much of the increase in serum triglycerides that occurs in adult life is caused by weight gain, lack of exercise, and a diet rich in simple carbohydrates and sugar-sweetened beverages. Weight loss is one of the most important and effective approaches to lowering triglyceride levels, regardless of the method used to achieve it. Reducing the intake of simple carbohydrates and increasing physical activity are essential. Thus, referral for medical nutrition therapy (Answer A) is the first step and the best choice for this patient before starting drug therapy.

Statins (Answer B) are primarily LDL-cholesterol–lowering agents, but they can cause modest dosage-dependent triglyceride reductions (10%-15%). Statins may be useful for the treatment of moderate hypertriglyceridemia when indicated to modify cardiovascular risk. High-intensity and potent statins, such as atorvastatin, 80 mg daily, or rosuvastatin, 40 mg daily, can lower plasma triglycerides by 25% to 30%. In this patient, drug therapy should be offered after lifestyle therapy is attempted.

Long-chain marine omega-3 fatty acids (Answer C) (eicosapentaenoic acid, C20:5n-3 [EPA] and docosahexaenoic acid, C22:6n-3 [DHA]) lower fasting and postprandial triglyceride levels in a dosage-dependent fashion. Approximately 3 to 4 g daily of EPA plus DHA are necessary to reduce hypertriglyceridemia by 20% to 50%. HDL cholesterol is mildly increased by about 5%. With reductions of triglyceride levels, there can be increased levels of LDL cholesterol due to increased conversion of VLDL to LDL. To date, use of high-dosage omega-3 fatty acids in patients with hypertriglyceridemia has not shown consistent beneficial cardiovascular outcomes. These agents are not first-line therapy, and there is no indication at this time.

Levothyroxine (Answer D) is indicated in clinical hypothyroidism. Hypothyroidism should always be considered in individuals with dyslipidemias. The patient in this vignette has a TSH value that is slightly above the upper normal limit, which implies subclinical thyroid disease. However, she is asymptomatic and there is no indication for starting levothyroxine replacement therapy at this time. Hypothyroidism has minimal to no effect on triglyceride levels. Untreated hypothyroidism can result in increased total and LDL-cholesterol levels, occasionally to very high levels as seen in familial hypercholesterolemia.

Fenofibrate (Answer E) is the drug of choice in patients with severe hypertriglyceridemia and should be considered in patients with moderate hypertriglyceridemia. The lipid-modifying effects of fibrates are mediated via interaction with peroxisome proliferator–activated receptor α. Fibrates decrease triglyceride levels by 30% to 50% and sometimes increase HDL cholesterol. In patients with high triglyceride levels, LDL-cholesterol levels may increase, whereas in mild hypertriglyceridemia, LDL-cholesterol levels may decrease. There is inconsistency in the evidence base for cardiovascular risk reduction using fibrates. The primary indication for fibrates as monotherapy is to decrease the risk of pancreatitis in the setting of severe hypertriglyceridemia.

This woman meets the criteria for the metabolic syndrome based on levels of triglycerides, HDL cholesterol, and fasting glucose. Her BMI is 27.9 kg/m^2, which puts her in the overweight category using criteria for persons of white ancestry. In persons of Asian ancestry, a BMI greater than 27.5 kg/m^2 is considered obese. This patient was encouraged to pursue lifestyle modification, and with weight loss, her triglycerides decreased to less than 250 mg/dL (<2.82 mmol/L).

Educational Objective
Manage moderate to severe hypertriglyceridemia in the absence of diabetes mellitus.

UpToDate Topic Review(s)
Hypertriglyceridemia

Reference(s)

Duntas LH, Brenta G. The effect of thyroid disorders on lipid levels and metabolism. *Med Clin North Am*. 2012;96(2):269-281. PMID: 22443975

Reiner Z. Hypertriglyceridaemia and risk of coronary artery disease. *Nat Rev Cardiol*. 2017;14(7):401-411. PMID: 28300080

112 ANSWER: A) Complete tumor resection

Anaplastic thyroid cancer is a malignancy with a dismal prognosis. Although recent studies have shown some improvement in survival with aggressive multimodality therapy, mean survival is only approximately 1 year. Several studies have examined outcomes based on patient characteristics, tumor characteristics, and therapy used. However, because of small patient numbers and lack of randomized controlled trials, many analyses provide divergent results. Some observations can, nevertheless, be made. With regard to patient characteristics, male sex and older age are negative prognostic indicators in some, but not all, studies.

Regarding tumor characteristics, anaplastic thyroid cancer is thought to arise from differentiated thyroid cancer that has progressively accumulated chromosomal alterations. However, due to the multiple pathogenic variants that may be present and the heterogeneity of the pathogenic variants among patients, targeted therapy has not yet been developed, although it is likely to be available in the future. Common pathogenic variants seen in anaplastic thyroid cancer include those in the *TP53*, *RAS*, and *BRAF* genes. None of these pathogenic variants, including the presence of *BRAF* pathogenic variants, has yet been linked to prognosis (thus, Answer D is incorrect). As anaplastic thyroid cancer arises from well-differentiated thyroid cancers, it is common to see areas of papillary or follicular thyroid cancer within anaplastic thyroid cancer. Although some studies suggest that a predominantly well-differentiated thyroid cancer with small areas of anaplastic transformation may have a better outcome than tumors that are largely anaplastic, most studies do not show improved outcomes if there are small areas of coexisting differentiated thyroid cancer in the setting of anaplastic carcinoma (thus, Answer B is incorrect).

Anaplastic thyroid cancer can have several different histologic growth patterns. These include spindle-cell pattern, pleomorphic giant-cell pattern, and squamoid pattern. Although some study findings suggest that the histologic subtype may have prognostic significance, most do not (thus, Answer C is incorrect). Data regarding the impact of tumor size on patient prognosis vary. Some studies suggest a worse prognosis for tumors larger than 5 or 7 cm, while others do not. However, a tumor smaller than 5 cm is not the most significant prognostic indicator (thus, Answer E is incorrect).

Advanced tumor stage and metastatic disease at presentation adversely affect prognosis. Most studies show a beneficial effect of complete tumor resection (Answer A). Radiation therapy and chemotherapy can then be used. Findings from a recent study suggest that the best outcomes result from aggressive "trimodal" therapy consisting of surgery, radiation, and chemotherapy. Patients receiving such therapy at one institution had a survival of 22 months vs 6.5 months in those who received dual therapy with radiation and chemotherapy.

Educational Objective

Explain the influence of tumor characteristics and tumor resection on survival in patients with anaplastic thyroid cancer.

UpToDate Topic Review(s)

Anaplastic thyroid cancer

Reference(s)

Bonhomme B, Godbert Y, Perot G, et al. Molecular pathology of anaplastic thyroid carcinomas: a retrospective study of 144 cases. *Thyroid*. 2017;27(5):682-692. PMID: 28351340

Molinaro E, Romei C, Biagini A, et al. Anaplastic thyroid carcinoma: from clinicopathology to genetics and advanced therapies. *Nat Rev Endocrinol*. 2017;13(11): 644-660. PMID: 28707679

Rao SN, Zafereo M, Dadu R, et al. Patterns of treatment failure in anaplastic thyroid carcinoma. *Thyroid*. 2017;27(5):672-681. PMID: 28068873

Smallridge RC, Ain KB, Asa SL, et al; American Thyroid Association Anaplastic Thyroid Cancer Guidelines Taskforce. American Thyroid Association guidelines for management of patients with anaplastic thyroid cancer. *Thyroid*. 2012;22(11):1104-1139. PMID: 23130564

Sugitani I, Miyauchi A, Sugino K, Okamoto T, Yoshida A, Suzuki S. Prognostic factors and treatment outcomes for anaplastic thyroid carcinoma: ATC Research Consortium of Japan cohort study of 677 patients. *World J Surg*. 2012;36(6):1247-1254. PMID: 22311136

113 ANSWER: A) Spironolactone

Nonclassic congenital adrenal hyperplasia (CAH) due to 21-hydroxylase deficiency is the cause of hirsutism in about 4% of cases worldwide and is commonly misdiagnosed as polycystic ovary syndrome. Especially in a woman with severe hirsutism, it is appropriate to screen for this condition by measuring 17-hydroxyprogesterone, ideally tested in the early morning in the early follicular phase if a woman has regular menses. In this vignette, the random 17-hydroxyprogesterone was only mildly elevated, which led to the need for a diagnostic stimulation test. The diagnosis of nonclassic CAH is made with any 17-hydroxyprogesterone value greater than 1000 ng/dL (>30.3 nmol/L). If this patient's random 17-hydroxyprogesterone level had been similar to the baseline value drawn during her stimulation test, the stimulation test would not have been necessary. Cortisol levels are simultaneously tested to determine whether there might be sufficient 21-hydroxylase enzymatic impairment to decrease adrenal reserve.

Because treatment with corticosteroids in nonclassic CAH often leads to adverse effects of cortisol excess (weight gain and metabolic consequences), they should be reserved for consideration in women presenting with infertility and adolescent girls with precocious puberty or rapidly accelerating bone age. Especially in this patient with severe insulin resistance, dyslipidemia, and strong family history of type 2 diabetes, the use of corticosteroids would be more likely to cause harm.

Corticosteroid treatment in classic CAH should ideally prevent the morning rise in ACTH to more effectively decrease 17-hydroxyprotesterone, androgen, and progesterone concentrations that interfere with ovulation and implantation. For this reason, longer-acting corticosteroids such as dexamethasone, prednisone, or prednisolone, might be prescribed in a "reverse diurnal" pattern with the higher dose at night. However, in nonclassic CAH, studies have shown that shorter-acting and physiologic hydrocortisone therapy can improve ovulatory frequency. Compared with hydrocortisone, dexamethasone (Answer D) is typically associated with more adverse effects of cortisol excess and would need to be stopped as soon as pregnancy is diagnosed because it can cross the placenta into the fetal circulation. For patients with classic CAH, hydrocortisone with a reverse diurnal pattern with higher doses at night (Answer B) might be used to prevent the morning ACTH rise that increases 17-hydroxyprogesterone and conversion to androgen precursors. This regimen has not been used specifically in studies of nonclassic CAH.

Although lowering insulin concentrations can improve hyperandrogenemia, metformin (Answer E) has not been shown to have a greater effect on hirsutism than oral contraceptives or antiandrogen therapy or in combination with oral contraceptives. Metformin could be considered for the prevention of type 2 diabetes in this woman who has risk factors for developing diabetes (prediabetes and significant family history of type 2 diabetes), as studied in the Diabetes Prevention Program trial. However, lifestyle changes lead to greater reductions in the incidence of type 2 diabetes than does metformin, even in that trial.

Oral contraceptives are first-line therapy for the treatment of hirsutism in premenopausal women who are not planning to conceive due to the multiple effects of suppressing LH secretion and ovarian androgen production while also increasing hepatic production of SHBG, which will lower serum free androgen concentrations. Because this patient is already on oral contraceptives, the addition of antiandrogens would be the next step. Spironolactone (Answer A) is an aldosterone antagonist that also acts as a competitive inhibitor of the androgen receptor. Spironolactone for the treatment of hirsutism can be initiated at a dosage of 50 mg twice daily. If the desired effect is not seen after 6 months, the dosage could be increased to 100 mg twice daily. After initiation or change in dosage, potassium should be tested to screen for hyperkalemia, although this is rare with normal renal function. Women should be counseled to avoid trying to conceive while on spironolactone, and the use of oral contraceptives or a progesterone-releasing intrauterine device would also prevent the other potential adverse effect, irregular spotting or menstrual bleeding.

Flutamide (Answer C) is a potent antiandrogen developed for the treatment of prostate cancer that interferes with androgen uptake by cells and blocks androgen receptor binding at target tissues. It can be as effective as spironolactone for the treatment of hirsutism. However, because of flutamide's association with hepatic toxicity (which can be fatal), spironolactone is a better choice.

Educational Objective
Determine the best treatment strategy for hirsutism in a woman with nonclassic congenital adrenal hyperplasia.

UpToDate Topic Review(s)
Diagnosis and treatment of nonclassic (late-onset) congenital adrenal hyperplasia due to 21-hydroxylase deficiency

Reference(s)

Carmina E, Dewailly D, Escobar-Morreale HF, et al. Non-classic congenital adrenal hyperplasia due to 21-hydroxylase deficiency revisited: an update with a special focus on adolescent and adult women. *Hum Reprod Update*. 2017;23(5):580-599. PMID: 28582566

Martin KA, Anderson RR, Chang RJ, et al. Evaluation and treatment of hirsutism in premenopausal women: an Endocrine Society clinical practice guideline. *J Clin Endocrinol Metab*. 2018;103(4):1233-1257. PMID: 29522147

114 ANSWER: E) Observation with occasional monitoring of serum thyroglobulin and neck ultrasonography

The follicular variant of papillary thyroid carcinoma (FVPTC) is the most common, accounting for approximately 30% of all papillary thyroid carcinomas (PTC). FVPTC was previously considered clinically to be a single entity with a biology that straddled the classic PTC and follicular thyroid carcinoma. These tumors were subclassified into 2 subgroups according to their growth pattern: infiltrative (IFVPTV) and encapsulated (EFVPTC), the latter being further subdivided as invasive if capsular and/or vascular invasion is present or noninvasive if the tumor lacks these features. Noninvasive EFVPTC is histologically similar to follicular adenoma but with nuclear features of PTC. Invasive EFVPTC resembles follicular carcinoma with nuclear features of PTC.

The incidence of thyroid cancer has increased significantly in most countries worldwide and has tripled in the United States over the past 3 decades (from 4.9 per 100,000 in 1975 to 14.7 per 100,000 in 2013). The rise in incidence is mainly attributed to an increase in PTC diagnosis secondary to increased imaging, increased detection of incidental thyroid tumors, and introduction of high-sensitivity ultrasonography detecting small subcentimeter lesions. Mortality rates, however, have remained static during the same period, and the problem of overtreating indolent tumors has been increasingly recognized. The long-term prognosis of EFVPTC is nearly universally excellent, supporting the notion that these tumors are indolent. In 2016, the findings from an international working group who had re-examined the terminology for encapsulated FVPTC were published. The term noninvasive follicular thyroid neoplasm with papillary-like nuclear features (NIFTP) was introduced to recognize the indolent behavior of noninvasive FVPTC. By eliminating the word "carcinoma," the principal intent is to decrease overtreatment of these tumors. Subsequent studies have confirmed the indolent behavior of this tumor clinically, and the term has been included in the most recent World Health Organization Classification of thyroid tumors (fourth edition) and has been endorsed by the American Thyroid Association.

The histologic diagnosis of NIFTP is stringent: the tumor must demonstrate encapsulation or circumscription, a purely follicular architecture, and the presence of nuclear features of papillary thyroid carcinoma, while lacking capsular and vascular invasion, a significant component of solid growth, and high-grade features (increased mitotic activity and necrosis). To ensure that these inclusion and exclusion criteria are met, the tumor should be sampled extensively, and the entire lesional capsule should be submitted for microscopic scrutiny. A nuclear scoring system was presented to provide criteria for the assessment of nuclear features that could assist in the diagnosis of NIFTP. In this system, nuclear features are grouped into 3 categories: size and shape (nuclear enlargement/overlapping/ crowding and elongation), nuclear membrane irregularities (irregular contours, grooves and pseudo-inclusions), and chromatin characteristics (clearing with margination/glassy nuclei). For each feature, a tumor can receive 1 point, and tumors scoring 0 or 1 are considered benign adenomas, whereas those scoring 2 to 3 are classified as NIFTP. Exclusion criteria include any capsular or vascular invasion, true papillae (exceeding 1% of the tumor), psammoma bodies, infiltrative interface, coagulative necrosis (except for ischemic FNA biopsy injury), increased mitoses (at least 3 per 10 high-powered field), features of other aggressive PTC variants (tall cell, columnar cell, cribriform-morular, hobnail, diffuse sclerosing, or dedifferentiated), and oncocytic (Hurthle-cell) lesions. The Figure illustrates some of the typical histologic features of NIFTP.

The patient in this vignette presents with a large thyroid nodule that would be classified as being of low suspicion for malignancy on the basis of ultrasonographic criteria (hyperechoic without microcalcification, irregular margin or extrathyroidal extension, or taller than wide shape). FNAB is indicated in such lesions if they are larger than 1.5 cm. Cytologic evaluation has indicated indeterminate findings and this is usually found in patients with NIFTP. Genetically, NIFTP lesions are frequently characterized by *RAS* pathogenic variants, although more rarely the *BRAF* K601E pathogenic variant and gene rearrangements in *PPARG* occur.

While long-term follow-up studies are awaited, it remains unclear how patients with NIFTP should be managed and monitored. On the basis of the low risk for recurrence, the 2015 American Thyroid Association guidelines recommend that thyroid lobectomy is sufficient for such tumors (thus, Answers A and B are incorrect). Remnant ablation is not recommended and since the patient in this vignette has not undergone total thyroidectomy, the administration of an ablative dose of ^{131}I (Answer C) is inappropriate. The TSH target should be 0.5 to 2.0 mIU/L for low-risk differentiated thyroid cancer and within the normal range for benign thyroid lesions (thus, Answer D is incorrect). Until further data are available, occasional monitoring with serum thyroglobulin and neck ultrasonography could be considered (Answer E), although this is not mandatory.

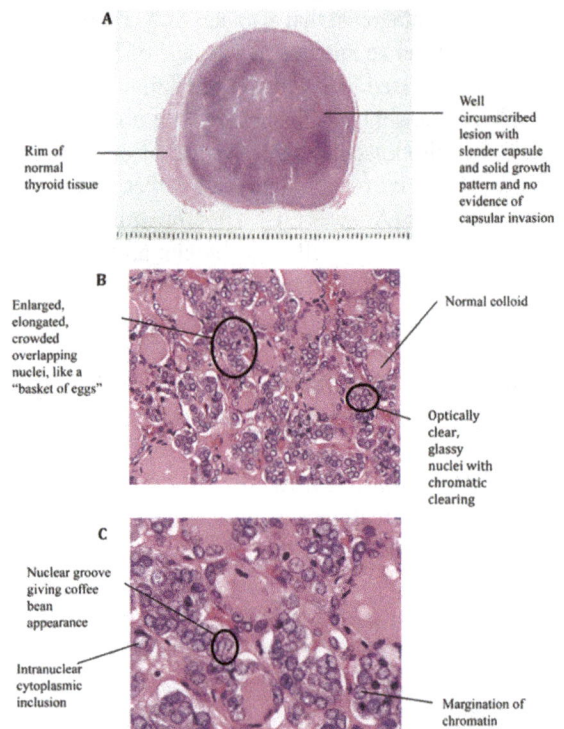

Histologic appearance of noninvasive follicular thyroid neoplasm with papillary-like nuclear features. A) Whole mount section following right hemithyroidectomy. B) Medium-powered hematoxylin and eosin stained section demonstrating nuclear features associated with papillary thyroid carcinoma. C) High-powered hematoxylin and eosin stained section demonstrating nuclear features associated with papillary thyroid carcinoma.

Educational Objective
Guide the management of a noninvasive follicular thyroid neoplasm with papillary-like nuclear features.

UpToDate Review(s)
Follicular thyroid cancer (including Hurthle cell cancer)

Reference(s)

Hung YP, Barletta JA. A user's guide to non-invasive follicular thyroid neoplasm with papillary-like nuclear features (NIFTP). *Histopathology*. 2018;72(1):53-69. PMID: 29239036

Haugen BR, Sawka AM, Alexander EK, et al. American Thyroid Association Guideline on the Management of Thyroid Nodules and Differentiated Thyroid Cancer Task Force Review and Recommendation on the Proposed Renaming of Encapsulated Follicular Variant Papillary Thyroid Carcinoma Without Invasion to Noninvasive Follicular Thyroid Neoplasm with Papillary-Like Nuclear Features. *Thyroid*. 2017;27(4):481-483. PMID: 28114862

Haugen BR, Alexander EK, Bible KC, et al. 2015 American Thyroid Association Management Guidelines for Adult Patients with Thyroid Nodules and Differentiated Thyroid Cancer: the American Thyroid Association Guidelines Task Force on Thyroid Nodules and Differentiated Thyroid Cancer. *Thyroid*. 2016;26(1):1-133. PMID: 26462967

Nikiforov YE, Seethala RR, Tallini G. Nomenclature revision for encapsulated follicular variant of papillary thyroid carcinoma: a paradigm shift to reduce overtreatment of indolent tumors. *JAMA Oncol*. 2016;2(8):1023-1029. PMID: 27078145

115

ANSWER: A) Postprandial glucose

This vignette highlights the ongoing debate regarding the sequence of medications to select in a patient already on metformin monotherapy. Monnier and colleagues studied daytime glucose profiles in 290 patients with type 2 diabetes who had a spectrum of diabetes control based on their hemoglobin A_{1c} levels. The authors found that the higher the hemoglobin A_{1c} level is above 7.0%, the more important the fasting glucose is to overall glycemia. In contrast, as the hemoglobin A_{1c} level approaches 7.0%, the postprandial glucose has a greater influence (*see figure*).

These results were confirmed by Woerle et al. On the basis of these studies, the correct answer is postprandial glucose (Answer A), not fasting glucose (Answers B and C). Although body weight (Answer E) and insulin resistance (Answer D) are important parameters to address, medications to alter these factors are slow in onset and only indirectly lower fasting glucose.

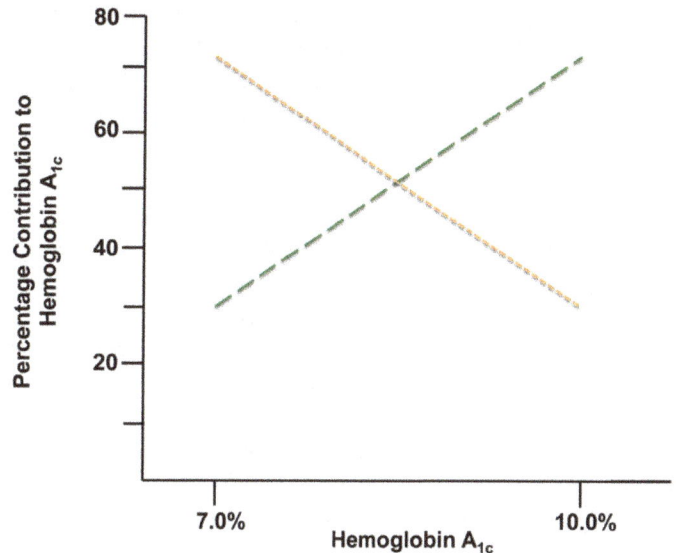

Relative contributions of fasting blood glucose (—) and postprandial glucose (- -) to overall dysglycemia as a function of hemoglobin A_{1c}. See listed references for individuals graphs.

Medications that specifically lower postprandial glucose are acarbose, thiazolidinediones, DPP-4 inhibitors, GLP-1 receptor agonists, meglitinides (eg, repaglinide), or prandial insulin. Any of these agents would be a valid second medication for this patient.

Educational Objective

Determine the most important factors to consider when adding a second diabetes medication to metformin monotherapy in a patient with diabetes mellitus.

UpToDate Topic Review(s)

Initial management of blood glucose in adults with type 2 diabetes mellitus

Reference(s)

Monnier L, Lapinski H, Colette C. Contributions of fasting and postprandial plasma glucose increments to the overall diurnal hyperglycemia of type 2 diabetic patients: variations with increasing levels of HbA(1c). *Diabetes Care*. 2003;26(3):881-885. PMID: 12610053

Woerle HJ, Neumann C, Zschau S, et al. Impact of fasting and postprandial glycemia on overall glycemic control in type 2 diabetes Importance of postprandial glycemia to achieve target HbA1c levels. *Diabetes Res Clin Pract*. 2007;77(2):280-285. PMID: 17240473

116

ANSWER: A) Refer to neuro-ophthalmology

Immunotherapy is being used more often in the treatment of many forms of cancer. Immune checkpoint proteins, such as the cytotoxic T-lymphocyte antigen-4 (CTLA4) and programmed death-1 (PD-1), maintain immune tolerance by down-regulating T-cell signaling. Humanized monoclonal anti-CTLA-4 has been shown to improve survival in metastatic melanoma. However, by reducing immune tolerance, it can cause immune-related adverse events, including rash, colitis, hepatitis, and several endocrinopathies (eg, hypophysitis, thyroiditis, adrenalitis, and insulitis). The most frequent endocrinopathy caused by the anti-CTLA-4 agent ipilimumab is hypophysitis, described in up to 15% of patients treated with this drug. The time to onset of ipilimumab-induced hypophysitis is typically 2 to 4 months (range, 7-20 weeks) after starting therapy. However, delayed presentations can occur. PD-1 inhibitors very rarely cause hypophysitis, but are more likely to cause thyroiditis, typically with a thyrotoxic phase followed by hypothyroidism.

In patients with ipilimumab-induced hypophysitis, MRI images show an enlarged pituitary gland, although such enlargement may be subtle and not obvious when a baseline MRI image is not available. The use of high-dosage glucocorticoids had initially been advocated in all patients with this form of hypophysitis, but it is becoming more clear that even with this treatment, while recovery of pituitary-thyroid and gonadal axes is not uncommon, very few patients are able to discontinue glucocorticoid replacement due to persistent secondary adrenal insufficiency.

Therefore, high-dosage glucocorticoid treatment is generally reserved for patients who have significant mass effect. This patient's headaches have improved and are responding to acetaminophen, and the only indication for high-dosage glucocorticoids would be neuro-ophthalmologic evidence of chiasmatic syndrome. Although the mass on imaging does not seem to cause obvious compression of the chiasm and visual fields are grossly normal, the MRI study is already 2 weeks old, and subtle vision abnormalities may only be picked up by an experienced ophthalmologist. Furthermore, even a normal exam will be useful as baseline for future follow-up. Therefore, referral to neuro-ophthalmology (Answer A) is needed.

A more difficult question is whether this adverse effect should trigger stopping ipilimumab treatment. This possibility must be discussed on a case-by-case basis with the oncologist, weighing the risk of possibly worsening hypophysitis vs the risk of cancer recurrence.

Pituitary metastasis can certainly occur in melanoma, but the temporal relation to ipilimumab and the lack of symptoms of diabetes insipidus (most often present in pituitary metastasis) make this diagnosis unlikely. Therefore, biopsy (Answer B) is not necessary now. As mentioned, high-dosage prednisone (Answer D) would only be needed for mass effect symptoms. Rituximab (Answer C) (a genetically engineered chimeric murine/human monoclonal IgG1 kappa antibody directed against the CD20 antigen) has been used occasionally in cases of primary lymphocytic hypophysitis not responsive to glucocorticoids, but it has never been used in immune checkpoint inhibitor–induced hypophysitis. Similarly, intravenous immunoglobulins (Answer E) have no role in treating this disease.

Educational Objective
Determine when high-dosage glucocorticoids are appropriate in the setting of ipilimumab-induced hypophysitis and when it is appropriate to refer to neuro-ophthalmology to assess for chiasmatic syndrome.

UpToDate Topic Review(s)
Patient selection criteria and toxicities associated with checkpoint inhibitor immunotherapy

Reference(s)

Torino F, Corsello SM, Salvatori R. Endocrinological side-effects of immune checkpoint inhibitors. *Curr Opin Oncol*. 2016;28(4):278-287. PMID: 27136136

Faje AT, Sullivan R, Lawrence D, Tritos NA, Fadden R, Klibanski A, Nachtigall L. Ipilimumab-induced hypophysitis: a detailed longitudinal analysis in a large cohort of patients with metastatic melanoma. *J Clin Endocrinol Metab*. 2014;99(11):4078-4085. PMID: 25078147

He W, Chen F, Dalm B, Kirby PA, Greenlee JD. Metastatic involvement of the pituitary gland: a systematic review with pooled individual patient data analysis. *Pituitary*. 2015;18(1):159-168. PMID: 24445565

117   ANSWER: E) Ophthalmoscopy and fundus examination by an eye specialist

In the Diabetes Control and Complications Trial (DCCT), the rate of diabetic retinopathy in patients with less than a 5-year duration of disease was about 50%. However, the rate of vision-threatening retinopathy was very low. The American Diabetes Association consensus statement therefore recommends screening for diabetic retinopathy within 5 years for a patient with type 1 diabetes. This should be followed by repeated evaluation every 1 to 2 years if there is minimal to no baseline retinopathy. Those with more significant disease should be followed more closely.

Adherence to national guidelines is about 50% to 60%. The screening rates are lower in rural areas and among minority populations. One study in North Carolina revealed that only 25% of eligible patients underwent screening in rural areas. Because screening and intervention can decrease the threat of significant vision loss by 98%, efforts to improve the screening rates are essential.

There is increasing interest in telemedicine technologies. To improve access to care, outreach clinics have been established that have (1) retinal photography, (2) a camera operated by a health care worker, (3) nondilated (nonmydriatic) examination, and (4) images interpreted at a distant site by a specialist. Although promising, these processes have not been standardized. Sensitivity and specificity when the images are gradable are reported to be as high as 98% and 100%, respectively. A meta-analysis of telemedicine technology showed specificity to be lower. The sensitivity and specificity for nonmydriatic digital stereoscopic photography (Answer B) in nonresearch settings remains unclear. The American Diabetes Association consensus statement still recommends a direct funduscopic examination (Answer E) for initial screening, and this is the best recommendation for this patient.

Because many patients require screening for diabetic retinopathy (according to NHANES 2008 data, 5 million patients have diabetic retinopathy, and there are an estimated 32 million annual evaluations required), there is increasing interest in automated technology (Answer C). Deep-learning algorithms are being studied to identify patients who may have "referable disease." Large sets of retinal images are used to train algorithms to identify moderate to severe retinal disease. These algorithms are then tested on other data sets. Although promising, the role of these algorithms as widespread initial screening methods is unclear.

Fluorescein angiography (Answer A) and optic coherence CT (Answer D) are specialized techniques that would not be useful as initial screening methods. Fluorescein angiography may be useful for assessment of retinal vein occlusion or extent of neovascularization. Optical coherence CT offers high-resolution imaging of the retina. It is useful in defining areas of edema and assessing retinal nerve integrity.

Educational Objective
Recommend initial screening options for diabetic retinopathy.

UpToDate Topic Review(s)
Diabetic retinopathy: Screening

Reference(s)

Solomon SD, Chew E, Duh EJ, et al. Diabetic retinopathy: a position statement by the American Diabetes Association. *Diabetes Care*. 2017;40(3):412-418. PMID: 28223445

Jani P, Forbes L, Choudhury A, Preisser JS, Viera AJ, Garg S. Evaluation of diabetic retinal screening and factors for ophthalmology referral in a telemedicine network. *JAMA Ophthalmol*. 2017;135(7):706-714. PMID: 28520833

Gulshan V, Peng L, Coram M, et al. Development and validation of a deep learning algorithm for detection of diabetic retinopathy in retinal fundus photographs. *JAMA*. 2016;316(22):2402-2410. PMID: 27898976

118 ANSWER: E) Add alirocumab

This patient presents for secondary prevention of progressive atherosclerotic cardiovascular disease. She has premature cardiovascular disease, having undergone surgical intervention at age 45 years, which suggests an underlying genetic dyslipidemia. She also has type 2 diabetes. When adequate LDL-cholesterol reduction is not achieved in an individual at very high cardiovascular high risk, such as this patient, additional therapy should be considered.

Alirocumab (Answer E) belongs to a new class of injectable drugs called PCSK9 inhibitors that work in conjunction with statins to significantly reduce LDL-cholesterol levels. It is a human monoclonal antibody that binds to PCSK9 and inhibits its interaction with the LDL receptor, resulting in increased receptor recycling and LDL clearance. Accumulating evidence suggests that PCSK9 inhibitors effectively (up to 60% from baseline without or with statin therapy) and safely lower LDL-cholesterol levels in individuals taking statins, without significant adverse effects. The first large cardiovascular outcome study of PCSK9 inhibitors, The FOURIER study (Further Cardiovascular Outcomes Research With PCSK9 Inhibition in Patients With Elevated Risk), evaluated the effect of evolocumab on major adverse cardiac events in individuals with atherosclerotic cardiovascular disease taking maximal tolerated statin dosage over the course of 2.2 years. Addition of evolocumab resulted in a 15% decrease in primary cardiovascular endpoints. A cardiovascular outcomes trial on alirocumab has been recently completed, and early reports suggest a reduction in cardiovascular outcomes in individuals with acute coronary syndromes. Currently, PCSK9 inhibitors are approved for use in patients with known cardiovascular disease who are on a maximum tolerated statin dosage and need further LDL-cholesterol lowering due to the presence of additional cardiovascular risk factors. PCSK9 inhibitor therapy does not appear to affect glycemic control. Despite the higher cost of PCSK9 therapy and burdensome prior authorization process, this patient should be offered treatment with alirocumab in combination with statin therapy due to her high-risk status. Fibrate therapy should then be discontinued, as there is no current evidence for benefit in combination with PCSK9 inhibitors.

This patient has progressive cardiovascular disease and needs further intervention to manage risk. Thus, no change in therapy (Answer A) is not the best choice. Atorvastatin is considered a high-potency statin because it can lower LDL cholesterol by more than 50% at higher dosages. On average, every doubling of the statin dose only provides an additional 6% reduction in LDL cholesterol ("rule of 6"). Although increasing the atorvastatin dosage to

80 mg daily (Answer B) could be beneficial to enable further LDL-cholesterol lowering, this approach would most likely not be sufficient in this woman with recurrent cardiovascular disease.

Ezetimibe (Answer C) is an intestinal cholesterol absorption inhibitor that localizes to the brush border of the intestine by binding to the Niemann-Pick C1-like 1 (NPC1L1) receptor. It inhibits the delivery of intestinal cholesterol to the liver by blocking absorption of both cholesterol and dietary sterols. The resulting decreased hepatic cholesterol leads to up-regulation of hepatic LDL receptors and increased clearance of cholesterol from the blood. Ezetimibe has modest LDL-cholesterol–lowering effects as a single agent, but in combination with statins, it results in up to a 25% LDL-cholesterol reduction. Current limited evidence suggests benefit for secondary prevention of cardiovascular disease in individuals at high risk based on results from the IMPROVE-IT study. Addition of ezetimibe would enable further decrease in LDL cholesterol, but more potent lipid-lowering therapy is indicated in this patient at high risk.

Nicotinic acid or niacin (Answer D) can decrease triglycerides and LDL-cholesterol levels and increase HDL-cholesterol levels. Early trials in the pre-statin era used immediate-release niacin monotherapy in men with previous myocardial infarction and showed reduced cardiovascular morbidity and mortality. However, 2 large cardiovascular disease outcome trials (AIM-HIGH [Atherothrombosis Intervention in Metabolic Syndrome with Low HDL/High Triglycerides: Impact on Global Health Outcomes] and HPS2-THRIVE [Heart Protection Study 2-Treatment of HDL to Reduce the Incidence of Vascular Events]), both with the use of extended-release niacin formulations added to statins, failed to show clinical benefit. These were conducted in individuals with known atherosclerotic cardiovascular disease on statin therapy to raise HDL cholesterol and highlighted several safety effects of niacin. Therefore, niacin cannot be recommended for this patient.

Educational Objective

Manage the care of a patient with progressive coronary artery disease who is at very high risk.

UpToDate Topic Review(s)

Management of elevated low density lipoprotein-cholesterol (LDL-C) in primary prevention of cardiovascular disease

Reference(s)

Sabatine MS, Giugliano RP, Keech AC, et al; FOURIER Steering Committee and Investigators. *N Engl J Med*. 2017;376(18):1713-1722. PMID: 28304224

Lloyd-Jones DM, Morris PB, Ballantyne CM, et al. 2017 focused update of the 2016 ACC Expert Consensus Decision Pathway on the Role of Non-Statin Therapies for LDL-Cholesterol Lowering in the Management of Atherosclerotic Cardiovascular Disease Risk: a report of the American College of Cardiology Task Force on Expert Consensus Decision Pathways. *J Am Coll Cardiol*. 2017;70(14):1785-1822. PMID: 28886926

119 ANSWER: A) Polycystic ovary syndrome

This patient presents with mild hirsutism and irregular menses or oligomenorrhea. Importantly, the symptoms are new (or acquired) since her mid-20s and her blood pressure is normal. Without a clear sense of the familial or genetic predisposition for body hair growth in this patient's family, it can be debated whether her clinical manifestations are severe enough to be consistent with hirsutism or clinical hyperandrogenism. However, she has a slightly elevated DHEA-S level, suggesting biochemical hyperandrogenism. The differential diagnosis is broad and includes neoplastic and functional etiologies of the ovary and adrenal. Adrenal and ovarian tumors are unlikely given the very mild elevation in DHEA-S, the normal total testosterone, and the absence of more marked virilization on clinical examination.

The biochemical studies show normal total testosterone and prolactin levels, gonadotropin levels in the reference range with an approximately 2:1 LH-to-FSH ratio, and a normal morning cortisol level and appropriate stimulation to cosyntropin. The morning 17-hydroxyprogesterone level is normal, and following stimulation with cosyntropin, there is little to no increase in this metabolite. Collectively, these findings exclude adrenal insufficiency and nonclassic 21-hydroxylase deficiency (Answer B). The absence of hypertension most likely excludes 11β-hydroxylase deficiency (Answer C) since it manifests with hyperandrogenemia and excess deoxycorticosterone, resulting in excessive mineralocorticoid activity. 17α-Hydroxylase deficiency (Answer D) also presents with excessive deoxycorticosterone, resulting in excessive mineralocorticoid activity and androgen deficiency.

3β-Hydroxysteroid dehydrogenase deficiency (Answer E) is a very rare form of congenital adrenal hyperplasia that can manifest with glucocorticoid and mineralocorticoid deficiencies and hyperandrogenemia in females. In cases of mild androgen excess such as this one, the nonclassic form of 3β-hydroxysteroid dehydrogenase deficiency is often considered; however, polycystic ovary syndrome (Answer A) is by far the more common diagnosis in these situations and true nonclassic 3β-hydroxysteroid dehydrogenase deficiency is extremely rare. Most patients with late-onset 3β-hydroxysteroid dehydrogenase deficiency present with abnormal pubarche and irregular menses and virilization in their teenage years at the latest. The diagnostic test of choice is demonstrating elevated 17-pregnenalone, particularly following a cosyntropin stimulation test where levels of 17-pregnenalone should exceed 5000 ng/dL (>150 nmol/L). Although this patient had a notable increase in 17-pregnenalone levels with cosyntropin stimulation, the increase was far less than the diagnostic threshold and this milder increase can frequently be seen in polycystic ovary syndrome. Studies have shown that some forms of polycystic ovary syndrome may present with a mild, nongenomic 3β-hydroxysteroid dehydrogenase insufficiency. Therefore, mild elevations of 17-pregnenalone should not be ascribed to congenital or genetic 3β-hydroxysteroid dehydrogenase deficiency.

This patient's mild hyperandrogenism, oligomenorrhea, and heightened LH secretion are consistent with the diagnosis of polycystic ovary syndrome and the exclusion of other potential diagnoses, such as congenital adrenal hyperplasia, provides reassurance that it is the diagnosis of exclusion.

Educational Objective
Distinguish between polycystic ovary syndrome and 3β-hydroxysteroid dehydrogenase deficiency on the basis of clinical and laboratory findings.

UpToDate Topic Review(s)
Diagnosis of polycystic ovary syndrome in adults

Reference(s)
Carbunaru G, Prasad P, Scoccia B, et al. The hormonal phenotype of nonclassic 3 beta-hydroxysteroid dehydrogenase (HSD3B) deficiency in hyperandrogenic females is associated with insulin-resistant polycystic ovary syndrome and is not variant of inherited HSD3B2 deficiency. *J Clin Endocrinol Metab*. 2004; 89(2):783–794. PMID: 14764797

Mermejo LM, Elias LL, Marui S, Moreira AC, Mendonca BB, de Castro M. Refining hormonal diagnosis of type II 3beta-hydroxysteroid dehydrogenase deficiency in patients with premature pubarche and hirsutism based on HSD3B2 genotyping. *J Clin Endocrinol Metab*. 2005;90(3):1287-1293. PMID: 15585552

120 ANSWER: B) Insulin detemir

This patient exhibits poor glycemic control, evidence of microvascular complications, and, most importantly, symptoms of both hyperglycemia and catabolism. In this circumstance, initiation of insulin (Answer B) is the best next step both for improving glucose control and providing symptomatic relief. In light of the recent 2018 American Diabetes Association Standards of Medical Care in Diabetes and the patient's hemoglobin A_{1c} level, it maybe reasonable to initiate dual or triple therapy with a noninsulin agent, especially with an agent that has proven cardiovascular benefit. However, in the presence of polyuria and unintentional weight loss suggesting catabolism, the combination of liraglutide and empagliflozin (Answer E) is not the best choice. If the patient did not have catabolic symptoms, both medications in combination may have been reasonable, assuming no other contraindications. This patient had pyelonephritis, making either empagliflozin alone (Answer C) or in combination with liraglutide an incorrect choice. Individually, liraglutide (Answer D) or empagliflozin would not achieve a reasonable glycemic target (hemoglobin A_{1c} <7% [<53 mmol/mol], for example). If her hemoglobin A_{1c} level were greater than 10% (>86 mmol/mol) or her blood glucose value were greater than 300 mg/dL (>16.7 mmol/L), it would be reasonable to initiate combination insulin injectable treatment. Glimepiride (Answer A) would be a poor choice as it does not provide adequate glycemic lowering and has no known cardiovascular benefit. Indeed, data suggest sulfonylureas may be associated with increased death from cardiac causes.

Educational Objective
In a patient with type 2 diabetes mellitus, determine when addition of insulin is a better choice than other noninsulin agents to achieve glycemic targets.

UpToDate Topic Review(s)
Insulin therapy in type 2 diabetes mellitus

Reference(s)
Standards of medical care in diabetes-2018. *Diabetes Care*. 2018;41(Suppl 1):S1-S153.

ENDOCRINE SELF-ASSESSMENT PROGRAM 2019

Part III

This question-mapping index groups question topics according to the 8 umbrella sections of ESAP (Adrenal, Bone-Calcium, Diabetes, Lipid-Obesity, Pituitary, Reproduction [Female], Reproduction [Male], and Thyroid). Relevant **question numbers** *follow each topic.*

ADRENAL

Adrenal incidentaloma: **86**
Adrenal insufficiency: **55, 92**
Adrenal venous sampling: **79**
Catecholamine-secreting tumors: **6, 26**
Cushing syndrome: **92, 104**
Hirsutism: **119**
HIV therapy: **92**
Hypertension: **1, 71, 79**
Myelolipoma: **86**
Pheochromocytoma: **6, 26**
Polycystic ovary syndrome: **119**
Primary aldosteronism: **1, 71, 79**
Radiographic characteristics of malignancy: **20, 46**
Salivary cortisol testing: **104**

CALCIUM-BONE

ALPL gene: **67**
Bariatric surgery: **51**
Chronic kidney disease–mineral and bone disorder: **12**
COL1A1, COL1A2 genes: **62**
Denosumab: **33**
Dual-energy x-ray absorptiometry: **17**
Fibrous dysplasia: **83**
Hypercalcemia: **58, 77**
Hypercalciuria: **90**
Hyperparathyroidism: **51**
Hyperparathyroidism, primary: **37, 58**
Hypocalcemia: **29, 105**
Hypomagnesemia: **105**
Hypoparathyroidism: **29**
Hypophosphatasia: **67**
Hypophosphatemia: **67, 94**
Lymphoma: **77**
McCune-Albright syndrome: **83**
Metastatic cancer to bone: **41**
Nephrolithiasis: **54, 90**
Osteogenesis imperfecta: **62**
Osteomalacia: **94, 100**
Osteoporosis: **2, 17, 33, 90, 100**
Paget disease: **41**
Vitamin D deficiency: **100**

DIABETES

Atypical diabetes: **43**
Cardiac ischemia: **87**
Cardiovascular risk: **87**
Continuous glucose monitoring: **3, 57**
Diabetes screening: **95, 103**
Diabetic amyotrophy: **53**
Diabetic ketoacidosis: **69**
Diabetic muscle infarction: **59**
End-stage renal disease: **35, 95**
Exercise: **82**
Factitious hypoglycemia: **49**
Hemoglobin A_{1c}: **9**
HIV treatment: **103**
HNF1A gene: **110**
Hybrid closed-loop insulin pump therapy: **3**
Hypoglycemia: **5, 30, 49, 75, 82**
Insulin therapy: **5, 82, 91, 120**
Insulin, U500: **91**
Insulinoma: **30**
Kidney transplant: **95, 98**
Malnutrition: **13**
Maturity-onset diabetes of the young: **110**
Metformin: **115**
Monogenic diabetes: **38, 110**
Neonatal diabetes: **38**
Neuropathy: **65**
Osteoporosis: **18**
Pancreas transplant: **98**
Posttransplant diabetes mellitus: **95, 98**
Pregnancy: **110**
Retinopathy: **107, 117**
Sickle cell disease: **9**
Type B insulin resistance: **22**
Type 1 diabetes mellitus: **3, 59, 69, 78, 82, 87, 98, 117**
Type 2 diabetes mellitus: **5, 9, 13, 18, 24, 35, 43, 53, 57, 65, 91, 107, 115, 120**

LIPID-OBESITY

Bariatric surgery: **48**
Cardiovascular risk: **8, 23, 42, 60, 74, 111, 118**
Chronic kidney disease: **60**
Contraceptive methods after bariatric surgery: **57**
Coronary artery calcium score: **42**
Diabetes mellitus: **74, 93, 102**
Familial hypercholesterolemia: **84**
Glucagonlike peptide 1 receptor agonists: **93**
Hypercholesterolemia: **84, 102, 118**
Hypertriglyceridemia: **111**
Lipid assessment: **23**
Lipoprotein (a): **8**
Night eating syndrome: **14**
Obesity: **34, 48, 56, 74, 93, 102**
Obesity, pharmacotherapy: **34, 93**
PCSK9 inhibitors: **60, 119**
Pregnancy: **84**
Statin therapy: **42**
Very low-calorie diet: **102**

PITUITARY

Acromegaly: **25, 96**
Apoplexy: **64**
Carcinoid syndrome: **73**
Craniopharyngioma: **7**
Cushing disease: **52**
Diabetes insipidus: **7, 15**
Growth hormone deficiency: **109**
Hypopituitarism: **40, 64, 99**
Hypophysitis: **116**
Hypothalamic-pituitary-adrenal axis: **52**
Immune checkpoint inhibitors: **116**
Neuroendocrine tumor: **73**
Nonfunctional macroadenoma: **15, 64**
Optic nerve glioma: **40**
Pregnancy: **96**
Prolactinoma: **36**

REPRODUCTION, FEMALE

Amenorrhea, secondary: **28, 101**
Congenital adrenal hyperplasia: **113**
Contraception: **101**
Hirsutism: **47, 63, 113**
Hyperandrogenism: **63**
Hyperprolactinemia: **101**
Hypogonadotropic hypogonadism: **39**
Infertility: **4**
Oral contraceptives: **63**
Ovarian hyperthecosis: **47**
Polycystic ovary syndrome: **4, 28, 63, 101**

Spironolactone: **113**
Transgender medicine: **19**
Turner syndrome: **39**

REPRODUCTION, MALE

Exercise: **80**
Gynecomastia: **21**
Hypogonadism: **11, 21, 45, 66**
Infertility: **89**
Prostate cancer: **66**
Semen analysis: **89**
Testosterone assays: **11**
Testosterone therapy: **66**
Testosterone therapy,
    cardiovascular effects: **45**
Transgender medicine: **32, 108**

THYROID

Anaplastic thyroid cancer: **112**
BRAF gene: **112**
Breastfeeding: **68**
Cysts: **106**
Differentiated thyroid cancer: **50**
Follicular variant of papillary
    thyroid carcinoma: **114**
Goiter: **16**
Graves disease: **27, 44, 68, 97**
Hyperthyroidism: **10, 27, 44, 68, 97**
Hyperthyroidism, subclinical: **85**
Hypothyroidism: **16, 70, 76**
Hypothyroidism, subclinical: **81**
Immune checkpoint inhibitors: **76**
Nonthyroidal illness: **31**

Ophthalmopathy: **44**
Papillary thyroid cancer: **85**
Pituitary adenoma: **16**
Postpartum thyroiditis: **72**
Pregnancy: **68, 72, 81, 97**
Radioiodine: **50, 97**
Sex hormone–binding globulin and
    thyroid status: **61**
Teratogen: **97**
TP53 gene: **112**
TSH receptor antibodies: **68, 72**
Thymoma: **27**
Thyroid storm: **10**
Thyrotoxicosis: **88**
Thyrotropinoma: **88**
Ultrasonography: **106, 114**